HORMONAL MANAGEMENT
IN BREAST CANCER

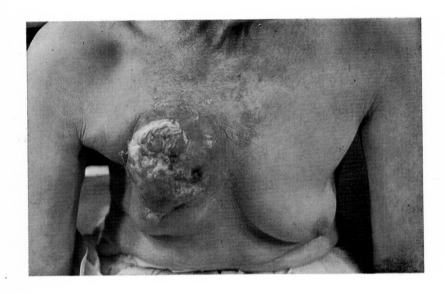

Patient VD. Photographs to show regression of malignant ulceration of the breast within nine months of stilboestrol therapy 5 mg tds
  Photographs taken 10 April 1959 and 4 January 1960

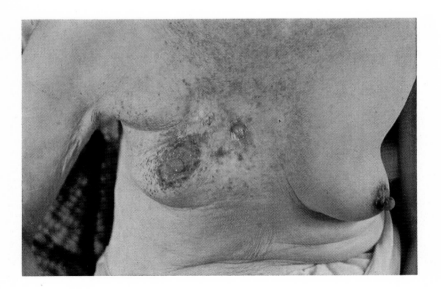

Hormonal Management in
BREAST CANCER

BASIL A. STOLL

*Honorary Consultant to the Radiotherapy Department
St Thomas's Hospital, London*

*Formerly
Consultant to Cancer Institute of Victoria
Melbourne, Australia,
Honorary Consultant to the Prince
Henry's Hospital, Melbourne, Australia,
and Consultant to the Radium Institute, Liverpool*

LONDON
PITMAN MEDICAL PUBLISHING COMPANY LIMITED

First published 1969

PITMAN MEDICAL PUBLISHING COMPANY LTD
46 Charlotte Street, London, W1

Associated Companies

SIR ISAAC PITMAN AND SONS LTD
Pitman House, Parker Street, Kingsway, London, WC2
P.O. Box 6038, Portal Street, Nairobi, Kenya

SIR ISAAC PITMAN (AUST.) PTY LTD
Pitman House, Bouverie Street, Carlton, Victoria 3053, Australia

PITMAN PUBLISHING CORPORATION (S.A.) PTY LTD
P.O. Box 7721, Johannesburg, Transvaal, S. Africa

PITMAN PUBLISHING CORPORATION
20 East 46th Street, New York, NY 10017

SIR ISAAC PITMAN (CANADA) LTD
Pitman House, 381–383 Church Street, Toronto, 3

THE COPP CLARK PUBLISHING COMPANY
517 Wellington Street, Toronto, 2B

SBN: 272 79311 6

Printed in Great Britain at the Pitman Press, Bath
21 3475 11

Contents

Plates

Preface

TODAY IN the Western world, breast cancer is the most commonly occurring malignant disease in women. Approximately one in thirty of all women will develop breast cancer, and the majority, even of those receiving treatment aimed at cure, will require palliative endocrine therapy later in the course of their disease. Furthermore, there is an increasing body of evidence to suggest that cancer of the breast is already disseminated in the vast majority of patients, even before an attempt at curative therapy is made, although the metastases may not manifest clinically for many years. It is therefore essential to crystallise the existing knowledge concerning the hormonal influences on the established tumour, as hormonal manipulation can either increase or decrease the resistance of the host to the disease.

Apart from its use in the management of breast cancer, endocrine therapy is well established in the management of prostatic cancer. It may not be so well known that in the last ten years endocrine therapy has been reported to have a place in the management of several other types of cancer—namely those of the uterus and ovary, kidney and testis, thyroid and melanocarcinoma.

Hormonal therapy of cancer has two major advantages over other methods of treatment such as surgery, radio-therapy, or cytotoxic therapy in this disease. First, systemic therapy by hormones does not damage the normal tissue of the host to a significant degree. Second, if administered to a patient with a hormone sensitive tumour, it is capable of palliating even a widely disseminated tumour in the late cancer patient.

The benefits from endocrine ablation therapy in the management of advanced breast cancer are well known, although the place of the various modalities, and the choice between them, are still the subject of considerable difference of opinion. The use of steroidal hormones in the management of breast cancer is more recondite. It has received considerable impetus from recent proliferation in the synthesis of new androgenic, oestrogenic, progestational, and adreno-cortical steroids, and over-optimistic claims have been made for some of these agents in the treatment of breast cancer. Unfortunately, the practice of hormonal therapy in breast cancer has been, for many years, based mainly upon empiricism, and therefore subject to individual judgements and to the possibility of misapplication. The thesis of this book is that it is possible to plan such therapy in a rational manner.

For the rational planning of hormonal therapy, there are three basic guide-lines; (1) *scientific* criteria of hormonal responsiveness, (2) the selection of suitable treatment for each patient by *individual* criteria, and (3) clinical criteria of *significant* response to hormonal therapy. Individualised treatment on a rational basis is essential when dealing with late breast cancer patients, of whom only a minority will benefit from treatment. In those not benefiting, not only has valuable time been lost, but even worse, the disease may be exacerbated by injudicious selection of therapy.

It must be emphasised that the scope of this work does not embrace the total management of advanced breast cancer. The day-to-day management of the patient, requiring as it does both symptomatic and psychological care of a high order, is not discussed. Techniques of endocrine ablation by surgery or radiation are mentioned only in relation to overall hormonal management, and the role of palliative surgery or radiation therapy is mentioned only in passing. On the other hand, a discussion of endocrine factors which may have a bearing on the development of hormone sensitive breast cancer is included, as is also a chapter on the place of cytotoxic chemotherapy in relation to hormonal therapy. Case reports are included at the end of some chapters in order to illustrate the problems inherent in the subject, rather than the occasional triumphs of therapy.

References are given to support observations derived from the work of the author and of many others. Apart from this, the author offers twenty years of specialised experience in this field as a basis for the opinions expressed. With such background, this book has been written for the practising physician, surgeon, gynaecologist, endocrinologist, or radiotherapist involved in responsibility for the care of the patient with advanced breast cancer. It is intended essentially as a *practical* handbook, describing the available means of selecting a suitable hormonal method for the palliation of each individual patient's disease. The biochemical tests which are finally recommended are not complex, and are within the scope of the average hospital laboratory.

Acknowledgment is gratefully made to the Management of the Cancer Institute, Melbourne, for ready permission to use illustrative case material from the records, and for the clinical opportunities provided during my term there as Consultant from 1952–67, upon which much of this work is based. To the managements of British Drug Houses Ltd, G. D. Searle and Co. Ltd, Imperial Chemical Industries Ltd, Lederle Laboratories Ltd, Organon Ltd, Schering Chemicals Ltd, and Upjohn Ltd, my thanks for financial assistance towards a research project mentioned in this book on the assay of steroid effects on breast cancer in organ culture.

My deep gratitude to my surgical colleague Mr T. H. Ackland for constant encouragement and close co-operation over many years, and to Dr W. J. Moon for numerous discussions, and for loving care in the revision of the text. To Dr T. Bates and Dr S. Campbell my gratitude for useful suggestions on the text, and to Mrs J. Farquharson, Miss B. Gallimore and Miss J. Dewe my thanks for painstaking help in bringing this book to completion.

London, 1969

Basil A. Stoll

Dedicated to the memory of my adored wife,

Gertrude Stoll,

whose inspiration in death, as in life,
gave me strength when I tired.

Part One

THE BASIS OF ENDOCRINE THERAPY IN BREAST CANCER

1

Hormonal Sensitivity

WHEN CELLS become malignant, they have a tendency to lose differentiation in their biological properties, as well as in their histological structure. In spite of this, some groups of malignant tumours may resemble their parent tissue, in that their continued growth will depend, to a greater or lesser extent, on the presence of specific circulating hormones. Not every tumour in these groups shows such hormone dependence, and the failure of a tumour to demonstrate a clinical response to specific endocrine therapy is regarded as evidence of autonomy.

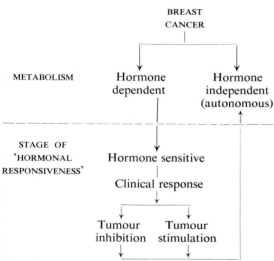

FIGURE 1.1

HORMONAL SENSITIVITY AND AUTONOMY

Above in Fig. 1.1., set out in relation to each other, are some of the terms used in this section. They refer to the need by some breast tumours for a specific hormonal environment for their active metabolism, and their consequent responsiveness to changes imposed on this hormonal environment. As shown in the above diagram, the initially hormone sensitive tumour tends eventually to lose this dependence. It continues to grow independently of changes in the hormonal environment, whether these are spontaneous or therapeutically induced.

The biological mechanism of this change is not clear. It is assumed by some that the tumour initially contains cells of both types—dependent and autonomous. The autonomous elements eventually replace the tumour when the dependent cells are eliminated, as a result of withdrawing the essential hormone. An alternative explanation for the development of autonomy is that the dependent tumour cells are able to adapt their metabolism to the altered hormonal environment, by the use of alternative enzymatic pathways.

About 30–40 per cent of breast cancers show clinical hormone sensitivity, as revealed by a significant measurable response to some form of endocrine manipulation. The responsiveness usually takes the form of tumour growth inhibition but, sometimes, of growth stimulation. After a period of inhibition lasting for months or years, the quiescent tumour finally reactivates, and losing its sensitivity to hormonal manipulation, its growth becomes autonomous.

About 60–70 per cent of tumours appear clinically to be autonomous from the start. It is possible that some of these tumours have a short period of hormonal sensitivity, which is not recognised by the usual clinical criteria. This can occur because most authorities set an arbitrary minimum period of three months for an acceptable significant tumour remission, while many even insist on a six months minimum period. If, however, there was a scientific criterion for identifying limited control of tumour growth by hormonal means, patients with such a response could progress to further selected hormonal therapy. This could well lead to an additional, and possibly longer, remission of tumour growth.

Thus, a scientific index of hormonal sensitivity and of its disappearance, is the first guide-line for individualised hormonal therapy.

OESTROGEN DEPENDENCE HYPOTHESIS

The following discussion, until Chapter 14, applies only to breast cancer in the female, a discussion of breast cancer in the male being reserved to a later chapter.

Both experimental and clinical evidence suggest that the oestrogenic hormone may provide a favourable environment for the *growth* of mammary cancer, once it is established. Although mammary cancer can be induced in the mouse by continuous administration of oestrogen, there is no direct evidence to implicate this hormone in the *induction* of breast cancer in the human (*see* p. 8). It has been found in the mouse that there is an optimum dosage of oestrogen for cancer induction, and doses either smaller or larger than this, are not as effectual. It has been assumed that such an observation may apply also to the growth control of human breast cancer once it is established, and this has been expressed in the 'oestrogen dependence' hypothesis.

In an attempt to create an unfavourable hormonal environment for disseminated breast cancer in the human, one of the theoretical aims has been the reduction of oestrogen levels in the body. This may be achieved by surgical or radiation ablation of specific endocrine glands. Such ablation therapy may fail to control tumour growth either because of tumour autonomy, or alternatively because the resulting withdrawal of oestrogenic hormones is incomplete. As an example, ovarian ablation will remove the major source of oestrogen, but homeostatic mechanisms (*see* p. 6) will subsequently cause increased secretion of pituitary gonadotropin which can then stimulate oestrogen secretion by the adrenal cortex.

Another example of incomplete withdrawal of ostrogenic hormone is the observation that pituitary ablation, even after previous adrenalectomy and oophorectomy, rarely leads to the complete abolition of urinary oestrogen excretion (Greenwood and Bulbrook, 1957). Apart from the ovary and the adrenal gland, therefore, there must be a third source for the oestrogens found in the body in such cases. This may be in accessory adrenal tissue, in dietary oestrogens, in conversion of androgens to oestrogens (West *et al.*, 1958) or in oestrogen synthesis by the tumour (Adams and Wong, 1968). These sources could account for persistent oestrogenic stimulation of the tumour after pituitary ablation. If reactivated tumour could at this stage be indentified as being hormone dependent and not autonomous, further selected steroid therapy is still possible.

Thus, the delineation of the hormonal environment of the tumour is the second guide-line for individualised hormonal therapy.

GUIDE-LINES TO INDIVIDUALISED HORMONAL THERAPY

Advancing knowledge now permits us to guide hormonal treatment for the individual patient on the following fundamental factors:

(i) Scientific criteria of 'hormonal responsiveness', i.e. of the activity of the tumour in relation to its hormonal environment. This requires knowledge of:

    (*a*) Indices reflecting tumour activity
    (*b*) Indices reflecting tumour sensitivity to hormones
    (*c*) Indices reflecting the hormonal environment of the tumour

(ii) Significant clinical criteria of hormonal response
(iii) Knowledge of the 'biological determinants' of hormonal response in the individual, i.e. the factors in the natural history of the disease which determine the hormonal response

The evaluation of these factors and their application to planned treatment of the individual are discussed sequentially in Chapters 10–13 of this book.

HORMONE COMBINATIONS

Therapy by oestrogens is well established in the treatment of both prostatic and breast cancer. Oestrogen treatment of prostatic cancer in the male is, in general, a more satisfactory method than similar treatment of breast cancer in the female. In both cases, secretion of pituitary gonadotropin is thought to be inhibited, but whereas the oestrogen may exert in addition, a direct inhibiting effect upon prostatic cancer tissue, it could, theoretically, exert a direct stimulating effect on breast cancer tissue. It is possible, therefore, that the observed effects in breast cancer under oestrogen therapy may result from two or more mechanisms acting at the same time, and that the resultant effects are not necessarily additive.

Our knowledge of the response by mammary cancer to combinations of hormones is still very limited, but relevant information is becoming available from two sources—chemically induced hormone sensitive mammary cancer in rats (*see* p. 72), and organ cultures of human breast cancer incubated with steroids (*see* p. 16). At present, there is some evidence that progestins may sensitise breast cancer in women to the effect of oestrogens in causing tumour regression (*see* p. 72). The use of selected combinations of hormones, or of a hormone with a cytotoxic agent, offers one possibility of improving the present results of hormonal management in advanced breast cancer.

CHOICE OF METHOD

At this point it may be useful to clarify the use of the terms *hormonal* therapy, *steroid* therapy, and *endocrine* therapy as applied in the hormonal management of breast cancer. Hormonal therapy embraces treatment by steroid hormones (e.g. androgens and oestrogens) and by non-steroid hormones (e.g. stilboestrol, and polypeptides such as prolactin). Steroid therapy embraces the use both of hormonal steroids (e.g. testosterone) and of non-hormonal steroids (e.g. testololactone). Endocrine therapy embraces treatment by all hormonal methods, including surgical or radiation ablation of endocrine glands. The various methods of treatment available are discussed in Chapters 4–9 of this book.

PRESENT LIMITATIONS OF HORMONAL THERAPY

Recently, with more exacting criteria of response, the proportion of patients showing objective evidence of tumour regression from any one of the methods specified in the preceding paragraph appears to be less than previously presumed. The best methods provide a 30–40 per cent likelihood of tumour regression, and the average duration of such a growth remission is twelve to twenty-four months. Furthermore, in patients responding favourably to endocrine therapy, the mean survival time is increased only by a period of six to ten months over that of untreated patients (Ratzkowski and Hochman, 1961; Hortling *et al.*, 1962). Treatment is therefore purely palliative in nature.

It was shown in a series of 843 patients that 65 per cent of responding cases survived two years, but only 25 per cent of non-responding cases (Escher and Kaufman, 1963). Scientific methods of treatment selection would not only increase the percentage of patients responding, but also with the use of suitable sequential therapy, could increase their survival time.

It might be suitable at this point to comment on the worth of palliative treatment of this type to the individual patient with inoperable or metastatic breast cancer. An increase of six to ten months life expectancy in responding cases is of course an average figure, and, in some cases, the survival time may be prolonged by two years or even longer. The value of an extra year or two of life to a woman with young children is obvious, but it should be emphasised that these months or years under endocrine therapy must not be a time of constant pain or of physical or mental grotesqueness.

By suitable methods of endocrine therapy in sequence, the use of morphine can often be postponed until the last month or two of life. Nevertheless, there finally comes a time to cease operations, transfusions and tubes, in order to give the patient who is now resigned to death, some final comfort and dignity. The choice of this moment requires great wisdom and understanding on the part of the attending physician, qualities which are achieved by experience and humility.

TO SUMMARISE

Whatever the endocrine method of palliation used, we must consider the result quantitatively, in terms of increased survival, and qualitatively in terms of the well-being enjoyed by the patient during that increased term of survival. In order to justify a method which offers a one in three likelihood of controlling tumour growth, and that only for a limited period, we must aim to reduce the side effects, the morbidity and mortality resulting from existing methods. Above all, we must aim to *select scientifically the method of treatment most likely to be successful in each individual patient*. Guide lines are available for the rational planning of hormonal therapy.

2

Hormonal Influences in Tumour Development

As EARLY as 1889, Schinzinger suggested castration as an aid to the treatment of young women with breast cancer. In 1939, Loeser suggested the trial of androgen therapy, and in 1943, Biden suggested the trial of oestrogen therapy for advanced breast cancer. Major endocrine ablation therapy in the disease was established with the introduction of bilateral adrenalectomy with cortisone replacement by Huggins and Bergenstal (1952), and of hypophysectomy by Perrault *et al.* (1952).

MULTIPLE HORMONAL RELATIONSHIPS OF BREAST CANCER

This chapter surveys the role of hormonal influences both in the induction and in the growth of breast cancer. It will be noted that on the subject of induction, most of our evidence in the human is deductive. Once the tumour is established, however, it is possible to directly observe objective evidence of hormone responsiveness. The clinical evidence of such a response may not always be clear cut, and this could

result from local stromal factors in healing which are involved, apart from direct and indirect hormonal effects on the tumour. A manifestation of the importance of these local healing factors may be the not uncommon observation of tumour regressing at one site, while progressing in another. For a similar reason, different steroids may appear more efficacious at specific metastatic sites because of their effect on these local healing factors (*see* p. 17).

The complexity of the hormonal relationships affecting the development of breast cancer is shown diagrammatically in Fig. 2.1. The growth of the tumour is thought to be influenced, not only by oestrogens and progesterone from the ovary, but also by similar hormones from the adrenal cortex. It is probably influenced by ovarian androgens, by adrenal glucocorticoids, and androgens, and possibly, also by the thyroid hormones. It is influenced directly by at least one pituitary hormone, prolactin, and possibly by growth hormone also. Finally, releasing factors for anterior pituitary hormones such as prolactin, adrenocorticotropic hormone (ACTH), gonadotropic hormone and thyrotropic hormone (TSH), are known to originate in the hypothalamic controlling centre which may be influenced by the cerebral cortex.

HOMEOSTATIC MECHANISMS

Associated with multiple hormonal control in the body is a tendency to homeostasis, whereby a fall in the blood concentration of a hormone will lead to increased secretion of its controller. Reciprocity between the gonadal and pituitary secretions was suggested by Moore (1935), and the pituitary gonadal relationship was compared by Huggins (1952) to a closed-cycle, feed-back electrical system (Fig. 2.2). In an analogy with this mechanism, a deficiency of the ovarian hormone, due either to the natural menopause or to castration, leads to an increased secretion of pituitary gonadotropin. Conversely, if

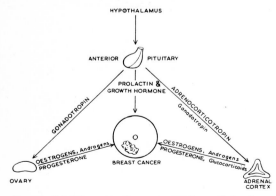

FIGURE 2.1 Diagrammatic representation of the hormonal factors which influence the growth of breast cancer in the female

→ denotes a controlling effect

one establishes an abnormally high oestrogen concentration in the blood as a result of its therapeutic administration, depression of gonadotropin secretion will result.

It follows, therefore, that whatever method is used to achieve a change in the hormonal environment of the tumour, the resulting imbalance will be of a temporary nature. If it is associated with regression

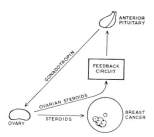

FIGURE 2.2 Diagrammatic representation of the pituitary-gonadal relationship in the female with breast cancer as a closed-cycle, feedback system

→ denotes a controlling effect

of tumour growth, this too will be temporary. Nonetheless, further episodes of tumour regression may follow subsequent endocrine manipulation, or even withdrawal of therapeutic hormone administration (*see* p. 43). In our present state of knowledge, endocrine therapy in breast cancer can be only a palliative and not a curative procedure.

HORMONAL INFLUENCES IN THE CAUSATION AND DEVELOPMENT OF BREAST CANCER

As we acquire further knowledge of the role of hormones in the induction and growth of breast cancer, it will be applied to diminish the future incidence of the disease. Such knowledge is also more immediately relevant to the application of endocrine therapy in the established disease.

It may be useful initially to review briefly our knowledge of certain physiological hormonal relationships in the female, both before and after the menopause. The anterior lobe of the pituitary gland secretes three gonadotropic hormones: (1) the follicle stimulating hormone (FSH), (2) the luteinising hormone (LH) and (3) the luteotropic hormone (LtH). In Fig. 2.3, is noted the increasing urinary oestrogen level during the first half of the menstrual cycle, following the development of an ovarian follicle which has been stimulated by FSH secretion. Ovulation, which requires LH stimulation, is then followed by a temporary fall in the oestrogen level. The development of a corpus luteum, which requires LH

and LtH stimulation, then leads to a rise in the systemic progesterone level and a concomitant second rise in the oestrogen level.

It was suggested by Henderson and Rowlands (1938) and by Severinghaus (1944) that, after the menopause, the excretion level of gonadotropin tends to rise as the oestrogen level falls. According to Albert (1956) the systemic level of gonadotropin

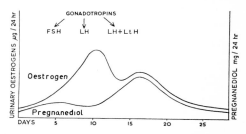

FIGURE 2.3 Diagrammatic representation of the variation in oestrogen and progesterone levels during the menstrual cycle, as reflected in urinary oestrogen and pregnanediol excretion respectively; also its control by anterior pituitary hormones

FSH = follicle stimulating hormone, LH = luteinising hormone, LtH = luteotropic hormone

reaches its peak at twenty years after the menopause, after which it begins to fall (Fig. 2.4). That the secretion of oestrogen at a low level persists during the early postmenopausal years was shown biochemically by Brown (1955) and in vaginal smear examination by Salmon and Frank (1956). The systemic oestrogen level tends to rise higher after the menopausal changes have subsided (Fig. 2.4).

Smith and Emerson (1954) suggested that postmenopausal oestrogen secretion is derived mainly from the adrenal cortex. Following bilateral oophorectomy in the premenopausal patient, there is usually a sharp fall in the oestrogen excretion level and following subsequent bilateral adrenalectomy, oestrogen excretion is almost completely abolished (Dao, 1953). Nathanson *et al.* (1951), West *et al.* (1958) and Sandberg *et al.* (1958) suggest that adrenocortical oestrogen secretion is stimulated by ACTH and probably also by FSH secretion from the pituitary, and is inhibited by corticosteroid administration.

Nissen Meyer (1964) has shown that a portion of the postmenopausal oestrogen excretion may originate also in the ovary, as shown by a fall in the level after ovarian ablation in the postmenopausal patient. The investigations of McBride (1957) do not agree with this conclusion, and this clinically important point is still undecided (*see* p. 25). Cyclical variations in the oestrogen excretion of postmenopausal patients, as suggested by Fluhmann and Murphy (1939) have been recently confirmed by Brown (1967).

Dexamethasone suppression fails to suppress all oestrogen excretion in a proportion of postmenopausal women (Schweppe *et al.*, 1967) suggesting an extra-adrenal source of secretion. This is, however,

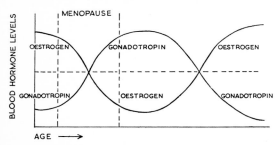

FIGURE 2.4 Diagrammatic representation of the fall in blood oestrogen level, and the rise in gonadotropin level which is associated with the menopause; also the reverse change in later years

(Figure modified from Scowen, 1955)

not necessarily the ovary, as it may also originate in dietary oestrogens, conversion of androgens to oestrogens, or in oestrogen synthesis by the tumour (*see below*).

ROLE OF OESTROGENS AND ORAL CONTRACEPTIVES

The classical experiments of Lacassagne (1936*a*) demonstrated that the presence of oestrogen is necessary for the development of mammary cancer in mice. This influence is effective only if other factors, such as hereditary predisposition, progesterone, and a specific virus, also coexist in the mouse.

Contrary to widespread belief, there is no concrete evidence that either natural or synthetic administered oestrogens are responsible for the *induction* of breast cancer in the human. This belief arose after the early reports of Allaben and Owen (1939) and of Auchinloss and Haagensen (1940), of breast cancer developing during, or soon after, the therapeutic administration of oestrogens to women. Such an association is probably coincidental, as it is suggested by Bulbrook (1966) that a latent period of five to fifteen years would usually be expected between a specific hormonal stimulus and the subsequent development of malignancy in a target organ. Nevertheless the possibility cannot be denied of exogenously administered oestrogen acting as a co-carcinogen or 'trigger factor' on a premalignant state of the breast.

Haddow *et al.* (1944), Nathanson (1947), and Taylor *et al.* (1948) were among the first to report cases of exacerbation by oestrogens of existing breast cancer growth in a proportion of young women. Oestrogen therapy is, therefore, best avoided in the treatment of menopausal symptoms in patients with a history of mastectomy for breast cancer. As a substitute, the use of parahydroxypropiophenone (which has gonadotropin depressant properties but is not oestrogenic), has been found useful in such cases (Stoll, 1956 *b*).

There is little evidence, if any, that the use of oral contraceptives may *induce* breast cancer in the human, and there may even be evidence to the contrary (Stoll, 1964*c*). However, the World Health Organisation (1966) has rightly cautioned against the use of oral contraceptives by patients with a history or suspicion of breast cancer, because their constituent hormones may exacerbate the growth of existing breast cancer.

Several large reported series, including those of Mustacchi and Gordon (1958), Wallack and Henneman (1959), Bishop (1960), and Wilson (1962), suggest that the incidence of breast cancer in patients taking oestrogens over a prolonged period of time is actually less than that in the general population. According to Pincus *et al.* (1959), Cook *et al.* (1961), and Rice Wray *et al.* (1963) this applies also to patients taking oral contraceptives for a prolonged period. However, as stated previously, a latent period of up to fifteen years should be allowed when observing correlation between specific hormonal stimulation and the subsequent development of malignancy. This time period had not elapsed in most of the patients included in the series enumerated above.

It has been noted by Sommers *et al.* (1952, 1953) that hyperplasia of the ovarian cortical stroma is found at autopsy in 83 per cent of patients with breast cancer compared to 38 per cent in the general population. Such pathology is suggestive of an abnormally high level of oestrogen production in such cases during life. They also noted a longer average survival after removal of hyperplastic ovaries in breast cancer patients than that noted for normal ovaries.

The range of oestrogen excretion in normal women is wide, and contrary to early reports, it is now believed (Jull *et al.* 1963; Segaloff, 1967*a*), that there is no evidence of gross abnormality in *total* urinary oestrogen excretion in premenopausal women with breast cancer. However, not only pre- but also postmenopausal patients with breast cancer show a relatively higher excretion of urinary oestriol, relative to oestrone and oestradiol, than does the normal population (Marmorston, 1966). Disturbed thyroid function is one possible cause for such an abnormality (*see* p. 10), or alternatively, it has recently been suggested that breast cancer tissue is capable of secreting oestriol (Adams and Wong, 1968).

It is of interest to note here that repeated pregnancy, with its associated high blood levels of natural oestrogen and progesterone, tends to protect from, rather than favour, the development of breast cancer (*see* p. 11).

ROLE OF ANTERIOR PITUITARY HORMONES

The relative roles of the anterior pituitary and the ovarian hormones in the development of breast cancer are not clear. It has been suggested that the former may be more important in the postmenopausal patient, and the latter in the premenopausal patient, and this hypothesis is based upon the difference in their response to oestrogen therapy (*see* p. 55). Nevertheless, it is also possible that the pituitary role is the major one, and that oestrogens influence the development of breast cancer merely by an indirect effect through the pituitary gland.

Furth and Clifton (1958) and Kim *et al.* (1963) suggest that *small* doses of oestrogen are capable of stimulating the mammotropic cells of the anterior pituitary to secrete prolactin. Prolactin is thought by many to be a major stimulant of breast cancer development (*see* p. 15). Although difficult to separate from prolactin, the role of growth hormone is more uncertain in this respect (*see* p. 109). Gonadotropin is considered to be incriminated in the stimulation of breast cancer development by Lazarev (1960), and like prolactin, its secretion can be stimulated by small doses of oestrogen (Riddle, 1963).

The newly recognised role of the hypothalamus in controlling pituitary function has suggested a possibly important role for the cerebral cortex in the initiation and maintenance of hormone sensitive tumours. Recent knowledge of hypothalamic controlling mechanisms is reviewed by Montemurro (1966). Releasing factors for gonadotropin, ACTH, and TSH have been isolated in extracts of hypothalamic tissue. Damage to the hypothalamus in animals can lead to hyperoestrinism, which may possibly result from interference with LH releasing factors. Release of prolactin also is controlled by the hypothalamus, and according to Khazan *et al.* (1962) can be influenced by the administration of tranquilising drugs. The effect of the higher brain centres upon the growth of breast cancer is, therefore, a subject for investigation.

Metastases from breast cancer are not uncommonly found in the pituitary fossa. If extensive, they may lead to a 'spontaneous hypophysectomy' and cause unexpected regression of advanced tumour, as reported by Gurling *et al.* (1957).

ROLE OF THYROID ACTIVITY

In recent years, many authors including Loeser (1954), Repert (1952), Sommers (1955), Ellerker (1956), Finley and Bogardus (1960), Humphrey and Swerdlow (1964), and Backwinkel and Jackson (1964) have reported a history of goitre, of thyroidectomy,

or signs of thyroid atrophy, in what they consider to be an abnormally high proportion of patients with breast cancer. A recent experimental report by Grice *et al.* (1966) has a bearing on these observations. They noted that the previous induction of hypothyroidism will increase the incidence of hormone sensitive, chemically induced, mammary cancer in rats, but only in the presence of the ovaries.

A relationship between the development of breast cancer and the presence of hypothyroidism has been

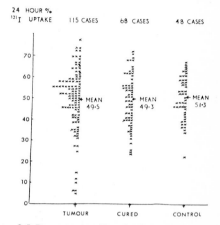

FIGURE 2.5 Percentage radioactive iodine uptake of thyroid gland at twenty-four hours, comparing active breast cancer and 'cured' breast cancer groups, with normal controls. Variance ratio tests on the 'spread' of the values show a significant difference between the active tumour and the control groups (F = 1·964, p < 0·01)

Stoll, 1967 (courtesy, Editor, *Cancer*, Philadelphia)

investigated by a number of authors including Rawson (1956), Edelstyn *et al.* (1958), Hortling *et al.* (1959), Marques *et al.* (1959), Carter *et al.* (1960), Reeve *et al.* (1961), and Dargent *et al.* (1962). Their findings, based upon radioactive iodine uptake levels in the thyroid gland or on protein bound iodine levels in the blood, conflict on the existence of an association between the presence of breast cancer and biochemical evidence of hypothyroidism. Dargent *et al.* (1962) showed abnormally high iodine uptake by the thyroid gland, and high protein-bound iodine levels in the blood, in patients with breast cancer. These levels returned to normal after mastectomy, but rose again when metastasis occurred. This suggested a relationship to the growth of the tumour.

The author (Stoll, 1965c), assessing thyroid uptake of [131]iodine in 183 breast cancer patients, showed no significant difference in the mean uptake level between patients with active tumour, those with 'cured' tumour, and a control group. However, the 'spread' of the levels in patients with active cancer was found to be much greater than in the other groups (Fig. 2.5). The presence of growing tumour appears to modify the [131]iodine uptake level and this may possibly be due to iodine sequestration in the tumour, as it seems to vary with tumour size (Fig. 2.6). The author suggested (Stoll, 1965b) that

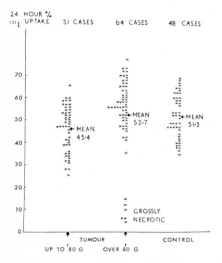

FIGURE 2.6 Percentage radioactive iodine uptake of thyroid gland at twenty-four hours, comparing breast cancer patients with tumours estimated up to 80 G with those over 80 G in size. Variance ratio tests on the 'spread' of the values show a significant difference between the 'over 80 G' tumour and the control groups (F = 2·658, p < 0·01)

Stoll, 1967 (courtesy, Editor, *Cancer*, Philadelphia)

different proportions of patients with large tumours may account for some of the conflicting biochemical results mentioned above in different series reported in the literature.

It has been suggested by Loeser (1954) that the prophylactic administration of thyroid hormone may exert a controlling effect on the growth of breast cancer. Nevertheless, Emery and Trotter (1963) have shown in a controlled trial that the administration of a course of tri-iodothyronine in doses of up to 120 μg daily did not influence the progress of breast cancer in their series.

However, the thyroid function of an individual has been shown to affect the total excretion level of androgens or of oestrogens. It also affects the relative proportion of the constituent oestrone, oestriol, and oestradiol fractions, according to Brown and Strong (1962) and Fishman et al. (1962). This may be of importance in the genesis of breast cancer, as it has been noted previously that a majority of patients

with this disease have a relatively higher urinary excretion of oestriol (Marmorston, 1966).

ROLE OF ADRENAL ACTIVITY

Warren and Witham (1933) and Lumb and Mackenzie (1959) have shown the presence of metastases in the adrenal glands of patients with breast cancer in 31 per cent and 39 per cent of cases respectively. The same authors noted also a high proportion of metastases in the ovaries of the same patients (*see* p. 31). The clinical significance of such observations is not clear. Nevertheless, it is possible that extensive replacement of the adrenal gland by metastases may account for the spontaneous regression of tumour seen occasionally in patients with advanced breast cancer. Similar regression may occur too as a result of pituitary fossa metastases (*see* p. 9).

It was shown by Dobriner et al. (1947) that abnormal steroids may be secreted by the adrenal cortex of patients with cancer, but later work showed that they are not specific to such patients. The presence of adrenocortical hyperplasia was reported in 7·7 per cent of autopsies of patients with cancer—a relatively high incidence according to Parker and Sommers (1956). This may be a response to, and not a cause of, the existence of the patient's tumour.

Bulbrook (1967) has shown that a low excretion level of androgen metabolites is found in a majority of women who subsequently develop breast cancer. Similar findings are noted in patients developing early recurrence after mastectomy, and in patients whose metastases do not respond to subsequent major endocrine ablation. A group of the latter patients were reported by Deshpande et al. (1967) to show a low level of 17 desmolase secreted by the adrenal cortex. This may be the enzyme abnormality responsible for the low excretion level of androgen metabolites.

Of possible relevance in this respect is the observation that the death rate from mammary cancer in Japan is about one fifth of that in the United Kingdom. Bulbrook et al. (1964b) reported a different pattern of androgen excretion in Japanese women compared to those in the United Kingdom, and this may reflect a different pattern of thyroid function (*see above*). It has previously been considered that prolonged lactation might be responsible for the low incidence of breast cancer in Japan (Fifth International Congress, 1954; Wynder et al., 1960).

ROLE OF PREGNANCY AND LACTATION

Apart from the effect of vascular engorgement, one might expect the hormonal changes occurring in pregnancy and lactation to influence the development of breast cancer. The first trimester of pregnancy is associated with a high level of circulating chorionic gonadotropin, which falls later when placental secretion of oestrogen and progesterone increases (Fig. 2.7). The levels of these steroids in the blood rise to their maximum in the second and third trimesters and then fall sharply at delivery. Increased secretion of prolactin from the anterior pituitary follows delivery and stimulates lactation.

There is a general impression of more rapid growth of breast cancer during pregnancy and lactation and an associated poor prognosis. Bloom (1955) has reported a higher proportion of more anaplastic

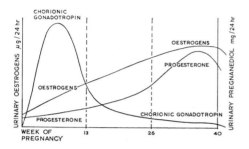

FIGURE 2.7 Diagrammatic representation of the variation in oestrogen, progesterone, and chorionic gonadotropin levels during each trimester of pregnancy as reflected in urinary oestrogen, pregnanediol, and gonadotropin excretion levels, respectively

tumours in 90 patients with cancer of the breast associated with pregnancy or lactation.

A series of 1,375 such cases in the world literature has been reviewed by White (1954) and demonstrates that the poor prognosis in breast cancer associated with pregnancy or lactation may be correlated with delay in diagnosis and treatment. White notes that patients treated in the second half of pregnancy carry a much worse prognosis than those treated in the first half of pregnancy or in lactation. The former group shows a greater delay between the first evidence of the tumour and subsequent treatment. As a result, a high proportion of patients are found to have advanced disease, at the time of coming to treatment.

Smaller personal series of breast cancer associated with pregnancy or lactation, such as those of Westberg (1946), Holleb and Farrow (1962), and Peters (1963), show little difference in their *overall* survival rate from that of an unselected group of women with breast cancer. In spite of this, such series also demonstrate a poor prognosis in patients treated in the second half of pregnancy. This is associated with a high proportion of advanced cases due to delay in diagnosis. The risk of tumour dissemination is presumably increased by delay when maximum physiological changes are present in the breast.

One conclusion which follows from review of the literature is that immediate mastectomy is indicated in the presence of early breast cancer associated with pregnancy or lactation. According to most reports, including that of White (1954) and Holleb and Farrow (1962), the interruption of pregnancy and the practice of immediate castration makes no difference to the prognosis in operable cases. If, however, the tumour is inoperable, both these procedures are indicated in the hope of delaying tumour growth.

The point is not proven, but it seems likely that the hormonal changes of pregnancy are not a determining factor in the curability of breast cancer. It is noted later (*see* p. 31) that there is no evidence that pregnancy increases the likelihood of reactivating 'cured' breast cancer.

ROLE OF PARITY AND AGE GROUP

Reports by Lane-Claypon (1926), Stocks (1939), Clemmesen (1951), and Smithers *et al.* (1952) agree that a history of multiparity is associated with a decreased likelihood of developing breast cancer. The risk of developing breast cancer is inversely proportional to the number of children borne. Again, we find no evidence that the repeated high levels of natural oestrogen and progesterone prevailing during multiple pregnancies, favour the development of breast cancer. In fact, a protective effect seems possible.

It is generally believed, and so stated by Cade (1950), Lewison *et al.* (1953), and Kleinfeld *et al.* (1963), that breast cancer in younger women is more often of a higher grade of malignancy and carries a poorer prognosis. Nevertheless, a prognosis similar to that for older women, has been claimed for young women with breast cancer by Richards (1948), Scarff (1948), Bloom (1950), and Treves and Holleb (1958), the last in a series of 549 patients under thirty-five years of age. In addition, Lees and Park (1949) concluded from studies on the histology of breast cancer in relation to age, that there was a similar distribution of histological grading in all age groups. The effect of pregnancy and lactation on the prognosis of the disease in the younger age group has already been discussed.

ROLE OF THE MENOPAUSE AND EARLY CASTRATION

Clemmesen (1948, 1965) and Anderson *et al.* (1950) have shown a decrease in the incidence of breast cancer in women between the ages of fifty and fifty-five. If we assume that the average age at the menopause is between forty-five and fifty, the disease seems less likely to manifest while oestrogen levels are falling and gonadotropin levels are rising after the menopause (Fig. 2.4).

Supporting this observation, Clemmesen (1948), Hadfield and Holt (1956), and the AMA Committee on Research (1960) suggest that the tumour growth in premenopausal women may be slowed up by the falling oestrogen level after the menopause. These reports note that when the menopause intervenes between mastectomy and the first recurrence, the average 'free interval' is found to be longer than in other age groups of patients with breast cancer. The author has noted that recurrence of breast cancer is rarely seen during the time that menopausal symptoms are severe. Finally, Richards (1948), Smithers *et al.* (1952), and Delarue (1955) have shown that survival rates in breast cancer are significantly higher for patients developing the disease between forty-one and fifty years of age.

A different interpretation by Hems (1967) is that the menopause marks a trough between two different types of breast cancer—the premenopausal and the late postmenopausal types. It was suggested by Jull (1958) that the former type would tend to be activated by oestrogen, but the latter inhibited (*see* p. 14).

With regard to the effect of castration on the development of breast cancer, several series including those of Herrell (1937), Lilienfeld (1956), and McMahon and Feinleib (1960), have shown a significantly greater proportion of previously castrated women in a control series than in a breast cancer series. It has also been shown by Olch (1937), Wynder *et al.* (1960) and the AMA Committee on Research Report (1960) that patients with breast cancer showed a higher proportion who were still menstruating compared with the normal population of the same age group. Both these observations suggest that the longer the premenopausal breast is exposed to cyclical hormonal changes, the greater the likelihood of developing breast cancer. It is possible that early castration may have a prophylactic value in decreasing liability to this disease.

TO SUMMARISE

Although there is no evidence that oestrogen administration causes the development of breast cancer in the human, there is indirect evidence that in the growth of the tumour the effect of oestrogens may be important. The protective effect of early castration, the predisposing effect of a late menopause and the decreased growth rate of the tumour at the time of the menopause in some cases may be examples of this effect.

There is evidence to suggest that premenopausal and postmenopausal breast cancer respond differently to endocrine manipulation as a result of their having originated in differing hormonal environments.

3

Rationale of Endocrine Therapy

ONLY ABOUT one third of breast cancer patients will respond to hormonal manipulation. The incidence of hormonal sensitivity is approximately the same in premenopausal women as in older postmenopausal women, although the methods of treatment involved may be quite different.

Ablation of ovarian secretion is, in the premenopausal patient, the simplest and most reliable endocrine method of obtaining tumour regression in late breast cancer. On the other hand, administration of oestrogen to premenopausal patients, or to patients whose tumour has responded favourably to castration, can lead to clinical evidence of stimulation of tumour growth, as reported early by Haddow *et al.* (1944), Nathanson (1947), and Taylor *et al.* (1948).

Basis of Hormonal Control in Breast Cancer

1. OESTROGEN DEPENDENCE

Based on the evidence noted in the last paragraph, it was suggested by Pearson *et al.* (1954) that the growth of breast cancer in women may be either oestrogen dependent or oestrogen independent. On this basis, it is assumed that the hormone sensitive tumour requires the presence of endogenous oestrogen for continued growth, and this hypothesis is widely quoted. Therapy based on this concept aims to eliminate, first of all, the major source of oestrogen —the ovary (Fig. 3.1). If castration is successful in causing objective evidence of regression of tumour growth, the neoplasm is categorised as being oestrogen dependent.

On the basis of this hypothesis, reactivation of tumour growth after control by castration has been ascribed to increasing oestrogen secretion derived from the adrenal cortex. Such secretion was suggested by Smith and Emerson (1954), and demonstrated biochemically by Bulbrook and Greenwood (1957). Hypertrophy, both of the adrenal and of the pituitary glands, has been observed after castration. Bilateral adrenalectomy at this stage therefore removes the second major source of oestrogen, and has been observed to cause further tumour regression in some cases.

Subsequently, when the tumour reactivates after control by adrenalectomy, hypophyseal ablation will eliminate secretion of both FSH and ACTH

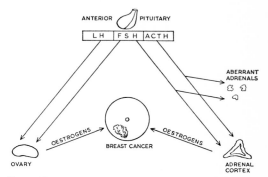

FIGURE 3.1 Diagrammatic representation of the oestrogen dependence hypothesis which has been suggested as a basis for the endocrine therapy of breast cancer in the female

→ denotes a controlling effect

which are capable of activating ectopic adrenal sources of oestrogen (*see* p. 8). Compensatory hyperplasia in these ectopic sources after bilateral

13

adrenalectomy was shown by Graham (1953) and Falls (1955). The assumption of oestrogen dependence thus appears to explain the clinical remission of tumour growth seen following endocrine ablation therapy in advanced breast cancer.

2. OVARY OR ADRENAL DEPENDENCE

The concept of oestrogen dependence was expounded first by Huggins and Dao (1953) who suggested, in addition, that oestrogen dependent breast cancer may be either ovary dependent or adrenal dependent in type. According to this hypothesis, specific oestrogens, derived either from the ovary or from the adrenal cortex, can stimulate the growth of hormone dependent breast cancer. Since the type cannot be determined beforehand, it is suggested that both oophorectomy and adrenalectomy are carried out simultaneously. The prolonged tumour growth remission seen to arise from oophorectomy alone in some patients, would suggest an ovary dependent tumour. Failure of such response but remission from subsequent bilateral adrenalectomy would suggest that the tumour growth is maintained by adrenal oestrogens.

Although useful to explain the tumour growth remissions from endocrine ablation therapy, the significance of oestrogen dependence as a theoretical basis for *all* endocrine control of breast cancer, may have been overestimated. Since the introduction of reliable biochemical methods of oestrogen assay, attempts have been made by numerous investigators to correlate a favourable clinical response to castration, bilateral adrenalectomy of hypophysectomy, with a decrease in subsequent oestrogen levels. Reports include those of Strong et al. (1956), Bulbrook et al. (1958), Gordon and Segaloff (1958), Scowen (1958), Hiisi Brummer et al. (1960), McAllister et al. (1960), Irvine et al. (1961), Swyer et al. (1961), Hortling et al. (1962), Palmer and Hellstrom (1962), and Jull et al. (1963).

Whether measured by biochemical estimation of oestrone, oestradiol or oestriol excretion, or by the cytohormonal evaluation of the vaginal smear, a correlation cannot be established to a significant degree between postoperative change in oestrogen level and the nature of the clinical response. Following castration, tumour regression breast cancer may be associated with either a higher, a lower, or an unchanged, oestrogen excretion level. Following bilateral adrenalectomy or hypophysectomy, tumour regression is often associated with little change in the oestrogen excretion level.

Reactivation of the tumour following a temporary favourable response to ovarian or adrenal ablation is rarely associated with an increase in the oestrogen excretion level. Furthermore, oestrogen administration does not appear to reactivate the tumour in the presence of regression following hypophyseal ablation (see p. 16).

The concept that the growth of hormone sensitive breast cancer is favoured by oestrogen is further unable to explain satisfactorily the tumour regression in breast cancer that is commonly seen following administration of either natural or synthetic oestrogens in postmenopausal women. This was first reported by Ellis and others (1944) and Nathanson (1946) and amply documented since (see p. 54). Moreover, such a response is seen occasionally also in *premenopausal* women with breast cancer given *very high* doses of oestrogen, according to Nathanson (1952) and Kennedy (1962a). According to the latter author, this applies both to the synthetic oestrogen diethyl stilboestrol, and to the natural oestrogens present in Premarin (see p. 55).

Difficult to explain is the report by Wilson et al. (1958) of occasional cases of tumour 'stimulation' after oophorectomy and bilateral adrenalectomy. A rise in calcium excretion levels following these operations was reported by these authors in some patients with bone metastases from breast cancer. It may be relevant that a transient rise in oestrogen excretion is common after oophorectomy (Bulbrook and Greenwood 1957) (see p. 25).

It is possible to explain some of these apparent contradictions on the basis that for every breast cancer, there is an optimal level of oestrogen favouring its growth. Either higher or lower concentrations may depress its growth activity (Segaloff, 1967a).

3. OESTROGEN OR PROGESTERONE DEPENDENCE

A hypothesis by Jull (1958) attempts to provide an explanation for some of the observations in the previous section. It suggests that hormone sensitive breast cancer is either oestrogen dependent or progesterone dependent, depending on the environment in which the tumour develops.

The oestrogen dependent type would would be more common in premenopausal women. Its tumour growth would be favoured by a high oestrogen/progesterone ratio, and antagonised either by reducing the oestrogen level or by increasing the progesterone level. The opposite would apply to the progesterone dependent type, which would be more common in postmenopausal women. Its tumour growth would be antagonised either by increasing the oestrogen level or by decreasing the progestin level.

Our experience of progestin therapy is still inadequate to lend support to this hypothesis (see p. 69). Nevertheless, the studies of Clemmesen (1948, 1965),

Anderson *et al.* (1950), and Hems (1967) lend support on a statistical basis to the suggestion that there are two types of breast cancer—a premenopausal and a postmenopausal type (*see* p. 12).

4. OESTROGEN OR ANDROGEN DEPENDENCE

A similar hypothesis to the previous one has been suggested which aims to explain the 'withdrawal response' sometimes seen after oestrogen or androgen therapy (*see* pp. 43 and 59). It is noted in 31 per cent of patients whose tumour has regressed under oestrogen therapy, and in 10 per cent of remissions under androgen therapy, that when the tumour eventually reactivates, withdrawal of the steroid may be followed by a further tumour regression. Furthermore, when the tumour then reactivates a second time, it may respond favourably once more to administration of the same hormone (*see* p. 62).

It is therefore suggested by Delarue (1955) that an optimal oestrogen/androgen ratio may exist at any one time, which favours the growth of hormone dependent tumour. Repeated change in the relative concentrations of the steroids, will cause an unfavourable environment for the tumour cells, and consequent tumour regression, until its metabolism adjusts to the new environment.

It should be noted that the observation of a 'withdrawal response' suggests that a *change* in the hormonal environment of the tumour may be more important than the actual nature of the steroid causing the change. This is confirmed by the commonly observed rise in serum alkaline phosphatase levels which occurs with every change of hormonal therapy in the presence of bone metastases from breast cancer (*see* p. 102).

5. PITUITARY DEPENDENCE

A hypothesis based upon pituitary dependence, postulates that breast cancer develops in an environment where prolactin levels are high. As a result, decrease in the prolactin level, by whatever method it is achieved, may cause regression of tumour growth. According to Furth and Clifton (1958) and Kim *et al.* (1963), the secretion of prolactin from the anterior pituitary is normally stimulated by physiological levels of oestrogen in the blood. Thus, ablation of oestrogen sources whether by castration or by bilateral adrenalectomy, will decrease prolactin secretion in the premenopausal woman.

Furthermore, according to Kim *et al.* (1963), administration of *high* doses of oestrogen can decrease prolactin secretion. This may be the basis of the control of advanced breast cancer by oestrogen therapy in the postmenopausal woman (*see* p. 16). Finally, hypophyseal ablation will eliminate secretion of prolactin (and also secretion of FSH and ACTH) in both premenopausal and postmenopausal women. The importance of suppressing prolactin secretion in the endocrine control of breast cancer was early emphasised by Pearson (1957) and by the author (Stoll, 1958*b*) (*see* p. 16).

MODE OF ACTION OF OESTROGEN THERAPY IN BREAST CANCER

As mentioned earlier, about one third of older postmenopausal women with breast cancer will show signs of tumour regression following oestrogen therapy. This applies both to synthetic oestrogens such as diethyl stilboestrol and to natural oestrogens such as Premarin. Their therapeutic action is not capable of direct explanation on the oestrogen dependent hypothesis of breast cancer growth. In fact, some would regard *failure* to respond to oestrogen therapy as a sign of oestrogen dependence (Kimel, 1957; Edelstyn *et al.*, 1965).

It is established that oestrogens have a wide range of action on the endocrine system in that they can affect the secretion of gonadotropin and prolactin from the anterior pituitary (*see* p. 16), and also hormonal secretion from the ovaries, adrenal cortex, and thyroid gland. Oestrogens can also cause calcium retention and can stimulate the reticulo-endothelial system.

The possible modes of action of oestrogen therapy in controlling breast cancer include:

(i) Direct inhibition of tumour growth
(ii) Suppression of pituitary hormone secretion
(iii) Body defence stimulation

More than one mechanism may be involved—the first and second being the most likely. If such is the case, their effects may not necessarily summate in the same direction (*see* p. 4).

1. DIRECT INHIBITION OF TUMOUR GROWTH

A direct action of oestrogen upon mammary tissue was suggested by MacBryde (1939). He demonstrated that the local application of an oestrogen to one mammary gland in castrated rats induced growth stimulation of the mammary gland under observation, but not of others. This refuted the suggestion of Gomez and Turner (1938) that the action of oestrogens on the mammary gland was an indirect one through the anterior pituitary. Mixner *et al.* (1942) suggested that physiological levels of oestrogen were merely increasing the vascularity of mammary stroma, so that access of other hormones (possibly prolactin) was facilitated. If this applies also to breast cancer in the human, then the role of endogenous oestrogen in stimulating the neoplastic growth in the premenopausal woman may not necessarily be a direct one upon the tumour. Physiological levels of oestrogen may at the same time stimulate prolactin secretion from the pituitary, and increase the access of prolactin to the tumour bed.

On the other hand, the action of oestrogen given as therapy for breast cancer may be quite different from its physiological effect. It has been shown by Huseby and Thomas (1954) that the stimulation of the normal breast epithelium that is seen in postmenopausal women with breast cancer receiving oestrogen therapy, cannot be related to the depression of activity which may be noted in the tumour. A similar observation has been made on a biochemical basis, by Rees and Huggins (1960). Oestrogen administration alters the activity of pyridine nucleotide linked dehydrogenase enzymes in hormone sensitive mammary carcinoma in rats. Inhibition by oestrogen of specific enzymes in mammary cancer may be associated with a raised level of those same enzymes in the adjacent normal mammary gland tissue. It has therefore been suggested that one effect of oestrogen therapy may be to increase the mitotic activity of the normal tissue cells at the expense of the malignant cells.

Specimens of human breast cancer have been incubated in organ culture with near pharmacological concentrations of steroids and a direct effect on tumour growth has been noted (see p. 106). However, this method measures the effect of the hormone itself, as distinct from its metabolites which occur in the body. This direct assay also obviates the influence of the other hormones of the body upon the tumour. Consequently, observed results *in vitro* need not necessarily be identical with the *in vivo* effects on the tumour resulting from therapeutic administration of the hormone.

Biochemical changes, reflecting inhibition or stimulation of metabolism in such tumour explants by oestrogens (and also by androgens), have been demonstrated by Rienits (1959), Heuson and Legros (1963), Altmann and Chayen (1967) and the author (Stoll, 1969). These observations were made at somewhat higher steroid concentrations than occur pharmacologically in the blood, but allowance must be made for concentration by the target organ. Morphological evidence of tumour stimulation or inhibition has been shown by Kellner and Turcic (1962), Rivera *et al.* (1963), Flaxel and Wellings (1963), Mioduszewska (1968) and Tchao *et al.* (1968) in organ cultures of mammary cancer incubated with either oestrogens, androgens, or progestins. Attempts to correlate the observed *in vitro* changes with clinical response to steroid therapy have been made by Hollander *et al.* (1958, 1959), Kellner and Turcic (1962), Heuson and Legros (1963), and by the author (Stoll, 1969).

In vitro observations suggest that the direct effect of oestrogen upon breast cancer may vary according to the nature of the stroma. Observed oestrogen effects may take the form either of stimulation or of inhibition of growth. This variation from one tumour to another may depend on the hormonal environment in which the tumour develops (*see* p. 14).

2. SUPPRESSION OF PITUITARY HORMONE

Tumour regression in breast cancer following oestrogen therapy has been explained on the basis of suppressing specific anterior pituitary hormones— probably prolactin, but possibly also gonadotropin. This is based on the pituitary dependent hypothesis for the growth of hormone sensitive breast cancer favoured by the author (Stoll, 1956*b*, 1958*b*). The following is evidence for the hypothesis (*see* p. 15).

(*a*) The effect of oestrogens on breast cancer is probably mediated through the intact pituitary gland. Several authors, including Pearson and Ray (1959), Lipsett and Bergenstal (1960), and Kennedy and French (1965) have now reported that after hypophysectomy, there is no observable effect upon the tumour from oestrogen administration, even in patients with previously hormone sensitive tumours. A similar observation has been made in hormone-sensitive rat mammary carcinoma by Kim *et al.* (1963).

(*b*) A mammotropic agent, probably prolactin, was noted by Hadfield (1957) in the urine of premenopausal and some postmenopausal women with breast cancer. He reported that favourable response of the tumour to hypophysectomy was associated with abolition of urinary prolactin. Similarly, tumour regression in breast cancer after high dose oestrogen therapy has been noted by Segaloff *et al.* (1954*b*) to be usually associated with a fall in the prolactin excretion level. (According to Kim *et al.* (1963), high dosage of oestrogen decreases the plasma prolactin level in animals while low dosage increases it.)

A report by Pearson (1957) suggests that the administration of prolactin to patients with breast cancer, after hypophysectomy, may induce clinical evidence of exacerbation of their disease. McCalister and Welbourn (1962) have reported that biochemical evidence of exacerbation of breast cancer by injections of ovine prolactin predicts a high likelihood of tumour regression resulting from hypophysectomy.

Because of the difficulties of prolactin assay, reports on its relationship to clinical hormonal response in breast cancer are difficult to interpret.

(*c*) Rowlands and Sharpey-Schafer (1940), Albert (1956), and Rosemberg and Engel (1960) have reported decreased gonadotropin secretion following high dosage of oestrogens such as oestradiol or Premarin (2·5–10 mg daily.) On the other hand, they observed stimulation of gonadotropin secretion following low dosage of Premarin (0·1–0·25 mg daily). A similar observation applies to synthetic oestrogens such as diethyl stilboestrol.

Stewart et al. (1965) have reported that tumour regression in breast cancer in postmenopausal patients after high dose oestrogen therapy is associated with a marked fall in the gonadotropin excretion in the urine. Reduced gonadotropin content of the pituitary gland was shown by Dekker and Russfield (1963) in male patients treated by oestrogen.

According to Riddle (1963) there is a close correlation between systemic prolactin and gonadotropin levels. Secretion of both hormones is related to oestrogen levels, being stimulated by low levels and depressed by high levels.

3. BODY DEFENCE STIMULATION

Recent cancer research suggests that the immune response of the body may be stimulated to destroy existing cancer (Southam, 1965). According to Nicol et al. (1964), oestrogenic compounds can stimulate the reticulo-endothelial system to raise body defences both in males and in females. Both natural and synthetic oestrogens have been shown to stimulate the activity of phagocytic cells and to raise the serum gamma globulin level in animals. High dosage of oestrogen, according to Maximow and Bloom (1952), also tends to encourage proliferation of fibroblasts and subsequent fibrosis.

It may be relevant that the existence of abnormal antigens has been reported in breast cancer patients by de Carvalho (1963). It has therefore been suggested by Nicol et al. (1964) that non specific stimulation of the reticulo-endothelial system may be one possible mode of action of oestrogen in breast cancer therapy. If oestrogen control of breast cancer involves such a mechanism, it is surprising that other steroids with a similar effect on breast cancer, such as testosterone and progesterone, are reported by Nicol and Bilby (1957) to have no specific effect on phagocytic activity, while corticosteroids are even strong depressants of such activity. Furthermore, it is reported that the depressing effect of corticosteroids can be reversed by the simultaneous administration of diethyl stilboestrol.

There appears to be no correlation between the stimulating effect of an oestrogen upon the reticulo-endothelial system, and its oestrogenicity as measured by its effect on the reproductive tract.

MODE OF ACTION OF ANDROGEN THERAPY IN BREAST CANCER

Androgen therapy leads to tumour regression in a proportion of women with breast cancer, particularly those in the postmenopausal age group.

Occasional regression of tumour results also in premenopausal patients (see p. 37). It is established that androgens can cause nitrogen and calcium retention, and also stimulation of erythropoiesis. They affect the secretion of pituitary gonadotropin and prolactin, and also hormonal secretion from the adrenal cortex and thyroid glands.

The possible modes of action of androgen in controlling breast cancer include:

  (i) Direct inhibition of tumour growth
 (ii) Suppression of pituitary hormone secretion
(iii) Anti-oestrogenic effect upon the target tissue
 (iv) Conversion of androgen to oestrogen

Although more than one mechanism may be involved, the first is the most likely. If more than one mechanism is involved, the effects may not necessarily summate in the same direction.

1. DIRECT INHIBITION OF TUMOUR GROWTH

A direct effect of androgen on mammary tissue was suggested by Ahren and Hamberger (1962). The local application of testosterone propionate to the mammary gland of a castrated male or female rat induced growth stimulation of the mammary gland under observation, but not of others. The suggestion of Gomez and Turner (1938) that steroidal agents exert their effect on mammary tissue via the anterior pituitary gland is therefore not substantiated in this case.

Biochemically, it has been shown by Rees and Huggins (1960) that androgen administration can alter the metabolism of hormone sensitive mammary carcinoma in rats, as reflected in the activity of pyridine nucleotide linked dehydrogenase enzymes in the tissue. As is the case with oestrogen administration, it is possible that the mitotic activity of the normal tissue cells may be increased by androgens at the expense of the malignant cells (see p. 16).

The direct effect of androgens upon the metabolism of organ cultures of human breast cancer has been discussed previously, together with that of oestrogens (see p. 16).

There may be additional direct effects from sex hormones upon stromal factors in healing and these may be specific for breast cancer metastases at certain sites. As stated above, androgens have a controlling effect upon protein anabolism and calcium deposition in bone, and also upon erythropoiesis. This may account for the high proportion of remissions observed from androgen therapy in the treatment of bone metastases (see p. 38). It may also account for the common observation of tumour regressing in one tissue under androgen therapy, while concomitantly progressing in another.

2. SUPPRESSION OF PITUITARY HORMONE SECRETION

Early reports suggested that the effect of androgen therapy in causing tumour regression of breast cancer was exerted via the anterior pituitary gland. However, case reports by Kennedy (1957), Beckett and Brennan (1959), Peck and Olsen (1963), and by the author (*see* p. 94), have demonstrated regression of tumour following fluoxymesterone therapy even in hypophysectomised patients. If ablation of pituitary tissue can be assumed complete in these cases, the presence of the pituitary may not be essential for androgen induced regression of breast cancer.

Segaloff *et al.* (1958) noted that tumour regression of breast cancer under therapy with the androgen, fluoxymesterone, is often associated with a rise in prolactin excretion levels (*see* p. 109). This is in contrast with oestrogen therapy where tumour regression is associated with a fall in prolactin excretion levels (*see* p. 109). Similarly, although oestrogens and the older effective androgens such as testosterone propionate and methyl testosterone caused a decrease in the gonadotropin excretion levels (Segaloff *et al.*, 1951, 1954*b*), this does not apply in all patients treated with fluoxymesterone (Segaloff *et al.*, 1958). It does not apply either to the newly introduced androgens, 2α-methyl dihydotestosterone propionate (Blackburn and Childs, 1959) and delta-1-testololactone (Segaloff *et al.*, 1962).

It may be noted here that fluoxymesterone and these newer compounds have also markedly decreased virilising tendencies compared to testosterone propionate, without detracting from their breast cancer controlling activity. In their virilising tendencies, there is also a qualitative difference between the older and newer androgens, as fluoxymesterone is relatively more likely to cause gross enlargement of the clitoris. The efficacy of each androgen in the treatment of breast cancer probably depends on the presence of specific metabolic end-products in the body.

3. ANTI-OESTROGENIC EFFECT

On the basis of the oestrogen dependence hypothesis, early reports on androgen therapy in breast cancer suggested that androgens might act by antagonising oestrogens at the tissue level. If this were the effective mode of action of androgens in breast cancer therapy, one might expect better results from androgen therapy in premenopausal patients than in post-menopausal patients, but the opposite is the case.

Blocking of oestrogenic activity at the target receptors by anti-oestrogens has recently been demon-strated (Jensen *et al.*, 1967). Dorfman *et al.* (1967) have reported that there is no correlation between the anti-tumour efficacy of androgens in the human and their anti-oestrogenicity in experimental animals. It was reported by Pearson *et al.* (1954) that given simultaneously with oestrogens to patients with bone metastases, androgens were incapable of preventing the tumour exacerbating influence of oestrogens in premenopausal women. A blocking action is further unlikely, because according to Kennedy and Brown (1965) a combination of androgen and oestrogen therapy gives no different a tumour regression rate to that of oestrogen therapy alone in breast cancer patients.

If androgens block the activity of oestrogens at the target receptors, it is difficult to explain the response of the same tumour to oestrogen and to androgens given successively (*see* p. 50). It is also difficult to explain on the same basis, the observation of a withdrawal response in some patients after cessation of androgen administration (Delarue, 1955; Kaufman and Escher, 1961) (*see* p. 43).

4. CONVERSION OF ANDROGEN TO OESTROGEN

It has been demonstrated that some androgens may be partly converted to oestrogens in the body and excreted as such (Steinach and Kun, 1937; Nathanson *et al.*, 1952; Baggett *et al.*, 1956). This may possibly explain the observation of Myers *et al.* (1955) of occasional cases of exacerbation of breast cancer growth following androgen administration. West *et al.* (1956) have demonstrated the conversion of testosterone to oestrogen in patients with breast cancer, who have previously been castrated and adrenalectomised. This conversion may possibly occur in the tumour (Adams and Wong, 1968).

TO SUMMARISE

The oestrogen dependence hypothesis has been adduced to explain the tumour regression seen in some breast cancers after castration, bilateral adrenalectomy, or hypophysectomy. However, existing biochemical methods of oestrogen determination fail to show a correlation between the nature of the clinical response and a quantitative change in oestrogen excretion. Furthermore the oestrogen dependence theory cannot explain regression of some tumours after oestrogen, androgen, or progestin therapy.

A combination of a direct effect by metabolic products of the steroid on the tumour, and an indirect effect via the pituitary, is therefore postulated in the steroid therapy of breast cancer. These two effects of a particular steroid, may not summate in their final effect upon a tumour. The individual steroid members of a group may yield different metabolic breakdown products in the body, and this may explain selectivity of effect. Different tumours may vary in their response to hormonal therapy, depending on the hormonal environment in which they have developed.

The choice of a suitable steroid for therapy in each patient is therefore difficult. The available methods of assessing the sensitivity of an individual tumour to particular steroids are considered later.

Part Two

METHODS OF ENDOCRINE THERAPY IN BREAST CANCER

4

Therapeutic and Prophylactic Castration

THE FIRST to report benefit from therapeutic surgical castration in advanced breast cancer was the Scottish surgeon, Beatson, in 1896. Following his preliminary report, Thomson (1902) and Lett (1905) reported pain control and objective evidence of tumour regression in 22 per cent and 23 per cent respectively, of large series of premenopausal breast cancer patients treated by surgical castration. However, because of the relatively high mortality rate associated with the operation, at that time, Halberstadter introduced castration by radiation in 1905. Early reports on its use in the palliation of breast cancer were by Wintz (1926) and Ahlbom (1930).

With improvements in anaesthesia and surgical technique, Adair et al. (1945) once again drew attention to the therapeutic usefulness of surgical castration in breast cancer. Since that date, there have been numerous reports on the use both of surgical and of radiation castration in the treatment of young women with inoperable or recurrent breast cancer (Table 4.1).

Therapeutic Castration

Therapeutic castration is, in the premenopausal patient, the simplest and most reliable endocrine method of achieving tumour regression in breast cancer. Objective evidence of tumour regression after surgical castration has been noted in between 24·5 per cent and 38 per cent of patients with breast cancer, in the larger series reported in recent years (Table 4.1). Taylor (1962) utilising the stricter criteria of the AMA Joint Committee, and Hall et al. (1963b) utilising those of the Co-operative Breast Cancer Group, reported the two lowest percentages of favourable response—29·7 per cent and 24·5 per cent respectively.

Between 14·8 per cent and 32 per cent of patients are reported to show objective evidence of tumour regression after radiation castration in the larger series (Table 4.1). Again, the wide range presumably reflects the degree of strictness in criteria of response.

No randomised controlled trial to compare the two methods of castration has yet been reported, but, in the long term, the objective tumour remission rate is probably similar in patients submitted to either procedure. It is clear from several reports that there is no difference in the residual oestrogen levels following castration in breast cancer patients, whether castration is carried out by surgery or by

TABLE 4.1

Major Reports of Favourable Clinical Response of the Tumour to Castration in Patients with Breast Cancer, in Relation to the Method Used

Author	Total cases	Percentage with regressing tumour	
Pearson et al. 1955	96	38%	Surgical castration
Treves and Finkbeiner, 1958	176	37%	
Dao, 1962	84	32%	
Taylor, 1962	398	29·7%	
Hall et al., 1963	282	24·5%	
Adair et al., 1945	304	15%	Radiation castration
Thayssen, 1948	99	32%	
Douglas, 1952	175	20%	
Stoll, 1964	162	14·8%	

radiation, or even if surgery is carried out after radiation. This is established in reports by Struthers (1956), Gordon and Segaloff (1958), Diczfalusy *et al.* (1959), and Nissen Meyer and Sanner (1963). However, whereas oestrogen levels fall sharply within two to three days after surgical castration, it may take as long as three to five months for them to reach comparatively low levels after a dose of 1,200 to 1,600 roentgens in four days to the ovaries (Nathanson *et al.*, 1940; Block *et al.*, 1958). It should be noted that symptoms of 'hot flushes' do not necessarily indicate low levels of oestrogen secretion.

Thus, the relatively lower tumour remission rate in breast cancer reported by some radiation castration series may reflect a failure to appreciate the slower and less dramatic nature of the response to this method. With any method of endocrine therapy in breast cancer, but especially after radiation castration, it may take as long as six months before a tumour growth remission capable of satisfying a strict protocol is apparent (*see* p. 112).

With regard to the minimum period necessary for clinical assessment after radiation castration, it should be taken into account that it usually takes from one to three months for menses to cease.

breast cancer series, objective signs of tumour regression followed oophorectomy, whereas previous ovarian radiation had failed to yield benefit. As pointed out by Gordon and Segaloff (1958), irradiation of the ovaries, as sometimes performed in past years, was inadequate for permanent castration either on account of dosage or of anatomical misdirection.

Tumour growth remission may also be associated with *temporary* depression of ovarian activity, as it is sometimes possible to achieve a second remission, from surgical castration in breast cancer patients previously responding to radiation castration. The attempt is worth while if there is evidence of persisting or returning ovarian function, as shown by high oestrogen excretion levels, or cycling in serial urinary oestrogen estimations (Moon, 1968).

In the author's experience, a fractionated total dose of 1,200 roentgens in one week to the ovaries is adequate to ensure permanent cessation of menses in almost all women over forty years of age. It should be taken into account that the interstitial cells of the ovary are probably more radio resistant than is the follicle. In addition, as was reported by Nathanson and Kelley (1952), the ovaries of younger women are probably more resistant to radiation than are those

TABLE 4.2

Favourable Clinical Response of the Tumour to Radiation Castration in 127 *Patients with Breast Cancer. Results in Relation to the Dose and Overall Time of Ovarian Irradiation* (Author's Series)

Calculated dose at ovary	Overall treatment time	Cases with regressing tumour	Percentage with regressing tumour	Significance
500 to 1,500 roentgens	1 to 7 days	2 of 39	5·0%	Difference
600 to 2,000 ,,	8 to 12 ,,	4 of 45	8·9%	sig.
1,000 to 2,000 ,,	13 to 26 ,,	7 of 43	16·5%	$p < 0·05$
950 to 1,050 ,,	1 to 10 ,,	2 of 44	4·5%	Difference
950 to 1,050 ,,	11 to 17 ,,	6 of 40	15·0%	sig. $p < 0.05$

Nevertheless, the author has seen the onset of tumour regression in some cases even before the menses cease (*see* p. 33). This suggests that *complete* ablation of ovarian function may not be necessary for tumour control in all cases (*see below*).

SURGICAL VERSUS RADIATION CASTRATION

Treves and Finkbeiner (1958) suggest that surgical castration may be more effective than radiation castration, because in a small percentage of their

of women over forty years of age, and a higher dose is advisable in the former group.

Gordon and Segaloff (1958) have suggested that apart from total dosage, the overall time of ovarian irradiation also may be important in determining effective castration. Table 4.2 shows the duration of the X-ray therapy course and the dose delivered to the region of the ovaries in 127 women in the author's series of therapeutic castration in breast cancer. The data suggest that the tumour remission rate may be significantly greater when the same radiation dose is spread over a more prolonged time period.

Because of the slower response to radiation, surgical castration is advised by the author in case of clinical urgency. This category would include the presence of painful bone metastases, or of lung, pleural, brain or liver metastases from breast cancer. Surgical castration is also advised in all cases where the tumour growth rate is rapid, as evidenced by a short 'free interval' between mastectomy and recurrence.

A disadvantage of surgical castration is the operative mortality rate. A further possible disadvantage is that any procedure causing 'acute stress' leads to an outpouring of ACTH, which as suggested by Nathanson et al. (1951) can stimulate increased oestrogen secretion from the adrenal cortex. Thus, Bulbrook and Greenwood (1957) reported an immediate *increase* in oestrogen excretion following oophorectomy in some cases, presumably due to operative stress.

Comparison of the two methods in respect of the stress factor has not been reported, but on a theoretical basis 'acute stress' is probably greater from surgical than from radiation castration. This may account for the observation by Wilson et al. (1958) of occasional exacerbation of breast cancer activity after oophorectomy. Such an observation would lend support to the suggestion of Nissen Meyer and Vogt (1959), that corticosteroids be prescribed after castration in breast cancer for the purpose of counter-acting increased ACTH secretion.

INDICATIONS FOR THERAPEUTIC CASTRATION

It cannot be emphasised too strongly that for all pre-menopausal patients with recurrent or inoperable breast cancer, castration is indicated as the initial method of treatment. 'Medical' castration by androgen therapy carries with it the complication of virilisation and does not provide as high a proportion of remissions or as prolonged remissions (*see* p. 37). It is advised in premenopausal patients only if there is a specific contra-indication to surgical or radiation castration. Surgical castration is worth while even in premenopausal patients with liver, lung, or cerebral metastases, and may gain one or more years of useful life in a proportion of cases.

For postmenopausal patients within five years of the clinical menopause, cytohormonal evaluation by serial vaginal smears is suggested. If persistent oestrogenic activity is noted, series of biochemical estimations of oestrogen excretion levels in the urine are carried out. If the levels are high, or if they show cyclical fluctuation in level (Brown, 1967), or if the levels are not suppressed by dexamethasone administration (Castellanos et al., 1963), castration is advised as initial endocrine therapy also in these patients. The use of the vaginal smear as a method of selecting treatment for such cases has been suggested by Munguia et al. (1960), Hortling et al. (1962), Donegan (1967), and the author (Stoll, 1967b).

Postmenopausal secretion of oestrogens by the adrenal cortex is well recognised, but Nissen Meyer (1964) has shown that the ovary also may continue oestrogen secretion for some years after the menopause (*see* p. 8). Block et al. (1960) have shown that postmenopausal patients with a high oestrogen excretion level before castration, are more likely to benefit from the operation. In a series reported by Munguia et al. (1960), the tumour remission rate of breast cancer after castration was 51·8 per cent in pre-menopausal, as against 38·8 per cent in recently postmenopausal patients. However, when the patients were sub-divided on the basis of vaginal smear examination, the tumour remission rate was 72·7 per cent in those with a highly oestrogenised smear as against 21·7 per cent in those with a poorly oestrogenised smear. If an unselected group of patients past the menopause, both recent and long-standing, is submitted to castration the tumour remission rate of breast cancer is less than 10 per cent, according to Treves and Finkbeiner (1958).

Cytohormonal evaluation of the vaginal smear is suggested by the author (Stoll, 1967b) also in deciding whether castration is necessary for the younger patient with breast cancer who has had a hysterectomy in the preceding five years, and in whom it is uncertain whether ovarian activity persists. It is generally believed that the ovaries atrophy rapidly in such cases, due to interference with their vascularity, but persistent oestrogenic activity after several years has been demonstrated in some of these patients. If oestrogenic activity is demonstrated in the serial vaginal smear, biochemical estimations to determine its source are carried out as described at the beginning of this section.

PALLIATIVE RESULTS OF CASTRATION

The mean duration of tumour regression is between ten and fourteen months in the majority of therapeutic castration series reviewed by Lewison (1965). The average period before reactivation of breast cancer in the author's series was 20·9 months and in the series of Hortling et al. (1962) was as long as twenty-five months. Such average periods of tumour regression are as long as those reported from bilateral adrenalectomy or from hypophyseal ablation (*see* p. 91) and are certainly longer than the average period of tumour growth remission following androgen therapy.

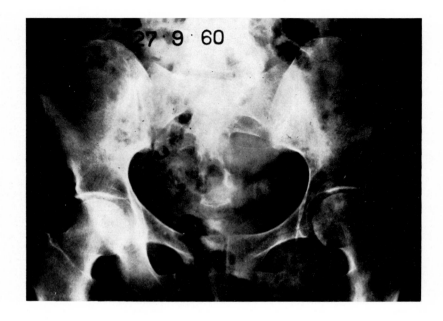

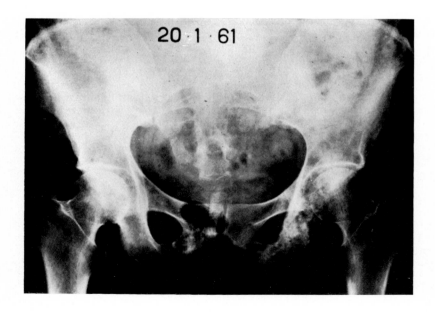

FIGURE 4.1 Patient M.G. Radiographs to show recalcification of metastases from breast cancer in the ischium and acetabulum within four months of surgical castration

Radiographs taken 27 September 1960 and 20 January 1961

Castration also prolongs life in hormone sensitive cases. An average survival of 31·3 months following castration is noted in favourably responding cases of breast cancer in Taylor's series (1962) compared to only 8·8 months in non-responding cases. The corresponding figures in the author's series are 32·1 and 13·7 months respectively—a considerable extension of survival. It has been suggested that this prolonged survival in responding cases may reflect the natural history of a slower growing tumour, such as responds to castration. Nevertheless, the author's series shows no significant difference in response to castration between a group of patients with a short recurrence-free interval following mastectomy compared with those with a long recurrence-free interval (Table 4.3).

Objective evidence of tumour regression following castration in breast cancer includes significant shrinkage of a breast tumour (Plate 1), or of metastatic nodes or nodules, or significant regression of visceral metastases in liver, brain or lungs. Delay in reaccumulation of serous effusions and recalcification in lytic bone metastases are also observed radiographically in some cases (Fig. 4.1). It should be noted that patients often fail to show regression of metastatic lesions in all systems or their control for the same period. Existing lytic lesions in bone may develop sclerotic changes even while new lytic lesions are appearing, or pleural metastases may appear while bone lesions are healing.

Subjective benefit is also seen following castration in advanced breast cancer. Some patients who show no radiographic evidence of healing in bone metastases, may nevertheless obtain subjective benefit in the form of rapid relief of pain, improvement in appetite, gain in weight or return to near normal activity. Changes in haemoglobin or in serum calcium levels are not generally accepted as objective evidence of tumour regression in patients with bone metastases.

FACTORS INFLUENCING RESULTS OF CASTRATION

Favourable response to castration by patients with recurrent breast cancer seems likely to be associated with a longer recurrence-free interval since mastectomy (Table 4.3). This characteristic cannot however be linked with any specific histological picture (*see* p. 117). In the series of Treves and Finkbeiner (1958) the mean recurrence-free interval is twenty-four months for favourably responding cases, but fourteen months for non-responding cases. In Taylor's series (1962) the figures are thirty-two and 20·9 months respectively. Remarkably enough, Table 4.3 shows that there is no significant difference in the recur-

rence-free interval between the two groups in the author's series.

There is a site selectivity governing the likelihood of response to oophorectomy according to Taylor (1962). Bone metastases respond favourably in 38·7 per cent of cases, breast and soft tissue tumour in

TABLE 4.3

Reports of Favourable Clinical Response to Castration in Patients with Breast Cancer. The Average Length of Free Interval Between Mastectomy and First Recurrence, in Those with Regression of Tumour as Against Those Without

| Author | Total cases | Average recurrence-free interval if: | |
		Regression of tumour	No regression of tumour
Treves and Finkbeiner, 1958	191	24 months	14 months
Taylor, 1962	398	32 months	20·9 months
Stoll, 1964a	162	20·3 months	20·9 months

22·6 per cent and visceral metastases in 18·6 per cent of cases. It has also been noted by Taylor (1962), that younger premenopausal patients with breast cancer show a lower tumour remission rate after surgical castration than do older premenopausal patients. He showed tumour regression in 16·3 per cent of patients under 35, but in 31·6 per cent of patients over thirty-five years of age. A significant difference in tumour remission rate was, however, not found between premenopausal patients under forty and those over forty years of age, in the author's series of 162 patients, treated by X-ray castration. The tumour remission rate was 18·7 per cent of patients in the younger age group and 12·6 per cent in the older group (Table 4.4).

As noted previously (*see* p. 14), the change in oestrogen excretion levels in breast cancer patients following castration cannot be related to the likelihood of tumour regression from castration. Associated with remission of tumour growth following castration, oestrogen excretion may either decrease, increase, or remain unchanged in level.

Escher (1958) reported that remission of tumour growth in breast cancer following castration is associated with a 30 per cent likelihood of a similar response later to androgen therapy. Hall *et al.* (1963b) have analysed the relationship between a favourable response to castration, and subsequent similar response to either androgen or oestrogen therapy. In a review of three collected series totalling

282 patients, they conclude that of the patients responding favourably to castration, 23 per cent will respond similarly to subsequent hormonal therapy, while of the patients not responding to castration, only 7 per cent will respond favourably to subsequent hormonal therapy (Table 4.5).

COMBINED CASTRATION WITH CORTICOSTEROIDS

It has been suggested by Nissen Meyer and Vogt (1959) that after X-ray castration for breast cancer, the ACTH stimulated oestrogen secretion of the adrenal cortex should be suppressed by the administration of cortisone 50 mg daily. Nevertheless, it must

In their breast cancer series, objective evidence of tumour growth remission was noted by Nissen Meyer and Vogt (1959) in 51 per cent of patients for an average duration of eighteen months following the combination of X-ray castration and corticosteroid therapy. They suggest that this treatment is as effective as bilateral adrenalectomy or hypophysectomy in this disease. Similarly a report by Brinkley and Kingsley-Pillers (1960) noted that the administration of prednisolone 20 mg daily after oophorectomy yields improved palliative results over those from oophorectomy alone.

It is of interest that Eley and Riddell (1960) find no correlation between clinical benefit in cases treated by corticosteroids after castration and the

TABLE 4.4

Clinical Response to Radiation Castration in Patients with Breast Cancer. Results in Relation to Age Group, and in Relation to Whether Androgen was Added Concurrently (Author's Series)

		Cases with regressing tumour	Percentage with regressing tumour	Significance
Age group	Up to 39	11 of 59	18·7%	Difference
	Over 40	13 of 103	12·6%	not sig.
Method used	Castration alone	15 of 95	15·8%	Difference
	Castration with added androgens	9 of 67	13·4%	not sig.

TABLE 4.5

Favourable Clinical Response to Hormonal Therapy by Patients with Breast Cancer. Results in Relation to the Response to Previous Therapeutic Castration (after Hall *et al.*, 1963b)

	Cases	Percentage
Tumours previously regressing after castration:		
Now regress after hormonal therapy in	16 of 69	23%
No reponse to hormonal therapy in	53 of 69	77%
No previous regression after castration:		
Now regress after hormonal therapy in	14 of 213	7%
No response to hormonal therapy in	199 of 213	93%

be taken into account that this will be only one of several possible relevant endocrinological effects from such therapy. This corticosteroid administration will also cause increased secretion of luteinising gonadotropin, according to Lemon (1957).

degree of adrenal suppression as shown by keto-steroid or oestrogen excretion levels. Therefore, the benefit from corticosteroid therapy in such cases may be from a local effect on the tumour, as the administration of 20 mg prednisolone daily in postmenopausal patients with breast cancer often leads to decrease in oedema around a tumour mass, relief of pain from bone metastases, and a subjective feeling of well-being (*see* p. 77).

Because of the side effects following prolonged prednisolone dosage the combined treatment is not recommended by the author as a routine procedure after castration. Nevertheless, there is no doubt that a *short* course of prednisolone after castration may be beneficial subjectively in a very ill patient. Corticosteroid therapy is combined with radiation castration also in the case of hormone insensitive tumours (*see* p. 121).

COMBINED CASTRATION WITH ANDROGENS OR THYROID HORMONE

Castration is always to be preferred to androgen therapy as the initial endocrine treatment in the premenopausal patient with recurrent or inoperable breast cancer, even in the presence of visceral metastases (*see* p. 25). However, it has been suggested by Poppe and Gregl (1961) and by Hortling *et al.* (1962) that the clinical benefits of castration may be improved by the concomitant administration of androgens. In the author's breast cancer series (Stoll, 1964*a*), and in the series of Donegan (1967), there was no significant difference in the overall tumour remission rate after castration, whether or not androgens were added (Table 4.4). Nevertheless, it was noted by the author that in patients with bone

metastases, the proportion showing recalcification was higher when androgens were added, probably because of a specific controlling effect of androgens upon calcium deposition in bone. It may also be useful to add androgen therapy to castration in patients under thirty-five years of age with advanced breast cancer, because of the poorer results from castration alone in this age group, as shown by Taylor (1962).

Except for patients with bone metastases, and those aged thirty-five or less, it is therefore better to reserve androgens until tumour activity recurs after castration. At this stage objective evidence of tumour regression is said by Escher (1958) to result from androgen therapy in 30 per cent of those patients previously responding favourably to castration—a much higher tumour remission rate than that which occurs in those previously not responding to castration. However, in the group of patients within two years of the menopause, the author finds objective evidence of favourable response to androgen therapy to be rare, whether or not there has been a previous response to castration. Nonetheless, relief of pain from bone metastases is commonly achieved.

Beatson (1896) suggested that thyroid extract be prescribed as an adjuvant to the effect of castration in young women with breast cancer, and this advice was repeated by early authors such as Boyd (1900) and Herman (1900). The value of tri-iodothyronine administration in controlling breast cancer was not proved in a clinical trial by Emery and Trotter (1963) (*see* p. 10).

Prophylactic Castration

This term describes castration carried out at the time of radical surgical treatment of the primary breast cancer. It had been suggested as early as 1889 by Schinzinger, and its results were first examined by Taylor (1939). The value of the procedure was not clearly established until Siegert (1952) demonstrated a fifteen months longer delay before the onset of recurrence, in a prophylactically castrated group compared with a non castrated group. Treves's series (1957) also confirmed that recurrence was delayed in patients castrated prophylactically, especially those castrated surgically.

With regard to the beneficial effect of prophylactic castration upon five year survival there have been several reports since that of Horsley (1954) (Table 4.6). The first *randomised* control trial was of prophylactic X-ray castration in patients with breast

cancer, who were premenopausal or up to two years postmenopausal. A single dose of 450 roentgens was given to the ovaries. This report by Paterson and Russell (1959) notes an increase in the five year survival in Stage 2 following prophylactic castration, although just below the usually accepted level of statistical significance (Table 4.6). The results might have been more significant if analysis had been confined to premenopausal patients only, and those up to two years postmenopausal excluded.

A later analysis of the same patients by Cole (1964) suggests that at ten years following castration there was a significant difference ($p = 0.007$) between the survival rates of castrated and non-castrated groups. Another randomised control trial was reported by Nissen Meyer (1964) which demonstrated a decreased recurrence rate in premenopausal women treated by prophylactic X-ray castration, compared to non-castrated women.

In an earlier study McWhirter (1957) had noted identical five year survival rates in breast cancer, whether or not prophylactic X-ray castration was given, both pre- and postmenopausal patients up to 69 years of age being included in the trial. Nevertheless, in a randomised series of *post*menopausal women up to seventy years of age with breast cancer, Nissen Meyer (1964) has more recently shown an improved four year survival and decreased recurrence rate, in those given prophylactic irradiation to the ovaries

patients subjected to the prophylactic procedure the interval *before* recurrence was longer than in those subjected to therapeutic castration. On the other hand survival *after* recurrence was shorter for prophylactic castration than for therapeutic castration (Table 4.7). The group of women castrated prophylactically suffered from recurrent disease for only 21·3 per cent of their survival time after mastectomy, although the *total* survival time was not significantly different between the two groups.

It should be taken into account that Kennedy's figures include both Stage 1 and 2 cases. It is in the

TABLE 4.6

Reports of Improvement in Five Year Survival Following Prophylactic Castration at the Time of Mastectomy for Breast Cancer

	Percentage 5 year survival in:				
	Stage 1		Stage 2		
Author	Castrated	Control	Castrated	Control	
Smith and Smith, 1953	82%	76%	74%	31%	Surgical
Horsley, 1957	88%	80%	45%	36%	castration
Treves, 1957	91%	77%	76%	39%	
Treves, 1957	80%	77%	43%	39%	Radiation
Paterson and Russell, 1959	83%	76%	55%	47%	castration
McWhirter, 1956	64%	64%	Stages 1 and 2 combined		

at the time of mastectomy, compared to non-irradiated women. Ovarian secretion of oestrogens was shown to continue after the menopause, as in each five year age group up to 70, the urinary output of oestrogen was found to be lower in the castrated than in the control group.

On this basis, Nissen Meyer (1964) advises prophylactic ovarian radiation in all breast cancer patients up to seventy years of age. In the author's opinion, it would be more logical to restrict such irradiation to those patients showing oestrogenisation in the vaginal smears, and then only if biochemical estimations suggest that this is likely to be of ovarian origin (*see* p. 25).

PROPHYLACTIC VERSUS THERAPEUTIC CASTRATION

Kennedy *et al.* (1964), in a retrospective study on 213 patients with breast cancer, compares the effect on survival time of prophylactic castration, with that of therapeutic castration delayed until metastases were manifest. The two series of women were carefully matched before analysis. He noted that in the

latter group that one would expect considerable advantage from castration, and the inclusion of the former group will tend to decrease the significance

TABLE 4.7

Benefit from Prophylactic Castration Compared to That from Therapeutic Castration in Breast Cancer (after Kennedy *et al.*, 1964)

Surgical or radiation castration in Stages 1 and 2 combined	Mean interval for:	
	Prophylactic castration	Therapeutic castration
Mastectomy to recurrence	38·2 months	24·6 months
Recurrence to death	13·7 ,,	23·4 ,,
Mastectomy to death	56·2 ,,	47·3 ,,

of the results. Nevertheless, it appears that the effect of prophylactic castration, like that of the spontaneous menopause (*see* p. 11), cannot be regarded as curative, but merely as a temporary retarding influence upon recurrence of tumour (Fig. 4.2).

When considering the justification of advising prophylactic castration at the time of mastectomy, it should be taken into account that only about one patient in three in Stage 1 (axillary nodes found free of tumour), will develop tumour recurrence. In this stage, therefore, the disadvantages of prematurely terminating ovarian function should be carefully weighed against the possible advantages. Castration of the premenopausal patient may lead to increased

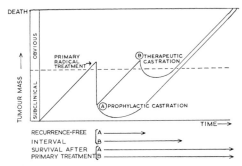

FIGURE 4.2 Diagrammatic representation of the effect of prophylactic castration in prolonging the 'recurrence-free' interval after mastectomy for breast cancer; also the effect of therapeutic castration in delaying tumour growth

(Figure modified from Nissen Meyer, 1964)

susceptibility to cardiovascular disease and may predispose to early osteoporosis, apart from causing thinning of the hair, dryness of the skin and loss of libido (Ansfield, 1967). Coming after a mutilating operation and a tiring course of irradiation, the psychological and physical burden of prophylactic castration needs to be justified by a high likelihood of benefit.

Although on a theroretical basis the hormonal changes following castration may lead to failure to survive of cells liberated at mastectomy, there is no evidence of an increased *cure* rate by adding castration to the primary treatment. Prophylactic castration therefore, is not usually advised in Stage 1 cases, except in the case of a highly anaplastic tumour which would carry a poor prognosis. In Stage 2 cases on the other hand, the likelihood of recurrence is high. It is in such cases that there is a high likelihood of prophylactic castration postponing recurrence and giving the patient a longer period free from anxiety, even if not providing a longer survival.

A disadvantage of therapeutic castration is that being postponed until recurrence occurs, it may find the patient too ill from pulmonary, hepatic, or cerebral metastases to benefit at that stage. Prophylactic castration may therefore be preferred in the

patient for whom regular follow up examination is likely to be difficult. On the other hand, prophylactic castration has the disadvantage that it deprives the medical attendant of an indicator of hormone sensitivity—the results of therapeutic castration later. This reason is of minor importance if biochemical indices are used to help determine hormone sensitivity to steroid administration. Such indices are discussed in Chapter 10.

EFFECT OF PREGNANCY ON 'CURED' BREAST CANCER

The prevention of future pregnancy has been quoted as one of the advantages of prophylactic castration in breast cancer. Although it is usual to advise postponement of pregnancy for two to three years after mastectomy, while watching for early recurrence, there is no evidence that the high natural oestrogen and progesterone levels of pregnancy will reactivate breast cancer which is under control after radical treatment (*see* p. 11).

In a review of the literature, White (1954) reported a five year survival rate of 49 per cent in 208 patients permitted to undergo pregnancy following radical treatment for breast cancer. This was comparable to the gross survival rate in a control series with breast cancer, in whom pregnancy did not occur. A similar finding was reported by Holleb and Farrow (1962) and by Peters (1963). Nevertheless, if pregnancy is postponed for a few years after radical treatment (as it usually is) such a series would naturally eliminate patients with more active tumours. The point is therefore not conclusively proven.

OVARIAN PATHOLOGY AND CASTRATION

It was suggested by Sicard (1948) that the presence of unsuspected ovarian metastases in a high proportion of women with advanced breast cancer, justifies prophylactic castration as a routine. Larger reported series, Warren and Witham (1933), Abrams et al. (1950), and Lumb and Mackenzie (1959) showed an incidence of ovarian metastases, varying between 9 per cent and 29 per cent of cases, according to the stage of the disease at which examination was carried out—laparotomy or autopsy. The significance of these observations is not clear but, in any case, the presence of ovarian metastase is usually indicative of widespread disease, and their removal could not be regarded as curative.

It has been shown by Sommers and Teloh (1952, 1953) that hyperplasia of the ovarian cortical stroma is found in 82 per cent of autopsies in patients with breast cancer—very much more frequently than in the normal population. This has been suggested as a reason for surgical removal of the ovaries as opposed to radiation menopause, because the ovarian stroma which is relatively radio-resistant compared to the follicle, is capable of secreting oestrogens. Nevertheless, biochemical evidence of excessive oestrogen secretion is not found in premenopausal patients with breast cancer according to Jull *et al.* (1963), and Segaloff (1967*b*). Nor is there a correlation, as pointed out previously (*see* p. 14), between the nature of the tumour response to castration, and the change in oestrogen excretion levels after such treatment. An advantage for surgical over radiation menopause on this basis, is therefore not obvious.

TO SUMMARISE

Therapeutic castration, whether by surgery or radiation is the initial method of choice and will induce objective evidence of tumour regression in over 30 per cent of premenopausal patients with advanced breast cancer. Prolongation of survival has been demonstrated in patients showing favourable response to castration. In a further proportion, there results evidence of subjective improvement, which is unassociated with objective signs of tumour regression. Castration is worth a trial even in patients with large visceral metastases, such as those in the lungs or liver.

Some postmenopausal patients with breast cancer, will also benefit from this procedure, if evidence of oestrogen secretion suggests persistence of ovarian activity. Short-term administration of corticosteroids may dampen down ACTH mediated increase in adrenal oestrogen production after castration.

Prophylactic castration at the time of mastectomy is justified in Stage 2 cases of breast cancer, as a means of postponing recurrence, and thus giving the patient a longer period free from anxiety.

Castration Therapy

ILLUSTRATIVE CASE SUMMARIES

Patient A.C.R. Recalcification of Bone Metastases for Three and Half Years following X-ray Castration and Androgen Therapy. Subsequent Bilateral Adrenalectomy Ineffective

A premenopausal woman aged forty-five, presented in November 1952 with a carcinoma of the right breast. Primary treatment was by radical mastectomy but thirty months later, bone pain appeared and radiographs showed the presence of multiple lytic areas of metastases in bone. Endocrine therapy was initiated by carrying out X-ray castration, delivering a dose of 1,500 roentgens in twenty-two days to the region of the ovaries. At the same time, a course of testosterone propionate 100 mg intramuscularly three times a week was begun.

Bone pain was quickly relieved and the patient was returned to near normal activity. Testosterone injections were continued for a period of eight months, and then replaced by implants of testosterone 800 mg every three months over a period of twenty-two months. The radiographs showed recalcification of previously lytic areas in bone, and no new areas of destruction appeared. Pain relief lasted altogether for three and a half years and was then lost. At the end of that time, a parasternal tumour appeared, presumed to be a metastasis arising in the internal mammary nodes. Bilateral adrenalectomy and oophorectomy were advised and carried out, but without any resulting clinical benefit, and the patient died four months later.

Patient P.S.H. Regression of Soft Tissue and Bone Metastases for Twenty-four Months following X-ray Castration and Androgen Therapy

A premenopausal patient aged forty-one presented in November 1954 with a cancer of the breast, and metastatic axillary node enlargement. Bone pain was found to be associated with multiple lytic areas of skeletal metastasis. In view of the widespread metastases, endocrine treatment was initiated by carrying out X-ray castration, delivering a dose of 1,500 roentgens in twenty days to the ovaries. At the same time a course of testosterone propionate 100 mg intramuscularly three times a week was begun. It was continued for sixteen months after which Primoteston depot 250 mg intramuscularly was given at one to two weeks intervals for five months. The former androgen was found more effective in relieving pain.

Within two months of castration, evidence of tumour regression was seen in the breast and axillary nodes. The pain from the bone metastases was relieved for a total period of twenty-four months, and the patient was able to maintain full activity during that time. The radiographs showed recalcification of previously lytic areas, and no new areas of destruction appeared. After twenty-four months, however, bone pain recurred, and six months later irregular enlargement of the liver was palpable. The patient died five months later.

Patient E.T.H. Castration-induced Regression of Lung Metastases for Eighteen Months. No Subsequent Control of Bone Metastases after Androgen or Corticosteroid Therapy or Bilateral Adrenalectomy

A premenopausal patient aged fifty-two, presented in August 1954 with a Stage 2 carcinoma of the left breast. Primary treatment was by radical mastectomy, followed by a prophylactic course of X-ray therapy to the axillary and supraclavicular draining node areas. At ten months after operation the patient complained of cough and dyspnoea, and radiographs showed multiple nodular opacities of metastasis in the lung fields.

Endocrine therapy was initiated by carrying out an X-ray castration, delivering a dose of 1,200 roentgens to the ovaries in a period of fourteen days. The lung opacities decreased in size and density in the ensuing months and dyspnoea was considerably relieved. However, after fourteen months the patient developed bone pains found to be associated with the presence of lytic areas of skeletal metastasis. A trial of testosterone propionate 100 mg intramuscularly three times a week was prescribed for two months. There was no clinical evidence of favourable response and it was therefore followed by a trial of prednisolone 10 mg tds for two months, and a trial of fluoxymesterone 10 mg tds for two months. As there was still no clinical remission, bilateral adrenalectomy and oophorectomy were carried out, but again without relief of pain. The patient died three months later.

Patient F.M.C. Castration-induced Regression of Soft Tissue and Pleural Metastases for Fifteen Months

A premenopausal female aged thirty-two, presented in December 1954 with a Stage 2 carcinoma of the left breast. Primary treatment was by radical mastectomy, followed by a prophylactic course of X-ray therapy to the mastectomy scar, axillary, and supraclavicular draining node areas. At the end of thirty-three months, the patient complained of dyspnoea on exertion, and this was found to be associated with the presence of a malignant right pleural effusion. In addition, new tumour growth soon appeared in the right breast, axillary and supra-clavicular nodes.

Endocrine therapy was initiated by carrying out X-ray castration, delivering to the ovaries a dose of 1,000 roentgens in eleven days. The soft tissue

tumour showed regression in size within a month (although menstruation persisted for two months), and the effusion did not require paracentesis for fifteen months. However, after this time, new metastatic nodes appeared in the left axilla, and the effusion began to reaccumulate. A course of the corticosteroid, dexamethasone 1·6 mg qid, was then prescribed for three months. The corticosteroid administration yielded no control of either of the disease manifestations, and the patient died two months later.

Patient E.P.O. Castration-induced Recalcification of Bone Metastases for Nineteen Months. Subsequent Subjective Benefit from Corticosteroid Therapy

A premenopausal patient aged forty-six, presented in November 1955 with a Stage 2 carcinoma of the right breast. Primary treatment was by radical mastectomy, but eighteen months after the operation, she developed tumour recurrence in the right axilla. This was followed soon after by bone pain found to be associated with multiple lytic areas of skeletal metastasis.

Endocrine therapy was initiated by carrying out X-ray castration, delivering to the ovaries a dose of 1,000 roentgens in nine days. Relief of bone pain resulted in a few weeks, and recalcification of the destroyed areas was seen in the radiographs within three months. Pain relief lasted altogether nineteen months, after which new bone metastases appeared, of a lytic-sclerotic type. At this stage treatment by a course of prednisolone 5 mg qid was prescribed for nine months, yielding relief of pain, but no objective evidence of tumour control. The patient died nine months later.

Patient M.J.E. Castration-induced Regression of Soft Tissue Tumour for Twelve Months. Subsequent Subjective Benefit from Corticosteroid Therapy but Bilateral Adrenalectomy Ineffective

A premenopausal patient aged forty-two, presented in March 1957 with a carcinoma of the right breast. Primary treatment was by radical mastectomy but seven months after the operation, she developed bone pains found to be associated with the presence of lytic areas in a skeletal survey. Soon after, there appeared also metastatic enlargement of the right supraclavicular nodes.

Endocrine therapy was initiated by carrying out surgical castration. This resulted in regression in size of the enlarged nodes, recalcification of the bone metastases and relief of bone pain for a period of twelve months. When pain recurred, a trial of testosterone propionate 100 mg intramuscularly three times a week was found to cause aggravation of the symptoms. Subsequently, a course of prednisolone 10 mg tds was prescribed for a period of three months, with partial control of the pain. For this reason, bilateral adrenalectomy and oophorectomy were advised and carried out, but without clinical evidence of benefit and the patient died two months later.

Patient N.H.E. Short-term Control of Bone Metastases following Surgical Castration

A premenopausal woman aged twenty-eight, attended in May 1957 with a Stage 2 carcinoma of the right breast. Primary treatment was by radical mastectomy but eleven months after operation, the patient developed bone pains found to be associated with lytic areas of skeletal metastasis. Endocrine therapy was initiated by carrying out surgical castration. Pain relief was rapid, and radiographs showed sclerosis of the previously lytic areas of bone metastasis.

No new areas of bone metastases appeared, but within six months of castration bone pain recurred. A course of Sublings testosterone 10 mg qid, was prescribed for eight months without relief of pain. At this stage, malignant ascites developed, and a mass of tumour was found to be palpable in the soft tissues of the pelvis. A single intravenous dose of the cytotoxic agent, Endoxan 50 mg/kilo, resulted only in subjective improvement, and the patient's condition deteriorated until death seven months later.

Patient A.F.E. Castration-induced Recalcification of Bone Metastases for Sixteen Months. Subsequent Androgen Therapy Caused Pain Exacerbation

A premenopausal patient aged thirty-four, presented in March 1960 with cancer of the left breast. Primary treatment was by radical mastectomy but twenty-four months following the operation she complained of skeletal pain, found to be associated with multiple areas of metastasis in bone. Endocrine therapy was initiated by carrying out surgical castration and this resulted in immediate relief of pain. In the following months, recalcification of the bone metastases was visible in the radiographs.

At sixteen months following castration, pain recurred and new areas of bone metastases were visible in the radiographs. Separate attempts to institute testosterone propionate therapy and fluoxymesterone therapy, caused pain exacerbation. On the other hand, a trial of prednisolone 10 mg tds, yielded relief of pain for a month. For this reason, the patient was referred for adrenalectomy but she died postoperatively.

Patient R.K.E. Healing of Bone Metastases for Nine Months following X-ray Castration and Androgen Therapy. Liver Metastases Developed Under Treatment

A premenopausal woman aged forty, presented in December 1951 with cancer of the breast. It was associated with the presence of metastatic supraclavicular node enlargement, and multiple lytic areas of metastasis in the spine. The breast, axillary, and supraclavicular areas were treated by a palliative course of X-ray therapy to a minimum dose of 4,000 roentgens in thirty-five days. Regression of the soft tissue tumour followed X-ray therapy and was maintained until death.

Endocrine therapy was initiated by carrying out X-ray castration, delivering to the ovaries a dose of 2,000 roentgens in fourteen days. At the same time, androgen therapy was instituted—at first testosterone propionate 100 mg intramuscularly three times a week, and later methyl testosterone 25 mg qid. As a result, bone pain was relieved and the previously lytic areas of metastases in bone assumed a sclerotic appearance. Androgen therapy was maintained for twelve months, but in spite of this, the liver was found to be grossly enlarged and irregular, when examined nine months after X-ray castration. The patient died three months later.

Patient E.S.Y. Recalcification of Bone Metastases for Fourteen Months following X-ray Castration and Androgen Therapy. Subsequent Subjective Benefit from Corticosteroid Therapy

A premenopausal woman aged thirty-seven, presented in August 1953 with a Stage 1 carcinoma of the right breast. Primary treatment was by radical mastectomy, followed by a prophylactic course of X-ray therapy to the mastectomy scar, axillary, and supraclavicular draining node areas. At thirty-three months after the operation, she developed bone pain and this was found to be associated with lytic areas of metastasis in the skeleton. Shortly afterwards, new tumour growth appeared in the left breast and left axilla.

Endocrine therapy was initiated by carrying out X-ray castration, delivering to the ovaries a dose of 900 roentgens in four days. At the same time, a course of fluoxymesterone 10 mg tds was begun. Bone pain was relieved very rapidly and the X-rays showed recalcification of previously lytic areas of metastasis after about three months. After fourteen months of androgen therapy, however, the bone pain increased and treatment by fluoxymesterone was stopped. A urinary calcium suppression test was carried out using prednisolone, and when this caused a fall in calcium excretion levels, a course of prednisolone 10 mg tds was prescribed for a period of three months. During this time there was pain relief, but progression of bone metastases in the radiographs. The patient died eight months later.

Patient L.L.A. Failure of Favourable Response to X-ray Castration, Surgical Castration, Androgen Therapy, Prednisolone Therapy, and ThioTEPA Administration

A premenopausal patient presented in October 1957, with a Stage 1 carcinoma of the left breast. Primary treatment was by radical mastectomy, followed by a prophylactic course of X-ray therapy to the axillary, supraclavicular, and internal mammary draining node areas. At twenty-eight months after the operation, recurrent tumour appeared in the left parasternal area, presumed to be arising in the internal mammary nodes. Later, enlarged metastatic nodes appeared above the clavicles.

Endocrine therapy was initiated by carrying out X-ray castration, delivering a dose of 1,200 roentgens in four days to the region of the ovaries. Regression in the soft tissue tumour did not follow, and therefore five months later, oophorectomy was carried out. At the same time, a trial of fluoxymesterone 10 mg tds was prescribed for two months. Again, there was no remission of tumour growth and, after an interval, a two months trial of prednisolone 10 mg tds was prescribed. This was associated with an intramuscular course of the cytotoxic agent, thioTEPA, given to haemopoictic tolerance levels. Nevertheless, the soft tissue tumour grew progressively, and the patient died thirteen months after developing the first recurrence.

Patient M.D.U. Favourable Response to X-ray Castration and Androgen Therapy, Delayed Six Months in the Case of Soft Tissue and Liver Metastases

A premenopausal patient aged forty-three, presented in July 1955 with a carcinoma of the right breast. Primary treatment was by radical mastectomy, but eight months after the operation, she developed nodular recurrence in the scar, and metastatic enlargement of the axillary and supraclavicular nodes. Later, new tumour growth appeared in the left breast.

Endocrine therapy was initiated by carrying out X-ray castration, delivering to the ovaries a dose of 1,000 roentgens in eleven days. At the same time, a course of methyl testosterone 25 mg qid was prescribed for three months. At five months after castration, the liver was found to be grossly enlarged and irregular, and new nodular recurrence had appeared near the mastectomy scar. In addition, the patient complained of bone pain, and this was found to be associated with multiple lytic areas of metastasis in bone.

Arrangements were being made to carry out bilateral adrenalectomy when, one month later, the bone pain was spontaneously relieved. A month after that the skin nodules had flattened, and the liver enlargement had decreased. In spite of this, the radiographs showed increase in bone destruction, and the patient died three months later, of bone marrow replacement.

5

Androgen Therapy

THE BASIS for the treatment of human breast cancer by androgen therapy was the observation by Lacassagne (1936*b*), that the growth of mammary carcinoma in female mice could be inhibited by the administration of testosterone propionate. As a consequence, androgens were suggested in the treatment of advanced breast cancer by Loeser (1939) and by Ulrich (1939) independently.

The place of androgen therapy in the steroid treatment of breast cancer has been debated somewhat emotionally in the literature. The androgen most widely used until about ten years ago was testosterone propionate, early reports on its use in breast cancer being those of Adair (1947) and the author (Stoll, 1950). Effective treatment with this androgen was often associated with a considerable degree of virilisation, and for this reason, a large body of opinion considered its use unjustifiable in the treatment of breast cancer in women. In spite of numerous reports in the last 10 years of newer, equally effective, but less virilising androgens (*see* p. 46), a deprecatory attitude against the androgen therapy of breast cancer is still maintained by authorities such as Juret (1966) and Pearson (1967).

FREQUENCY OF RESPONSE TO ANDROGENS

The AMA Committee on Research (1960) in a retrospective survey of 420 assembled cases of postmenopausal breast cancer who had been treated with androgens, reported objective evidence of tumour regression in 21·9 per cent of cases. A collective survey of 521 patients by the Co-operative Breast Cancer Group (1964) reported tumour regression in 21·5 per cent of cases treated by testosterone propionate (Table 5.1.) The author (Stoll, 1964*a*), reported a personal series of 434 patients treated with androgens, and noted objective evidence of tumour regression in 15 per cent of cases (Table 5.2).

Until recently, doubts were expressed as to whether androgen therapy could actually prolong survival in advanced breast cancer. However, in 1960 the report of the AMA Committee on Research quoted an average survival after treatment of 19·1 months for favourably responding cases, compared to 9·7 months for non-responding cases—a considerable extension of survival. The report of the

TABLE 5.1

Favourable Clinical Response to Testosterone Propionate Therapy, in Relation to Menopausal Age Group, and in Relation to the Dominant Site of Metastasis (Co-operative Breast Cancer Group, 1964*a*)

		Total cases	Percentage with regressing tumour
Age group	Postmenopausal <1 year	92	8·7%
	,, 1–5 years	100	17%
	,, 5–10 ,,	82	25·6%
	,, >10 ,,	247	26·7%
Site	Breast	127	31·5%
	Bone metastases	189	18·5%
	Visceral metastases	205	18%
	Total	521	21·5%

Co-operative Breast Cancer Group (1964) quotes corresponding figures of twenty-three and nine months respectively. The possibility has been suggested (*see* p. 38) that hormone sensitive breast cancers, as a group, may be more slowly growing than the autonomous group.

The average duration of clinical remission from androgen therapy (testosterone propionate or fluoxymesterone) is 10·9 months in the author's series. The Co-operative Breast Cancer Group (1964) reports a median period of remission of eight months from testosterone propionate therapy. A relative

36

preponderance of bone metastases in the author's androgen treated series may explain the somewhat longer average period of remission in his cases. Whereas the average duration of regression of soft tissue lesions is only 6·9 months, that of bone metastases from breast cancer is 13·2 months in the author's series.

TABLE 5.2

Favourable Clinical Response to Androgen Therapy in Relation to the Menopausal Age Group, and in Relation to the Dominant Site of Metastasis (Author's Series)

		Total cases	Percentage with regressing tumour
Age group	Postmenopausal 0–5 years	212	10%
	,, > 5 ,,	222	24%
Site	Local soft tissue	149	16%
	Bone metastases	204	19%
	Visceral metastases	81	11%
	Total	434	15%

The duration of tumour regression after androgen therapy is, in general, shorter than that after castration or oestrogen therapy. Nevertheless, growth remissions for over five years, such as those reported by Raven (1954) are not uncommon in breast cancer following androgen therapy, especially in the case of patients with bone metastases.

FACTORS INFLUENCING THE RESULTS OF ANDROGEN THERAPY

Androgen administration to premenopausal patients will cause temporary amenorrhea. Reports by Pearson *et al.* (1955), Peters (1956), and the AMA Committee on Research (1960) noted tumour regression in between 11 per cent and 20 per cent of premenopausal breast cancer patients treated by androgen therapy. The author, on the other hand, found no objective evidence of tumour regression in a series of twenty-two premenopausal patients so treated, although subjective benefit was common (*see* p. 52). Because of the likelihood of a more frequent and prolonged remission from castration, and the absence of virilisation, practically all authorities prefer it to androgen therapy as the initial treatment in premenopausal patients with disseminated breast cancer. Nonetheless, in patients under the age of thirty-five, or in the presence of bone metastases, androgen therapy may usefully be added to castration,

because of the poorer results from castration alone in this age group shown by Taylor (1962).

In the first two years after the menopause, the tumour remission rate in a group of patients treated by androgen therapy was a disappointingly low 6 per cent in the author's series. Similarly the Co-operative Breast Cancer Group (1964) reports a tumour remission rate of 8·7 per cent from androgen therapy in women castrated less than one year. If androgens acted in breast cancer on an anti-oestrogenic basis, one would expect a greater success in the younger patient, but the reverse is the case (Table 5.1 and 5.2).

With regard to site selectivity, Fig. 5.1 represents the experience of the Co-operative Breast Cancer

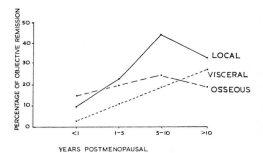

FIGURE 5.1 Clinical response of breast cancer to testosterone propionate therapy in relation to the number of years postmenopausal, and according to the dominant site of metastasis

(Figure modified from *Co-operative Breast Cancer Group Report*, 1961)

Group (1962) in the treatment of metastatic breast cancer by testosterone propionate 100 mg intramuscularly three times a week. Patients with predominantly local soft tissue tumour, have a somewhat higher tumour remission rate than those with predominantly osseous or visceral metastases. The author's series, on the other hand, shows a somewhat higher tumour remission rate in the case of bone metastases (Table 5.2).

Age dependency of response is well established for androgen therapy, as it is for oestrogen therapy (Tables 5.1 and 5.2). The remission rate from androgen therapy increases with increasing postmenopausal age for local and visceral metastases, although age dependency is much less marked in the cases of bone metastases (Fig. 5.1). This may reflect a non-specific role of androgens on calcium metabolism in bone, apart from an effect upon the tumour. In the case of local soft tissue tumour, patients who are more than five years postmenopausal, show tumour regression in between 34–44 per cent of cases, while patients with similar lesions in the first year after the menopause, show similar response to androgen therapy in less than 10 per cent of cases.

INDICATIONS FOR ANDROGEN THERAPY

In breast cancer patients more than five years postmenopausal, there is little doubt that the *overall* results of oestrogen therapy are superior to those of androgen therapy. This was confirmed by Kennedy (1965*a*) in a randomised trial in such patients (*see* p. 54). Nevertheless, there still remain some groups of postmenopausal patients with breast cancer for whom androgen therapy is preferred.

1. AFTER FAILURE OF RESPONSE TO THERAPEUTIC CASTRATION

A trial of androgen therapy may be worthwhile in such cases, because of the low likelihood of a favourable response to major endocrine ablation

to androgen therapy is more likely, and was noted in 17 per cent of patients up to five years postmenopausal (Table 5.1). Subjective benefit, with relief of pain from bone metastases and sometimes improvement in anaemia, is noted in a further number.

According to Escher and Kaufman (1963), the longer the free period between mastectomy and tumour recurrence, the greater the likelihood of favourable reponse to hormone therapy. This observation helps to select suitable patients after castration for androgen therapy, as well as for other forms of endocrine therapy.

2. PRESENCE OF BONE METASTASES

As mentioned previously, the tumour remission rate of bone metastases to androgen therapy appears to be less dependent on age group, than that of the other types of metastasis (Fig. 5.1). In addition, the relatively better overall tumour remission rate of bone metastases to androgen therapy than to oestrogen therapy in the author's experience (Table

TABLE 5.3

Favourable Clinical Response to Androgen Therapy Compared to that from Oestrogen Therapy, in Relation to the Dominant Site of Metastasis in Breast Cancer. (Figures from Author's Series and AMA Committee on Research, 1960)

Site of metastasis	Percentage with regressing tumour after:			
	Androgens		Oestrogens	
	Author's series	AMA series	Author's series	AMA series
Local	16%	23%	36%	38%
Bone	19%	24%	7%	27%*
Visceral	11%	29%*	28%	40%*
Overall regression rate	15%	21%	31%	37%
Cases	434	266	407	166

* represents small series of cases

therapy (*see* p. 88). Oestrogen therapy is not advisable in recently postmenopausal patients until the vaginal smear ceases to show evidence of oestrogenic activity, for fear of exacerbating the disease. Thus, most of this group is best treated by androgens according to Segaloff (1958), although the salvage rate is small (*see* p. 37). Objective evidence of favourable response to androgen therapy was obtained in three, and subjective benefit in a further four, out of thirty-two such cases treated within one year of the menopause by the author.

If patients less than one year postmenopausal are excluded, objective evidence of favourable response

5.3), suggests a trial of androgens in such cases. Such treatment has also been recommended by Huseby (1958).

In patients with bone metastases, androgen therapy is certainly advisable before bilateral adrenalectomy or hypophysectomy are considered, except in the presence of hypercalcaemia. In such a case, major endocrine ablation is the preferred treatment of the disease after initial control of the serum calcium level is established. This frequently requires the use of corticosteroid therapy (*see* p. 43).

A recent randomised trial reported by Dao and Nemoto (1965) illustrates the importance of individualising endocrine therapy. It compares the overall results of bilateral adrenalectomy with those of fluoxymesterone at a dose of 20 mg daily, in the therapy of a group of postmenopausal patients. The former treatment yielded an *overall* tumour remission rate of 45 per cent, the latter of only 16 per cent. However, if patients are selected for androgen therapy from among those with bone metastases and those more than five years postmenopausal, objective evidence of tumour regression is found in 26 per cent in the author's series. The corresponding figure of 24 per cent is noted by the Co-operative Breast Cancer Group (1962) using testosterone propionate. Operation can thus be postponed in such a selected group of patients and bilateral adrenalectomy would still be possible in these cases after control from androgens has been lost (*see* p. 126). It is important to state that in the patients failing to respond favourably to such a trial of androgen therapy in this group, operation is postponed for only about 6 weeks.

3. SECONDARY THERAPY

Postmenopausal patients who have previously shown favourable tumour response to castration or to oestrogen therapy may be given a trial of androgen therapy as long as the patients' symptoms are not urgent. In the author's series, there is a 22 per cent likelihood of favourable response to secondary androgen therapy after previous oestrogen therapy has lost its control. According to Escher and Kaufman (1961), clinical benefit from androgen therapy is seen in 30 per cent of castration or oestrogen responders.

It has been emphasised by Hortling *et al.* (1962) that androgen therapy, given as the secondary treatment in breast cancer, is less efficacious than when given as the first treatment. Nevertheless, after previous hormone therapy has been found ineffective, there is still a 15 per cent likelihood of favourable response to secondary androgen therapy, according to Witt *et al.* (1965). Osseous metastases, in patients more than five years postmenopausal, which have previously failed to show favourable response to oestrogens, are more likely to respond favourably to secondary androgen therapy than are soft tissue lesions with the same history.

Secondary androgen therapy appears in general, to be somewhat more efficacious in breast cancer than is secondary oestrogen therapy (Table 5.4). Furthermore, unlike oestrogens which are not effective after failure of hypophysectomy (Escher and Kaufman 1961), fluoxymesterone therapy has been shown by Kennedy (1958), Beckett and Brennan (1959), and the author (*see* p. 94), to cause tumour regression even in patients regarded as completely hypophysectomised.

TABLE 5.4

Favourable Clinical Response to Second Hormonal Trial After Initial Hormonal Therapy has Lost Control in Breast Cancer (Author's Series)

	Now regress after androgens in:	
Previous tumour regression after oestrogen	22%	Overall in 7 of 47 = 15%
Previous failure of oestrogen	12%	

	Now regress after oestrogens in:	
Previous tumour regression after androgen	20%	Overall in 5 of 46 = 11%
Previous failure of androgen	8%	

RECOGNITION OF ANDROGEN RESPONSE

The earliest signs of regression in the breast tumour, skin nodules or metastatic nodes, are not usually seen until about six weeks after starting androgen therapy. Approximately half the potential regressions are present by eight weeks according to the Co-operative Breast Cancer Group (1964). Nevertheless it should be emphasised that regression of soft tissue tumour may occasionally be delayed for three months, and recalcification of bone metastases for three to six months, after initiating androgen therapy. A course of such therapy should therefore not be abandoned under two months, unless there are urgent manifestations of advancing disease or urgent side effects necessitating termination of treatment. The form of androgen can be changed if it is not being tolerated, as the tolerance of patients seems to vary to different members of the group.

If after the original two months treatment, the tumour appears *static* in size and activity, further androgen trial for one month is continued. 'Arrested' growth is not usually accepted as objective evidence of favourable response (*see* p. 112). A common problem in the decision to discontinue therapy is the patient whose bone pain is relieved by androgen therapy, but whose soft tissue tumour manifestations continue to grow slowly (*see* p. 53). Each case must be judged on its own merits.

If tumour regression occurs, administration of

androgens is generally continued until evidence of reactivation occurs (*see* p. 46). Nevertheless, if androgen therapy is suspended when the tumour regression is maximal, and reactivation occurs later, a second or third period of tumour regression is possible from further courses of androgen therapy.

PALLIATIVE RESULTS OF ANDROGEN THERAPY

The author (Stoll, 1950) early described the disappearance of smaller nodules of breast cancer under androgen therapy with a tendency for the larger nodules to unbilicate, and become covered with a

tissue lesions from breast cancer is only 6·9 months in the author's series. Healing of large ulcerated areas, such as is seen not uncommonly following oestrogen therapy, is rare after androgen therapy (Plates 2 and 3*a*). It is not uncommon to see the primary tumour regress under treatment, while metastatic nodes remain unchanged in size.

Subjective benefit, in the form of pain relief from bone metastases, follows androgen therapy in the majority of cases, occurring in 82 per cent of patients receiving fluoxymesterone therapy in the author's series (Stoll, 1958*b*). It often appears after one or two weeks treatment, but only in a minority of cases is it associated with objective evidence of tumour

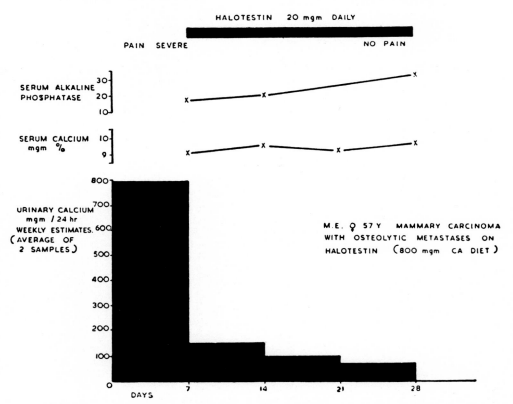

FIGURE 5.2 Patient M.E. The effect of fluoxymesterone (Halotestin) therapy on the urinary calcium excretion and on the serum calcium and alkaline phosphatase levels in a patient with bone metastases from breast cancer

Stoll, 1959 (courtesy, Editor, *Medical Journal of Australia*)

dark, greasy scab. In the case of widespread distribution of nodules, greasy scabbing tends to persist over the whole area. Regression of skin nodules or of metastatic nodes tends to be slower and less well marked in areas previously subjected to radiation therapy. The average duration of regression in soft

regression. Decrease in raised serum calcium levels associated with bone metastases may also occur within a few days of initiating androgen therapy (Fig. 5.2).

Recalcification of bone metastases is less common, and when it does occur is commonly delayed for at

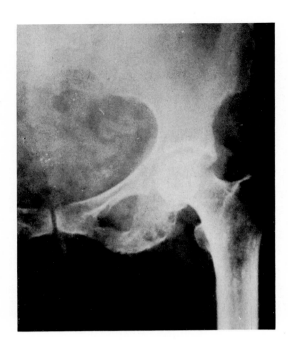

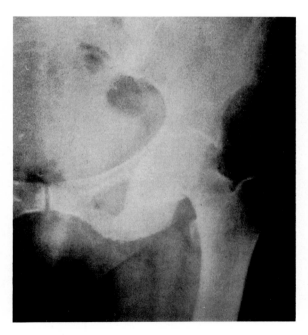

FIGURE 5.3 Patient E.F. Radiographs to show recalcification of metastases from breast cancer in the ischium within six months of instituting fluoxymesterone therapy 10 mg tds. Radiographs taken 26 February and 23 August 1957

Stoll, 1959 (courtesy, Editor, *Medical Journal of Australia*)

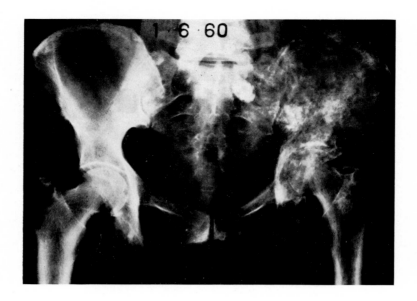

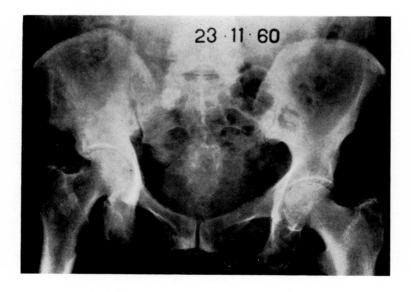

FIGURE 5.4 Patient M.C. Radiographs to show recalcification of metastases from breast cancer in the ilium, ischium, and pubis within five months of instituting fluoxymesterone therapy 10 mg tds

Radiographs taken 1 June and 23 November 1960

least three months after therapy is initiated. Its first manifestation is a ring of sclerotic bone around a previously lytic area, and often the whole skeleton shows increased density after androgen therapy. In occasional cases sclerosis of a metastasis may even be followed by reconstitution of bony trabeculae (Figs 5.3 and 5.4). There is no close correlation between the likelihood of healing of bone metastases and the regression of soft tissue or visceral metastases in the same patient (*see* p. 53).

Androgen therapy is usually continued without break until evidence of reactivation is noted (*see* p. 46). The average duration of control of bone metastases, without new metastases appearing, is 13·2 months in the author's series. Yet, control of metastatic bone pain by androgens for several years is not uncommon, and is one of the most satisfying experiences associated with the use of steroid therapy in breast cancer. Relief of pain from bone metastases is usually followed by increase in appetite and gain in weight. The haemoglobin level rises with androgen therapy, due as much to a stimulating effect on erythropoiesis (Gardner and Pringle, 1961), as to a reduction in bone marrow replacement by tumour.

Regression of visceral metastases from breast cancer, as a result of androgen therapy, is less common, but regression in lung and pleural metastases has been recorded by the author (Stoll, 1950). In general, subjective benefit in the form of gain in weight and increase in appetite and well-being may be associated with the anabolic effect of androgen therapy.

WITHDRAWAL RESPONSE AFTER ANDROGEN

After androgen therapy in breast cancer has lost its control, two months interval should be allowed to elapse before starting on new endocrine therapy. An exception is made in the presence of rapidly advancing disease, when immediate corticosteroid therapy or major endocrine ablation is advised. The reason for this delay is the possibility of achieving a 'withdrawal response'—a further tumour regression after cessation of steroid administration (Segaloff *et al.*, 1954; Delarue, 1955). According to Kaufman and Escher (1961), such a response occurs in 10 per cent of those responding favourably to androgen therapy. Its average duration is ten months, according to their report but, in the author's experience, its duration is always shorter than that of the original favourable response. In occasional cases, a second favourable response to androgen administration may be achieved after the withdrawal response has been lost.

The cause for such a withdrawal response is unknown, but an increase in serum alkaline phosphatase level usually follows initiation, change, or cessation of steroid therapy in the presence of bone metastases from breast cancer (*see* p. 102). This rise in enzyme level is thought to indicate an attempt at healing of destroyed bone following a change in the hormonal environment of the tumour. Such an attempt may or may not be successful, depending on the activity of the tumour. The existence of a withdrawal response suggests that repeated change in the hormonal environment of a tumour may be more important in hormonal therapy than the actual nature of the steroid causing the change (*see* p. 15). According to Kaufman and Escher (1961) a withdrawal response may be seen also in 2·2 per cent of patients *not* responding to androgen therapy.

HYPERCALCAEMIA

Hypercalcaemia is known to occur spontaneously in patients with bone metastases from breast cancer, according to Kennedy *et al.* (1955) and Jessiman *et al.* (1963) in 12–15 per cent of such patients. Certain steroids capable of osteolysis, such as 7-sitosteryl acetate and stigmesteryl acetate, have been found in the tumour and plasma of patients with breast cancer (Segaloff, 1967*b*) and these may be responsible for the appearance of hypercalcaemia. Nevertheless, hypercalcaemia appears just as commonly in the presence of bone metastases from other types of primary tumour (Thalassinos and Joplin, 1968) and the condition may also appear occasionally in the absence of bone metastases.

Hypercalcaemia should be suspected in the presence of rapidly developing headache, anorexia, nausea, vomiting and lassitude. Increasing dehydration, muscular weakness and drowsiness eventually progress to uraemia and coma. Treatment is by immediate cessation of any sex hormone therapy administered at the time (Fig. 5.5), by beginning a low calcium diet, intravenous sodium citrate (Kennedy *et al.*, 1955), inorganic phosphate therapy (Goldsmith and Ingbar, 1966), and care of hydration by glucose saline infusion. Prednisolone or prednisone therapy up to 100 mg daily is then prescribed if the serum calcium level has not fallen after these measures (*see* p. 77). Intravenous sodium citrate, or chelating agents such as sodium versenate (EDTA) act by temporarily increasing the urinary calcium excretion. Major endocrine ablation may be advised after the hypercalcaemic crisis has been controlled, and in fact, may be required before control is obtained in very severe and resistant cases (Thalassinos and Joplin, 1968; Moon, 1968). The use of methotrexate 2·5 mg daily may also be useful in such cases (Nevinny *et al.*, 1960; Hall *et al.*, 1963*a*).

EXACERBATION BY ANDROGENS

Although said to occur, exacerbation of the growth of breast cancer by androgen therapy is difficult to prove. The development of hypercalcaemia in breast cancer patients treated by androgens is often quoted as an example of exacerbation. However, Hall *et al.* (1963) note the incidence of hypercalcaemia in 102 androgen treated cases to be only 11 per cent and in some of these, clinical evidence of tumour healing occurred later with persistence of androgen therapy.

of breast cancer in 12 per cent of 208 cases treated by testosterone propionate or by Durabolin. An initial flare-up in bone pain, sometimes associated with fever, is not uncommon in the first few weeks after instituting androgen therapy (or oestrogen therapy—*see* p. 59). Its significance is not clear, as some of these patients go on to tumour healing. Such systemic reaction is sometimes, without sufficient evidence, interpreted as a sign of tumour exacerbation.

The author has never seen convincing evidence of

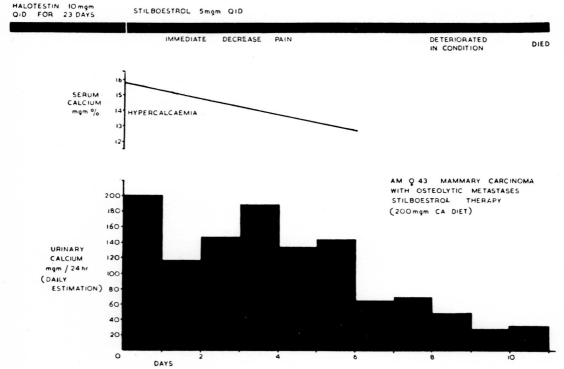

FIGURE 5.5 Patient A.M. Relief of hypercalcaemia and pain following cessation of fluoxymesterone (Halotestin) therapy, and institution of stilboestrol therapy; the patient died of uraemia

Stoll, 1959 (courtesy, Editor, *Medical Journal of Australia*)

It seems to be generally agreed that hypercalcaemia is somewhat more commonly seen during androgen therapy than during oestrogen therapy (Kennedy *et al.*, 1955; Myers *et al.*, 1955; Jessiman *et al.*, 1963; Hall *et al.*, 1963a). This may be due to a specific effect by androgens on tumour metabolism in bone. Whatever the causative mechanism of hypercalcaemia during steroid therapy, repeated serum calcium estimations are an essential procedure in the presence of bone metastases, especially when initiating or changing steroid therapy.

Bosboom *et al.* (1960) have reported exacerbation

exacerbation by androgens of local soft tissue metastases from breast cancer. The majority of cases claimed to be of this nature, are of autonomous tumour, showing continuing rapid progression of a lesion while on steroid therapy. Serial estimations of tumour volume as necessary to establish true exacerbation in such a case.

If true exacerbation does occur, it may be ascribed in the recently postmenopausal patient to partial conversion of androgens into oestrogens. That this occurs in the body has been shown by Steinach and Kun (1937), Nathanson (1952), West *et al.* (1956), and

Baggett *et al.* (1956). If exacerbation of tumour by steroid therapy can be proven, it is an indication of hormone sensitivity, and suggests that major endocrine ablation may be beneficial.

ANDROGEN COMBINED WITH RADIOACTIVE PHOSPHORUS

It has been shown by Hertz (1950) that pre-treatment of breast cancer patients by androgen or oestrogen, leads to a higher uptake by the tumour of radio-active phosphorus. For this reason, a combination of radioactive phorphorus and androgen has been suggested in the treatment of patients with bone metastases from breast cancer, whose pain has not responded to androgen therapy alone. Androgen pre-treatment has the added advantage of stimulating erythropoiesis in the marrow according to Gardner and Pringle (1961).

Testosterone propionate 50 mg or Durabolin 50 mg are injected intramuscularly daily for four days, and then continued at half dosage for a further eight days while 1·5 mc of radioactive phosphorus is given intravenously daily. Such dosage is usually followed later by leucopenia and thrombocytopenia, with bleeding tendencies in some patients, according to Huseby (1958). Repair of bone destruction is reported in 50 per cent of patients so treated, by Riordan and Browne (1961) and by Mandel and Chiat (1962), while pain was relieved in 87 per cent of patients for a period varying from two to eighteen months. Previous hormonal therapy or local X-ray therapy militate against a good response, according to Browne (1966). In the author's experience, pain relief was limited to a maximum of six months in a small series of patients treated with a combination of testosterone propionate and radioactive phosphorus, and severe thrombocytopenia was inevitable following therapy.

ANDROGEN COMBINED WITH ALKYLATING AGENTS

It was suggested by Watson and Turner (1959) and Cree (1960) that massive doses of the cytotoxic agent thioTEPA (*see* p. 134) could be given as a primary treatment for breast cancer, if a course of testosterone propionate was given previously and concurrently. It was suggested that the androgen protects the marrow, but not the tumour, against the toxic effects of the thioTEPA. This assumption has not been confirmed, as reports by Rider (1960), the author (Stoll, 1961, 1963*a*), and Lyons and Edelstyn (1962), describe deaths from toxicity in between 11 per cent and 63 per cent of patients treated by this technique (Table 5.5). Objective remission was noted

by Edelstyn *et al.* (1968) in 37 per cent of survivors, the mean duration of response being eight months. A combination of thioTEPA and deca-Durabolin has been reported to yield good clinical palliation in 68 per cent of late breast cancer cases, according

TABLE 5.5

Reported Incidence of Tumour Regression and Deaths from Toxicity Following Combined ThioTEPA and Testosterone Propionate Therapy

Author	Toxicity deaths in:	Tumour regression in:
Watson and Turner, 1959	0 of 23 cases	22 of 23 cases*
Cree, 1960	0 of 11 ,,	10 of 11 ,, *
Rider, 1960	7 of 11 ,,	3 of 11 ,,
Lyons and Edelstyn, 1962	5 of 46 ,,	17 of 46 ,,
Stoll and Matar, 1961	2 of 9 ,,	7 of 9 ,, †

* represents added oophorectomy in premenopausal patients
† represents half the recommended thioTEPA dosage

to Bond and Arthur (1966), compared to 35 per cent from the androgen alone.

Cyclophosphamide at a dose of 50 mg bd has been given for long periods in combination with androgen therapy for the treatment of bone metastases from breast cancer. Relief of pain is often dramatic and this alkylating agent is usually well tolerated, even by a damaged bone marrow (*see* p. 134). Such treatment is recommended especially if there has not been a response to previous endocrine therapy.

ANDROGEN FOR PROPHYLAXIS

The administration of androgens after mastectomy, to protect against recurrence, has been suggested by Prudente (1945) and later by Loeser (1954). The latter author advised its combination with thyroid extract for this purpose. The use of androgens for prophylaxis against recurrence fell into disrepute, however, because of the virilising effects of testosterone propionate at the dose recommended. A recent report by Bulbrook (1966), suggesting that a low androgen excretion is associated with a poor prognosis following mastectomy for breast cancer, has again encouraged trials of androgen prophylaxis at subvirilising doses.

Methods suggested in earlier reports were 250 mg testosterone oenanthate intramuscularly monthly for two years, or the instillation of 1 G of oily solution into the wound-bed at operation. The newer less virilising androgens which can be used instead are fluoxymesterone, by mouth, or methyl dihydro-testosterone, by injection (*see* p. 48).

The value of such prophylactic androgen therapy has not been established. On a theoretical basis, long continued administration of androgen could lead to the development of resistance by the tumour, so that when clinical recurrence of activity does occur, response to androgen therapy is less likely.

ANDROGEN COMBINED WITH OESTROGEN

A combination of these two agents has been suggested in the treatment of advanced breast cancer in an analogy with cytotoxic chemotherapy by multiple agents (*see* p. 131). On a theoretical basis, if the mode of action of each hormone is through a different channel, more than one enzymatic pathway in the tumour synthesis of DNA might be blocked at the same time.

Clinically, there is no evidence that such combined therapy yields any better palliation than does oestrogen therapy alone (Kennedy and Brown, 1965). Furthermore, if each hormone is used sequentially, a double remission can be achieved in some cases (*see* p. 39).

ANDROGEN: MODE OF ADMINISTRATION AND DOSAGE

Androgen therapy may be given either by continuous or by intermittent administration. In the former method, therapy is continued for as long as tumour regression persists. In the latter method, therapy is stopped when complete tumour regression has occurred in measurable lesions, and started again when reactivation of tumour is apparent. The author prefers the latter method.

In the continuous method, a withdrawal response in the tumour may be achieved when therapy is stopped (*see* p. 43), but only rarely is a second tumour regression obtained from a further course of therapy after withdrawal response has been lost. In the intermittent method, on the other hand, tumour regression may continue for some months following cessation of therapy, and when reactivation occurs, further regression of the tumour may follow further courses of androgen therapy (*see* p. 49). The intermittent method, by repeatedly varying the hormonal milieu of the tumour is thought to postpone the development of autonomy in the tumour. It has the added advantage of decreasing the degree of virilisation in the patient. There is an inclination with continuous therapy, for the therapist to decrease the androgen dosage, in order to minimise virilisation,

and a consequent danger of the dose falling below effective levels.

Natural *testosterone* (bull androgen) was the first androgen to be used clinically, but taken by mouth, testosterone is rapidly broken down by the liver into relatively inactive compounds such as androsterone. Injections of testosterone esters in oily solution have overcome the problem of rapid elimination, the propionate being the most widely used.

Until recently, treatment by intramuscular *testosterone propionate* 100 mg three times a week was accepted as the androgen of reference by the Co-operative Breast Cancer Group (1962). In Europe, implantation of crystalline *testosterone depot* 250–500 mg at two to three months intervals has been widely used. Both these agents cause gross signs of virilisation when their use is prolonged (*see* p. 47). In addition, the latter method has an indeterminate duration of action, and the implant has to be urgently removed if the serum calcium level rises.

ORAL ADMINISTRATION

While natural testosterone is inactivated when swallowed, *methyl testosterone* is actively absorbed by the buccal mucosa route. Given in this way, it has about one quarter the efficacy of testosterone propionate given intramuscularly. The recommended dosage of methyl testosterone is 150 to 200 mg daily. Although the danger is small, the use of the drug was reported by Foss and Simpson (1959) to carry a risk of hepatotoxic effects.

Fluoxymesterone (Halotestin, Ultandren) has been introduced in recent years for oral administration. It was reported by Kennedy (1967), Segaloff *et al.* (1958), and by the author (Stoll, 1958a, 1959a), to have the same clinical efficacy in the treatment of breast cancer as testosterone propionate, both objectively and subjectively, but with much reduced signs of virilisation (Plate 3b). The author's comparative results for the two parallel series are shown in Table 5.6.

It has been confirmed by the Co-operative Breast Cancer Group (1964) that the tumour remission rate, subdivided according to the site of metastasis and menopausal age, is no different from 20 mg fluoxymesterone daily than it is from testosterone propionate. There is no longer any basis for a statement such as that of Juret (1966), that oral androgen administration is less effective than parenteral administration. Pain relief from fluoxymesterone administration was achieved in 82 per cent of patients with bone metastases in the author's series (Stoll, 1959a). Kennedy (1962b) has shown that fluoxymesterone administration also stimulates erythropoiesis, as do other androgens found to be effective in the treatment of breast cancer.

Although a dosage of 15–20 mg fluoxymesterone daily is usually advised, it was shown by the author (Stoll, 1958a) that dosage between 25–40 mg daily yielded a higher tumour regression rate than did the lower dose. However, the increase in dose led to an increase in the number of patients virilised. Dosage

TABLE 5.6

Favourable Clinical Response to Fluoxymesterone Therapy Compared to that from Testosterone Propionate Therapy in the Treatment of Breast Cancer (Author's Series)

Androgen	Cases with regressing tumour	Percentage with regressing tumour	Significance
Fluoxymesterone	23 of 116	20%	Difference sig
Testosterone propionate	30 of 269	11%	$p < 0.05$

of 5–10 mg daily is rarely effective in causing tumour control except in premenopausal patients.

Whereas testosterone propionate almost always induces depression of gonadotropin secretion, fluoxymesterone does so in only about half the cases treated, according to Segaloff *et al.* (1958) and the same author reports that fluoxymesterone therapy often increases the prolactin level in the blood (*see* p. 109).

INTRAMUSCULAR ADMINISTRATION

The use of testosterone propionate was early recommended in the treatment of breast cancer by Herrmann *et al.* (1947) and by the author (Stoll, 1950), and practically all early reports on the use of androgens for this purpose adopted the dosage of 100 mg three times a week; it was accepted by the Co-operative Breast Cancer Group (1962) as a standard against which new androgens were measured both for efficacy and virilising tendency. Its prolonged use is nearly always closely associated with virilisation (*see below*) but, apart from occasional nausea, it is otherwise well tolerated. Unlike fluoxymesterone there is no evidence that when the recommended dosage is unsuccessful in achieving tumour regression, higher dosage is likely to be more efficacious. Neither is there any evidence that when testosterone propionate is ineffective, fluoxymesterone is likely to cause tumour regression, or vice versa. Nevertheless, in the author's experience, intramuscular

testosterone propionate is sometimes better tolerated in the occasional case when oral fluoxymesterone causes intractable nausea. It may also be useful in cases where the patient cannot be relied upon to take oral medication.

Long-acting androgens such as *Primoteston Depot* (250 mg fortnightly), and an anabolic norandrostenolone compound, *Durabolin* (25–50 mg weekly), have their adherents (Hortling *et al.*, 1961; Ford, 1959). The clinical efficacy of the latter in breast cancer and the incidence of virilisation and hypercalcaemia, are reported to be at the same level as from testosterone propionate. In the author's experience, while the efficacy of Durabolin in the presence of bone metastases is at a comparable level, its control of soft tissue and visceral lesions is inferior. In addition, attempts to change therapy from testosterone propionate to this agent was often associated with lessened control of the pain from bone metastases. Depot compounds are also much more dangerous in the event of the patient developing hypercalcaemia, because their action cannot be terminated abruptly.

SIDE EFFECTS OF ANDROGENS

Based upon earlier reports, it was stated by Segaloff (1957) that the clinical effectiveness of an androgen in the therapy of breast cancer, runs parallel with its androgenicity and gonadotropin inhibiting properties. The more recent results of fluoxymesterone, Δ-1-testololactone and 2α methyl dihydrotestosterone administration have changed this view (*see* p. 48).

Some side effects of androgen administration are beneficial—an increase in weight, and a feeling of well-being and increase in energy are particularly common in postmenopausal patients.

1. *Virilisation*

Increased hirsutism of the upper lip, chin, trunk and limbs develop to a greater or lesser extent in practically all women given the older effective androgens therapeutically for longer than six months at the dosage recommended. Coarsening or thinning of the scalp hair, acne over the shoulders, and seborrhoea of the skin are usually associated with it. These side effects may take several months to clear after cessation of androgen therapy. Increase in libido is sometimes an embarrassment but hypertrophy of the clitoris usually passes unnoticed by the patient. Hirsutism develops in only about one-third of breast cancer patients taking fluoxymesterone 20 mg daily for six to twelve months, and then only to a moderate degree. A trial of this hormone for two or three months only is usually free from such a complication.

With the older androgens, such as testosterone propionate and methyl testosterone, there was thought to be a correlation between the degree of clinical response and the degree of virilisation. This results from the fact that virilisation increases with prolonged androgen administration, and is therefore most obvious in responding patients who have been maintained on the steroid for long periods. Hirsutism decreases slowly after androgen therapy is withdrawn.

2. *Hoarseness*
This is due to decreased tension in the laryngeal muscles and thickening of submucous tissue in the larynx. Younger patients are more sensitive to small doses of androgens in this respect. Once established, restoration of normal voice is usually very slow after androgens are discontinued.

3. *Increased Libido, Irritability and Restlessness*
These symptoms are not uncommon, and the latter is sometimes a euphemism for increased libido. Tranquilisers and barbiturates are useful for their control, especially in postmenopausal patients. In the early postmenopausal patient, androgen has a beneficial effect in controlling hot flushes and similar symptoms of the climacteric.

4. *Fluid Retention*
Oedema of the ankles due to sodium retention and increase in weight are seen in about 25 per cent of all patients. Cardiac embarrassment due to fluid retention is less common than from oestrogen therapy, and only rarely necessitates cessation of treatment.

5. *Vomiting, Nausea, Dizziness or Pelvic Cramps*
These are occasional causes of temporary intolerance but are less commonly seen than with oestrogen therapy. It may be necessary to decrease the dose, and gradually build it up to the required level as the steroid becomes tolerated. In some sensitive patients, every dose of a long-acting ester such as Primoteston Depot or Durabolin is followed by about twenty-four hours of such upset.

6. *Hepatotoxic Effects*
As mentioned previously (*see* p. 46), certain androgenic steroids such as methyl testosterone may, in occasional cases, cause evidence of liver damage. The appearance of jaundice and biliary stasis was reported by Beckett and Brennan (1959) in one patient following treatment by fluoxymesterone.

NEWER ANDROGENS

Δ-1-TESTOLOLACTONE
This androgen, so far not available commercially, is claimed by Segaloff *et al.* (1962) to yield a similar tumour remission rate in breast cancer to that of testosterone propionate, without biological evidence of pituitary suppression or obvious signs of virilisation. Oral dosage has not yet been clarified, and doses of up to 1 G daily have been tried by Cantino and Gordon (1967) with no better results than from 150 mg. Although it is said to cause no depression of gonadotropin secretion, testololactone is said to stimulate the secretion of prolactin, according to Lerner and Hilf (1967).

Testololactone is claimed by Segaloff *et al.* (1962) to induce a higher tumour remission rate than does testosterone propionate in the poorly responding age group one to five years postmenopausal, but Bisel (1964) disagrees with this observation. The major interest of this compound is, that being relatively inert hormonally, its effect upon breast cancer may be mainly a direct one upon the tumour tissue.

2. METHYL DIHYDROTESTOSTERONE PROPIONATE (DROSTANOLONE)
This androgen has been reported by Blackburn and Childs (1959), Goldenberg and Hayes (1961), and Thomas *et al.* (1962) to be as effective in the treatment of breast cancer as testosterone propionate. At a dosage of 100 mg intramuscularly three times a week, it is said to lead to less virilisation than does testosterone propionate.

3. ANABOLIC ANDROGENS (Other than Durabolin)
These have also been claimed to have a controlling effect on occasional cases of advanced breast cancer. A norandrosterone derivative, Nilevar, has both anti-oestrogenic and gonadotropin inhibiting properties. Occasional examples of tumour regression following the use of this steroid were claimed in a small series of breast cancer by Pommatau *et al.* (1961), but a clinical trial with controlled protocol has yet to be carried out.

TO SUMMARISE

Androgen therapy will induce objective evidence of tumour regression in about 20 per cent of postmenopausal patients with advanced breast cancer. In these patients, prolongation of survival has been clearly demonstrated and, in addition, anabolic effects of androgens are beneficial in most patients. Objective evidence of tumour regression is best seen in the presence of soft tissue and bone metastases, especially in older patients, where over 30 per cent of the group may show response. Recalcification of bone metastases is common and in a further proportion, the pain of bone metastases is relieved without radiographic evidence of healing of metastases.

Virilisation is the main disadvantage of androgen therapy. Fluoxymesterone provides an orally administered androgen, which is efficacious and relatively less virilising than older effective compounds.

Δ-1-Testololactone and 2α methyl dehydrotestosterone are also said to be as efficacious and also relatively less virilising than testosterone propionate.

A change from one agent to another is worth a trial in the presence of intolerance but if the initial choice at effective dosage has failed to achieve tumour regression, benefit is unlikely to result from the use of an alternative androgen. It is possible, too, that some androgens such as testololactone exert more of a direct effect upon malignant cells than others.

Androgen Therapy

ILLUSTRATIVE CASE SUMMARIES

Patient A.W.R. Androgen-induced Recalcification of Bone Metastases and Control of Pleural Effusion over a Period of Three and a Half Years. Soft Tissue Metastases Appeared under Treatment

A woman aged sixty-eight, and eighteen years postmenopausal, presented in October 1957. She gave a history of a left radical mastectomy for breast carcinoma six years previously. She now presented with a malignant right pleural effusion, and bone pain found to be associated with multiple lytic areas of metastasis in bone.

Hormonal treatment was initiated with a course of Primoteston depot, 250 mg intramuscularly at one to two weeks intervals, and continued for a period of twelve months. Pain was rapidly controlled, and the radiographs showed recalcification of the previously lytic bone metastases. The pleural effusion required no paracentesis for a total period of twenty-eight months; nevertheless, metastatic supraclavicular node enlargement appeared while the patient was on androgen therapy. When pain again exacerbated at the end of twenty-eight months, androgen therapy with fluoxymesterone 10 mg tds was instituted. Control of bone pain was again achieved, but without control of soft tissue tumour, until the patient died fourteen months later as a result of bone marrow replacement.

Patient L.B.L. Androgen-induced Recalcification of Bone Metastases, and Control of Soft Tissue Tumour for over Three Years

A woman aged seventy-two presented in October 1955 with a large cancer of the breast, associated with bone pain and multiple lytic areas of metastasis in bone. Primary treatment was by a palliative course of X-ray therapy to the breast, axillary, and supraclavicular draining node areas, to a minimum

tumour dose of 4,000 roentgens in thirty-five days. At the same time, hormonal therapy was started with a course of methyl testosterone 20 mg qid which was continued for thirty-six months.

The breast tumour regressed after the radiation therapy and remained under control until death. The bone pain rapidly came under control of the androgen therapy, so that the patient was able to resume near normal activity. Radiographs showed recalcification of previously lytic areas in bone and no new areas of destruction appeared. The breast tumour and the bone metastases remained under control for a period of thirty-eight months, at which stage the patient's condition deteriorated suddenly.

Patient S.J.O. Androgen-induced Recalcification of Bone Metastases for Thirty-three Months

A woman aged sixty-eight, and twenty-three years postmenopausal, presented in February 1955 with a Stage 2 carcinoma of the right breast. Primary treatment was by radical mastectomy, followed by a prophylactic course of X-ray therapy to the mastectomy scar, axillary, and supraclavicular draining node areas. At only eleven months after the operation, she developed bone pain and radiographs showed the presence of multiple lytic areas of metastasis in bone.

Hormonal therapy was initiated with a course of fluoxymesterone 10 mg tds. This led to relief of pain within a few weeks, followed by recalcification in the radiographic appearance of the bone metastases. Androgen therapy was continued for twenty-one months, and pain control was maintained for a further twelve months after that. When pain subsequently recurred, a trial was attempted of testosterone propionate 100 mg intramuscularly three times a week, combined with thioTEPA intramuscularly continued to haematological tolerance levels. Control of pain did not result, and the patient died forty-three months after starting androgen therapy. The autopsy showed widespread sclerotic areas of bone replacement.

Patient E.L.E. Androgen-induced Regression of Skin Nodules for Twenty-two Months. Soft Tissue Metastases Appeared under Treatment

A woman aged sixty-seven, and twenty years postmenopausal, presented in December 1958 with an inoperable carcinoma of the left breast. It was fixed to the underlying pectoralis muscles, and associated with the presence of enlarged fixed nodes in the left axilla. A 'toilet' mastectomy was carried out, followed by a postoperative course of X-ray therapy to the mastectomy scar, axillary, and supraclavicular draining node areas. After only nine months, recurrent skin nodules appeared in the scar area.

Hormonal therapy was begun with a course of fluoxymesterone 10 mg tds and this was maintained for twenty-two months. The skin nodules regressed rapidly in size, and then remained under control until death. However, thirteen months after androgen therapy was initiated, enlarged metastatic nodes appeared in the opposite axilla, and continued to grow slowly in spite of androgen administration. The patient died two months after androgen therapy was stopped.

Patient J.M.K. Tumour Control by Oestrogen Therapy over a Period of Three Years. Therapy Caused Regression of Soft Tissue Tumour but Exacerbation of Bone Metastases, While Oestrogen Withdrawal had the Opposite Effect. Subsequent Androgen Therapy Controlled both until Death

A woman aged sixty-two, and twelve years postmenopausal, presented in August 1956 with a carcinoma in the left breast. Primary treatment was by radical mastectomy, but within nine months of the operation, recurrent skin nodules had appeared in the mastectomy scar and enlarged metastatic nodes were palpable above the clavicle. Hormonal therapy was initiated with a course of diethyl stilboestrol 5 mg tds and maintained for twenty-three months. Complete regression of soft tissue tumour resulted, but towards the end of that period, she developed pain found to be associated with multiple bone metastases of a mixed lytic/sclerotic appearance.

When diethyl stilboestrol administration was stopped at the end of twenty-three months there was rapid relief of bone pain, and previously lytic areas in bone began to show signs of recalcification in the radiographs. In spite of this, new skin nodules appeared, and enlarged in size during the period of ten months that the patient was not receiving oestrogen therapy. A course of diethyl stilboestrol was

prescribed again for four months, and once again the soft tissue tumour regressed, but at the same time, new lytic metastases appeared in the skeletal radiographs.

After an interval, a course of fluoxymesterone 10 mg tds was prescribed. This controlled both the bone pain and the soft tissue tumour until the patient died nine months later as a result of bone marrow replacement.

Patient M.M.I. Androgen-induced Regression of Soft Tissue Tumour for Twelve Months. Pleural Metastases Appeared under Treatment

A woman aged fifty-five, and four years postmenopausal, presented in January 1958 with a cancer of the breast, associated with metastases in the axillary and supraclavicular nodes. Primary treatment was by a palliative course of X-ray therapy to the breast, axillary, and supraclavicular area, to a minimum tumour dose of 4,000 roentgens in thirty days. At the same time irradiation of the ovaries was carried out to ablate residual ovarian function, delivering a dose of 1,000 roentgens in five days. Regression of the soft tissue tumour occurred with two months of the X-ray therapy and was maintained for twenty-five months, after which reactivation occurred.

Hormonal therapy was initiated with a course of fluoxymesterone 10 mg tds prescribed for twelve months. Regression of the soft tissue tumour occurred once again, but at the end of twelve months the patient complained of dyspnoea, found to be associated with the presence of a malignant pleural effusion. Androgen therapy was stopped and a trial of prednisolone 10 mg tds was prescribed for two months. In spite of this treatment, the patient died four months after developing pleural metastases.

Patient E.B.E. Tumour Control by Oestrogen Therapy of Pleural and Lung Metastases over a Period of Three Years Without Control of Bone Metastases. Subsequent Recalcification of Bone Metastases from Androgen Therapy

A woman aged sixty-seven, and twenty years postmenopausal, presented in May 1955 with a carcinoma of the right breast that was treated primarily by radical mastectomy. After fourteen months there was noted metastatic enlargement of the nodes above the clavicle and also a malignant pleural effusion on the opposite side to the mastectomy. Hormonal therapy was initiated with a course of diethyl stilboestrol 5 mg tds and maintained for thirteen months. During this time, the supraclavicular nodes regressed in size and the pleural effusion required no paracentesis.

Within eighteen months of diethyl stilboestrol being discontinued, the patient presented with increasing dyspnoea. This was found to be associated with multiple nodular opacities in the lung fields, presumed to be metastatic in nature. She soon after developed bone pain associated with multiple lytic areas of metastasis in bone. A further course of diethyl stilboestrol 5 mg tds was prescribed for a period of seven months. During this time, the lung metastases regressed in size and density, but there was no change in the radiographic appearance of the bone metastases.

After an interval, a course of fluoxymesterone 10 mg tds was prescribed. During its administration, there was no change in size of the lung metastases but recalcification appeared in the skeletal metases. Nevertheless, the patient's condition deteriorated and she died of her disease twenty months later, in spite of further unsuccessful attempts at therapy.

Patient V.W.A. Androgen-induced Recalcification of Bone Metastases. Subsequent Control of Pain by Oestrogen Therapy

A woman aged sixty-one, and thirteen years post-menopausal, presented in June 1957 with a large cancer of the breast. Bone pains were found to be associated with multiple lytic areas of metastases in bone. Serial estimations of urinary calcium excretion levels showed a fall to occur after androgen administration. Hormonal therapy was therefore begun with a course of Sublings testosterone 20 mg qid and yielded rapid relief of pain.

Androgen therapy was continued for eight months during which time there appeared recalcification in the radiographs of the bone metastases and no new areas of destruction appeared. At the end of this time pain relief was lost and, therefore, a course of ethinyl oestradiol 0·5 mg tds was prescribed after an interval. Oestrogen therapy was continued for three months and led to temporary relief of pain but the patient died two months later.

Patient D.W.J. Androgen-induced Recalcification of Bone Metastasis and Control of Pleural Effusion. No Subsequent Control by Oestrogen Therapy

A premenopausal patient, aged fifty-one, presented in October 1953 with a Stage 2 carcinoma of the left breast. Primary treatment was by radical mastectomy, followed by a prophylactic course of X-ray therapy to the mastectomy scar, axillary and supraclavicular draining node areas. At the same time, prophylactic X-ray castration was carried out, delivering a dose of 1,000 roentgens to the region of the ovaries in eleven days. Within twenty-nine months of the operation, she developed dyspnoea and bone pains, and was found to have signs of a malignant pleural effusion, and also multiple lytic areas of metastasis in bone.

Hormonal therapy was initiated with a course of testosterone propionate 100 mg intramuscularly three times a week, and maintained for seven months. Bone pain was rapidly relieved, and the pleural effusion was absorbed. Within three to four months, the bone radiographs showed recalcification in previously lytic areas. Control of bone pain was maintained for a total period of thirteen months and was then lost. At this stage, a course of ethinyl oestradiol 0·5 mg tds was prescribed for a period of three months, but control of pain was not obtained, and the patient died four months later.

Patient Q.A.M. Androgen-induced Regression of Soft Tissue Tumour after Failure of Oestrogen Therapy

A woman aged fifty-eight and seven years post-menopausal, presented in January 1956 with an inoperable advanced breast cancer invading all four quadrants, and associated with overlying peau d'orange of the skin. Primary treatment was by a course of ethinyl oestradiol 0·5 mg tds, continued for five months but with no evidence of tumour regression.

After an interval, a course of Sublings testosterone 10 mg qid was prescribed and maintained for five months. As a result of this therapy, rapid regression occurred in the size of the breast tumour and its skin infiltration. Virilisation was slight, and there was no evidence of fluid retention. Nevertheless, the patient's general condition then deteriorated and she died of widespread metastases three months later.

Patient F.B.L. Androgen-induced Recalcification of Bone Metastases. No Subsequent Control from Oestrogen or Corticosteroid Therapy

A woman aged sixty-two, and seventeen years post-menopausal, presented in November 1954 with a carcinoma of the left breast. This was treated, primarily, by simple mastectomy followed by a prophylactic course of X-ray therapy to the mastectomy scar, axillary and supraclavicular draining node areas. At twenty-two months following the operation, she developed bone pain associated with multiple lytic areas of bone metastases, and shortly after, recurrent skin nodules appeared near the mastectomy scar.

Hormonal therapy was begun with a course of testosterone propionate, 100 mg intramuscularly three times a week, and was maintained for thirteen months. Within a few weeks of starting therapy, bone pain was relieved, and within three months recalcification appeared in the skeletal metastases. However, after thirteen months therapy, bone pain recurred. Cessation of androgen therapy gave no withdrawal response in the pain, or decrease in the urinary calcium excretion.

A trial of diethyl stilboestrol for two months yielded some pain relief, but was discontinued because of complaints of constant nausea. A course of prednisolone 10 mg tds was prescribed for a period of six months, but it neither abolished the pain nor stopped spread of the bone metastases. The patient died five months later as a result of bone marrow replacement.

Patient D.C.O. Androgen-induced Regression of Soft Tissue Tumour after Failure of Oestrogen Therapy. Androgen Therapy had to be Discontinued because of Fluid Retention

A woman aged seventy-eight presented in April 1957 with a Stage 1 breast cancer. Because of her advanced age primary treatment by oestrogen therapy was decided on. A course of dienoestrol 0·5 mg tds was prescribed for a period of four months, but no tumour regression resulted. After an interval, a course of Sublings testosterone 10 mg qid was prescribed. As a result, rapid regression in the size of the breast tumour was noted, beginning within a few weeks of treatment.

Androgen therapy was continued for eight months and then had to be stopped because of the cardiac embarassment due to the fluid retention induced. When androgens were withdrawn, the tumour regrew rapidly and a 'toilet' mastectomy was therefore decided upon. Within five months of the operation, nodular recurrence appeared in the mastectomy scar. The tumour spread rapidly and the patient died within eleven months of the operation, after further unsuccessful attempts at therapy.

Patient J.C.R. Androgen-induced Relief of Pain from Bone Metastases. Androgen Withdrawal was followed by Regression of Soft Tissue Tumour but Hypercalcaemia Developed

A premenopausal woman, aged thirty-three, presented in July 1957 with a large carcinoma of the breast fixed to the underlying pectoralis muscles. Primary treatment was by a palliative course of X-ray therapy to a maximum tumour dose of 4,200 roentgens in twenty-seven days, delivered to the breast, axillary and supraclavicular draining node areas. Mastectomy was carried out ten months later, and endocrine therapy was begun at the same time with surgical castration.

Fourteen months after the operation there appeared recurrent skin nodules in the region of the scar, and a malignant pleural effusion, and soon after, the X-rays showed multiple lytic areas of metastasis in bone. A course of fluoxymesterone 10 mg tds was prescribed for a period of five months.

During this time, bone pains were relieved, but there was no sign of regression of skin nodules or recalcification of bone metastases.

When fluoxymesterone was stopped, there followed a withdrawal regression in the skin nodules. Nevertheless at the same time, hypercalcaemia appeared and the patient died within three months.

Patient F.D.A. Androgen-induced Hypercalcaemia, which did not Respond to Oestrogen, EDTA, or Corticosteroid Therapy

A premenopausal patient, aged fifty-three, presented in January 1958 with a Stage 2 carcinoma of the left breast. Primary treatment was by radical mastectomy, followed by a prophylactic course of X-ray therapy to the axillary, supraclavicular, and internal mammary draining node areas. At the same time prophylactic X-ray castration was carried out, delivering a dose of 1,200 roentgens in seven days to the region of the ovaries.

Twenty-two months after the operation, the patient complained of bone pain found to be associated with multiple lytic areas of metastasis in bone. A trial of testosterone propionate 100 mg intramuscularly three times a week was begun, but within one month, the patient developed hypercalcaemia. Treatment by prednisolone, sodium versenate (EDTA), and diethyl stilboestrol each caused a temporary fall in the serum calcium level, but it was never returned to normal, and the patient eventually died of uraemia.

Patient E.B.R. Androgen-induced Fall in Calcium Excretion in Premenopausal Patient, but No Recalcification of Bone Metastases and No Associated Relief of Bone Pain

A premenopausal patient, aged forty-five, presented in July 1957 with a Stage 1 carcinoma of the right breast. Primary treatment was by radical mastectomy followed by a prophylactic course of X-ray therapy to the axillary, supraclavicular, and internal mammary draining node areas. At six months after the operation, bone pain was complained of and radiographs showed multiple lytic areas of metastases in bone.

Serial estimations of urinary calcium excretion levels, showed a fall on fluoxymesterone administration. The patient was not castrated but hormonal therapy was begun with a course of fluoxymesterone 10 mg tds, and continued for three months. Relief of pain did not result, and the radiographic appearance of the metastases showed no recalcification. Because of the persistence of pain, oophorectomy was carried out at the end of three months. Still there was no relief of bone pain and the patient died one month later.

Patient E.E.V. Androgen-induced Recalcification of Bone Metastases but Soft Tissue Metastases Appeared under Treatment. Subsequent Oestrogen Therapy Partly Controlled New Soft Tissue Metastases

A woman aged fifty-three, and one year postmenopausal, presented in February 1960. Ten years previously, a right simple mastectomy had been carried out for breast cancer, and she now presented with bone pain due to multiple lytic areas of metastasis in bone. Hormonal therapy was begun with a course of fluoxymesterone 10 mg tds which was continued for seven months. Androgen therapy resulted in relief of pain, and also recalcification in the radiographs of the bone metastases.

However, while on therapy, enlarged nodes appeared in the right supraclavicular and axillary areas, and also recurrent skin nodules in the region of the scar. Androgen therapy was therefore discontinued and after an interval a course of stilboestrol 5 mg tds was prescribed. Oestrogen therapy was continued for nine months and yielded regression of the skin nodules, but not of the metastatic nodes. For this reason, an attempt was made to re-institute androgen therapy in the form of testosterone propionate 100 mg intramuscularly three times a week.

Within a month, hypercalcaemia developed, from which the patient died.

Patient T.G.O. Androgen-induced Hypercalcaemia Associated with Relief of Bone Pains. Relief of Hypercalcaemia by Oestrogen Therapy was Associated with Increase in Bone Pain

A premenopausal patient aged forty, presented in October 1958 with carcinoma of the left breast. She gave a history of a mastectomy for carcinoma of the opposite breast four and a half years previously. Left radical mastectomy was carried out, but within twelve months the first lytic areas of metastasis appeared in bone.

Surgical castration was carried out as the initial method of endocrine therapy. The metastasis remained solitary until nineteen months later, when further bone metastases appeared. A trial of testosterone propionate 100 mg intramuscularly three times a week, was begun at this stage. Pain was relieved, but hypercalcaemia appeared within two weeks of beginning treatment by androgens. Treatment by stilboestrol and sodium citrate infusions caused the serum calcium level to fall to normal. However, this change was accompanied by recurrence of bone pains and the patient died within two months.

6

Oestrogen Therapy

THE USE of oestrogen therapy in the management of advanced breast cancer in postmenopausal women was suggested by Biden (1943) and, in 1944, Ellis, and others reported tumour regression following oestrogen therapy in 25 per cent of a series of such patients. Further detailed reports of larger series by Nathanson (1946), Taylor *et al.* (1948) and the author (Stoll, 1950) followed in succeeding years.

FREQUENCY OF OBJECTIVE RESPONSE TO OESTROGENS

The AMA Committee on Research (1960) reported a retrospective review of 944 assembled cases of breast cancer treated by oestrogens or by androgens

TABLE 6.1

Favourable Clinical Response to Oestrogen Therapy Compared to that from Androgen Therapy in Breast Cancer, in Relation to Menopausal Age Group. (Figures from Author's Series and AMA Committee on Research, 1960)

| | Percentage with regressing tumour after: | | | |
| | Androgens | | Oestrogens | |
Years since menopause	Author's series	AMA series	Author's series	AMA series
0–5	10%	17%	9%	13%*
6–9	28%*	13%*	28%*	38%*
10 or more	22%	27%	36%	38%
Overall regression rate	15%	21%	31%	37%
Cases	434	580	407	364

* represents small series of cases

(Table 6.1). Objective evidence of tumour regression was seen in 21 per cent of androgen treated patients and in 37 per cent of oestrogen treated patients. A similar review of a personal series of 777 cases, treated by the author (Stoll, 1964a), reported objective evidence of tumour regression in 15 per cent of androgen treated cases, and in 31 per cent of oestrogen treated cases (Table 6.1). A randomised trial of

TABLE 6.2

Survival Rates in Patients with Intrathoracic Metastases from Breast Cancer. Comparison of Oestrogen Treated Cases with Untreated Cases (Stoll and Ellis, 1953)

Survival	Oestrogen treated group	Untreated group
Died within 3 months	29·5%	65%
Died within 6 months	50%	86%
Survival over 12 months	31%	7·5%
Survival over 18 months	18%	0
Total cases	61	66

hormonal therapy by Kennedy (1965a) in 114 post-menopausal women showed tumour growth remission in 10·1 per cent of patients treated by testosterone propionate, compared to 29·1 per cent of patients treated by diethyl stilboestrol.

The differences between the three series probably represent difference in criteria of benefit, and there is no doubt that, in postmenopausal patients, the overall results of oestrogen therapy are superior to those of androgen therapy. The average duration of objective response to oestrogens was 16·5 months in the author's series—longer than the average duration of response to androgens (10·9 months), but shorter than that to castration (20·9 months).

The effect of oestrogen therapy is not only to

palliate symptoms, but also to prolong life, in hormone sensitive patients with breast cancer. The mean survival after treatment was 27·3 months for patients responding favourably to oestrogen, compared to 10·4 months for non-responders, according to the AMA Committee on Research (1960). In the case of lung or pleural metastases, 31 per cent of oestrogen treated patients survived over twelve months in a series reported by the author (Stoll and Ellis, 1953) compared to 7·5 per cent of untreated patients (Table 6·2).

The possibility has been suggested (*see below*) that hormone sensitive breast cancers, as a group, may be more slowly growing than the autonomous group, and that this may account for prolonged survival. Nevertheless, this evidence of prolonged survival in oestrogen responsive cases is important, because of the early fears that prolonged oestrogen therapy would accelerate the development of cardiac failure in elderly patients.

INDICATIONS FOR OESTROGEN THERAPY

Oestrogen administration is not advised in premenopausal patients (Haddow *et al.*, 1944; Nathanson, 1947; Taylor *et al.*, 1948), or in recently postmenopausal patients until the vaginal smear ceases to show evidence of oestrogenic activity, because of the danger of exacerbating breast cancer. In spite of this warning, it has been shown by Nathanson (1952) and Kennedy (1962*a*) that very high doses of oestrogen, either synthetic or natural (diethylstilboestrol 400–1000 mg daily or Premarin 100–800 mg daily), may sometimes cause tumour regression in breast cancer also in premenopausal women (*see* p. 14).

It is now well recognised that the best results from oestrogen therapy in advanced breast cancer are obtained in patients more than five years postmenopausal (Table 6.1). It has therefore been suggested by Huseby (1958) that oestrogen therapy be instituted immediately in all inoperable cases of breast cancer in this older age group, whether or not symptoms are present, and whether or not localised manifestations of the disease can be controlled by radiation therapy.

The reasoning behind this advice is that if oestrogens are found ineffective at this stage, there is still time to try alternative therapy before the patient becomes too sick for any form of endocrine treatment. It will be noted that a similar reasoning has been applied to advise prophylactic castration in the premenopausal patient with breast cancer (*see* p. 31). Nevertheless, because of possible side effects from oestrogen therapy and the limited duration of oestrogen-induced control of breast cancer, the author prefers to follow a 'sequential' plan of therapy

(*see* p. 118). Oestrogen therapy is delayed until after local treatment has failed to control the disease.

FACTORS INFLUENCING OESTROGEN RESPONSE

It was early pointed out by the author (Stoll, 1950) that tumour remission rates from both oestrogen and androgen therapy in breast cancer tend to increase with increasing number of years since the menopause. In Table 6.1 it is noted that in the author's series, after the fifth postmenopausal year, oestrogens induced a somewhat higher tumour remission rate than did androgens (28–36 per cent for the former compared with 22–28 per cent for the latter). Within the first five years after the menopause, there was little difference between their tumour remission rates (9 per cent for oestrogens as against 10 per cent for androgens). However, in this younger age category it should be noted that the androgen and oestrogen treated groups are not strictly comparable, as androgens tend to be the only steroid prescribed in the immediate one to two years after the menopause (an unfavourable age group for hormone response), whereas oestrogen prescription is usually postponed for at least two years.

The author (Stoll, 1950) was among the first to report that both local soft tissue and visceral lesions showed a higher remission rate from oestrogen therapy than from androgen therapy. The tumour remission rate is 28–36 per cent for the former therapy, as against 11–16 per cent for the latter. (Table 5.3). In the case of bone metastases on the other hand, the figures suggested a higher tumour remission rate from androgens than from oestrogens—19 per cent as against 7 per cent. Thus, when both types of metastasis coexist, it is not unusual with oestrogen therapy to see soft tissue tumour regressing while bone metastases are uncontrolled; the reverse experience is more common with androgen therapy. Nonetheless, the highest tumour remission rates from steroid therapy in breast cancer are in the case of local soft tissue tumour.

A third factor deciding the tumour remission rate, apart from age and site, is the length of the 'free' interval between mastectomy and recurrence. That slowly growing tumours are associated with a greater likelihood of tumour growth remission from hormonal therapy was suggested by the author (Stoll, 1950). Escher and Kaufman (1963) reported objective evidence of tumour regression from steroid therapy in only 16 per cent of breast cancer patients with a recurrence free interval of less than two years compared to 22 per cent of those with a free interval over two years.

The administration of previous radiation therapy

to soft tissue deposits of breast cancer will militate against a good hormonal response, because of the decreased vascular supply which results from such treatment.

RECOGNITION OF OESTROGEN RESPONSE

The initial objective evidence of tumour regression in breast cancer is usually not seen until about four weeks after commencing oestrogen therapy, and often is delayed for a further two to four weeks. The author's experience does not support the opinion (Forrest, 1965) that if favourable response to oestrogen therapy does not occur within one month, further administration is unlikely to be of value. Although tumour regression from oestrogens is in general, more rapid than that from androgens, it should be emphasised that a trial of oestrogens should not be abandoned under two months, except in the presence of obvious exacerbation of the disease or of urgent side effects. Recalcification of bone metastases usually takes three to six months to appear.

If, however, the tumour is *static* in size and activity after the initial two months treatment, a further one month trial of therapy is worth while, before the condition is finally regarded as resistant to oestrogen therapy. 'Arrested' growth is not usually accepted as objective evidence of favourable response (*see* p. 112).

If tumour regression occurs, oestrogen administration is usually continued until evidence of tumour reactivation appears (*see* p. 60). Nevertheless, if oestrogen administration is suspended while the tumour is still under control, and reactivation then occurs, a second or even a third tumour regression with further oestrogen therapy is still possible (*see* p. 62).

The average duration of objective tumour remission from oestrogen therapy is 16·5 months in the author's series. The average duration of tumour remission for soft tissue lesions of breast cancer is longer than that for bone or visceral lesions, and five year remissions are occasionally seen (*see* p. 62), for soft tissue lesions. The longer remissions seen in the older patient may be a tumour characteristic of the disease in these patients.

PALLIATIVE RESULTS OF OESTROGEN THERAPY

Complete healing of large ulcerated areas of breast cancer is not uncommon with oestrogen therapy, especially in the elderly patient (*see* Frontispiece and Plate 4). A purple tinge in previously red skin and a flattening of the everted tumour edges are the initial signs of regression in such cases. When healing finally occurs in a primary breast cancer, scarring and shrinkage of the breast is evident, and the tumour may remain under control in this state for several years.

Regression of metastatic skin nodules or enlarged metastatic nodes is also seen following oestrogen therapy. Whether it occurs, bears no relationship to regression of bone or other metastases in the same patient (*see* p. 55). Regression, again, is not uniform in all soft tissue lesions. Sometimes the primary tumour heals, but the metastatic nodes show no sign of regression. Sometimes nodules regress in one area and spread in another. There is no relationship between the size of a lesion and the likelihood of its regression, and old nodules may regress before more recent ones. This is unlike the effect of corticosteroid therapy (*see* p. 74) where, in general, only the smallest nodules regress while the larger ones remain unchanged. Regression of metastatic skin nodules or nodes tends to be slower in appearing in areas previously subjected to radiation therapy, presumably because of the impaired vascular supply.

Regression of lung or pleural metastases following oestrogen therapy in breast cancer was recorded in sixteen out of sixty-one patients treated by the author (Stoll and Ellis, 1953). It was associated with a longer survival than in untreated cases (Table 6.2). Radiographic evidence of regression of lung metastases appeared within two to three months after initiating oestrogen therapy. All types of metastasis—rounded opacities, multiple mottling, or lymphatic permeation—appear susceptible to such therapy, although clearing of lymphatic permeation with its associated dramatic subjective benefit is usually very temporary. Decrease in size of a pleural effusion or delay for months or years in the reaccumulation of an effusion previously requiring repeated paracentesis, is a sign of tumour control (Fig. 6.1).

Subjective benefit from oestrogen therapy in breast cancer is less common than from androgen therapy. Relief of pain from bone metastases may occur after two to four weeks, but, in the author's experience, it is on the average of shorter duration than similar pain relief achieved from the use of androgens. Recalcification of bone metastases (Fig. 6.2) may eventually occur in a small proportion of the patients achieving pain relief from oestrogen therapy, but usually takes at least three months to appear. However, in spite of pain relief, a general feeling of well-being, and increase in energy such as is seen from androgen administration, is rarely associated with oestrogen therapy. In addition, the incidence of cardio-vascular embarrassment due to fluid retention, is greater with oestrogen therapy than

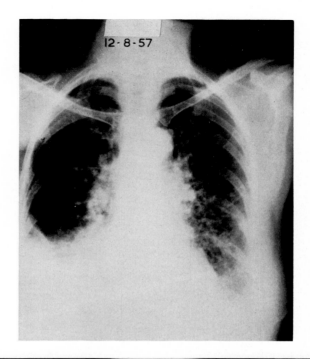

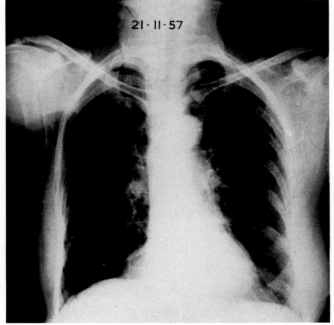

FIGURE 6.1 Patient E.B. Radiographs to show regression of malignant pleural effusion in a patient with breast cancer after three months therapy with ethinyl oestradiol 0·5 mg tds. The patient survived for nine years on hormonal therapy before final recurrence and death

Radiographs taken 12 August and 21 November 1957

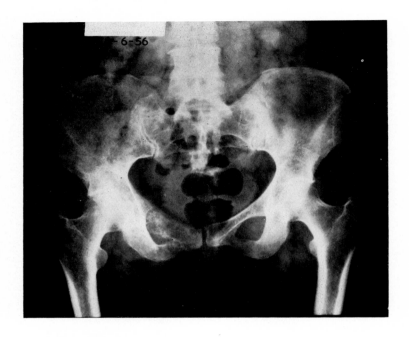

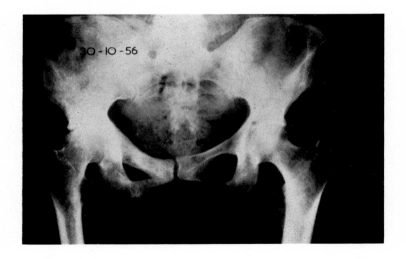

FIGURE 6.2 Patient M.C. Radiographs to show recalcification of metastases from breast cancer in ischium and pubis within four months of instituting ethinyl oestradiol therapy 0·5 mg tds

Radiographs taken 16 June and 30 October 1956

with androgen therapy at the usually recommended dosage.

HISTOLOGICAL EVIDENCE OF RESPONSE

The histological changes in breast cancer that is regressing under the influence of oestrogen therapy have been described by Koller (1944) and by Emerson *et al.* (1953, 1960). The initial change observed is a vacuolisation of the cytoplasm in the malignant cells, associated with a loosening of the connective tissue fibrils around the tumour cells. This is followed by an infiltration of the stroma with lymphocytes and plasma cells, while the malignant cells themselves show pyknosis and later fragmentation of the nuclei. Finally, the round cell infiltration subsides, leaving a mass of hyaline connective tissue, sometimes with a few clumps of surviving cancer cells in the interstices.

It is uncertain whether the effect of oestrogens on breast cancer is primarily on the epithelial elements or on the stroma of the tumour, as necrobiosis of the malignant cells and loosening of the connective tissue seem to proceed simultaneously. The connective tissue matrix of a target organ is known to be susceptible to the effect of oestrogens as manifested by increase in the turnover rate of chondroitin sulphate and hyaluronic acid (Sinohara and Sky-Peck, 1964). Collagen fibres have also been seen to change their physical characteristics under the influence of oestrogens.

SECONDARY OESTROGEN THERAPY

It has been emphasised by Hortling *et al.* (1962) that oestrogen therapy given as the first hormonal treatment in breast cancer yields a higher tumour remission rate than the same therapy given as a second or subsequent choice. The remission rate from secondary oestrogen therapy, after previous hormone therapy has lost control, is only 4 per cent according to Witt *et al.* (1963), and in the author's series is 11 per cent (Table 5.4). These figures are considerably lower than the author's 31 per cent primary tumour remission rate from oestrogen therapy. However, if assessment is restricted to patients with a previous favourable response to androgen therapy, the tumour remission rate from secondary oestrogen therapy is much higher—20 per cent in the author's series.

There is no evidence of clinical benefit from the use of oestrogen therapy in breast cancer after failure of hypophysectomy, according to Pearson and Ray (1959), Lipsett and Bergnestal (1960), and Kennedy and French (1960). This would suggest the importance of pituitary hormones in mediating oestrogen effects upon breast cancer, although Jessiman *et al.* (1959) reported possible exacerbation of tumour activity in one patient treated by oestrogen after hypophysectomy. A report by Landau *et al.* (1962) suggest the possibility of a direct steroid effect upon the growth of breast cancer. It reports objective evidence of tumour regression in several patients by treatment with a combination of progesterone and oestradiol after an attempt at complete hypophyseal ablation. It is possible that progesterone sensitises breast cancer to the effect of oestradiol (*see* p. 72).

WITHDRAWAL RESPONSE AFTER OESTROGENS

After oestrogen therapy in breast cancer has lost its control, no other attempt at endocrine therapy should be made for a period of two months, because of the possibility of a 'withdrawal response' (Segaloff *et al.*, 1954*b*; Delarue, 1955). An exception is made in the presence of rapidly advancing disease, when immediate corticosteroid therapy or major endocrine ablation is advised. Objective evidence of a withdrawal response is seen in 31 per cent of patients who have previously responded favourably to oestrogen therapy, and also in 3·6 per cent of those who have *not* responded, according to Kaufman and Escher (1961). Its cause is uncertain, but it is thought to reflect sensitivity of the tumour to changes in the hormonal environment (*see* p. 15).

Withdrawal response of this type has an average duration of ten months—a shorter duration than that of the average primary response. Huseby (1958) has noted that the extent and duration of withdrawal response in an individual is related to the extent and duration of the primary tumour regression in that patient. It is hardly to be expected in patients failing to respond favourably to primary oestrogen therapy. Occasionally a third period of tumour regression may be achieved if further oestrogen therapy is given after the withdrawal response has been lost (*see* p. 50).

EXACERBATION BY OESTROGENS AND HYPERCALCAEMIA

Oestrogen therapy is undoubtedly capable of exacerbating the growth of breast cancer in up to 50 per cent of premenopausal females (Pearson, 1957). Such exacerbation is also possible in postmenopausal females with evidence of persistent oestrogen secretion. It is generally agreed that exacerbation of breast cancer by oestrogens is extremely rare in patients more than ten years postmenopausal. According to Huseby (1958) it occurs in less than 1 per cent of women properly selected for oestrogen therapy (*see* p. 55).

An apparent showing up of tumour growth after withdrawing a hormone in a non-responding case *may* reflect the removal of an exacerbating influence. Nevertheless, exacerbation of tumour must be objectively demonstrated in order to be significant, and serial estimations of tumour volume are necessary to confirm it. General malaise, increase in bone pain or pyrexia have been described by Emerson and Jessiman (1956) as occurring in some cases after oestrogen administration. There is no evidence that such symptoms should, in themselves, be regarded as signs of tumour exacerbation, as some of these patients go on to tumour healing with continued oestrogen therapy (Lucchini *et al.*, 1962). Few of them benefit objectively by cessation of oestrogen therapy followed by oophorectomy.

Exacerbation of tumour is said to be manifest in the hypercalcaemia which sometimes follows oestrogen therapy in the presence of bone metastases, particularly if it disappears when oestrogen therapy is stopped (Escher, 1967). Hall *et al.* (1963a) showed that hypercalcaemia occurred in 5 per cent of 269 oestrogen treated patients. In the majority of these patients with hypercalcaemia, clinical evidence of tumour growth remission occurred if oestrogen was persisted with in spite of the hypercalcaemia. It should also be remembered that *spontaneous* hypercalcaemia occurs in 12 per cent of patients with bone metastases (Kennedy *et al.*, 1955).

It is evident that the danger of oestrogen exacerbation of the disease is low in older postmenopausal patients; it is probably exceeded by the danger of inducing cardiac failure from oestrogen therapy.

OESTROGEN COMBINATION WITH THYROID HORMONE OR CORTICOSTEROID

It was suggested by Bacigalupo (1959) and Luehrs (1961) that breast cancer which had ceased to respond favourably to oestrogen therapy might respond again if, in addition, tri-iodothyronine was administered. The author (Stoll, 1962b) prescribed the addition of tri-iodothyronine or thyroid extract throughout a course of oestrogen therapy, for patients whose tumour had failed to regress previously on oestrogen therapy alone. The investigation provided no evidence that thyroid hormone could sensitise breast cancer to the effect of diethyl stilboestrol therapy.

Larionov (1965) suggests that treatment with oestrogens must be accompanied by brief courses of cortisone therapy in order to prevent hyperproduction of progesterone by the adrenal cortex. He postulates on a theoretical basis that progesterone would counteract the beneficial effect of oestrogen therapy on cancer of the breast. This is contrary to the experience of Landau *et al.* (1962) in hypophysectomised patients (*see* p. 69).

OESTROGENS—MODE OF ADMINISTRATION

The administration of oestrogen therapy may be by one of two methods. It may be continuous, maintaining it for as long as control of tumour growth persists. In this case, a withdrawal response may occur, when oestrogen therapy is stopped on reactivation of the disease. Alternatively, treatment may be intermittent, stopping it as soon as complete regression has occurred in measurable lesions. In this

TABLE 6.3

Incidence of Intolerance to Oestrogen Therapy in Breast Cancer, According to the Preparation Used (Author's Series)

Oestrogen	Daily dose	% showing intolerance
Stilboestrol	1·5–15 mg	20%
Ethinyl oestradiol	1·5–3 mg	16%
Premarin	7·5–15 mg	3%

case, tumour regression is often maintained for many months after stopping therapy. When the disease reactivates, further tumour regression may occur, the oestrogen is reinstituted.

In the author's opinion intermittent administration, by alternating the hormonal environment of the tumour is more likely to postpone the development of autonomy. In general, however, the continuous method is more convenient in very old patients if serious side effects are absent, and it avoids the distressing complication of withdrawal uterine bleeding. The use of this method may necessitate incremental increases of the dose at intervals (*see* p. 61).

Diethyl stilboestrol is a synthetic non-steroidal oestrogen which has a high potency and is cheap in price. It has the added advantage of oral administration, and if complications arise, treatment effects are not prolonged when the steroid is discontinued. *Dienoestrol* has approximately one fifth of the oestrogenic potency of stilboestrol, and has no obvious advantages.

For patients who cannot tolerate diethyl stilboestrol, *ethinyl oestradiol*, also given orally but at one tenth of stilboestrol dosage, is sometimes better tolerated. Alternatively, *oestradiol monobenzoate* may be administered parenterally, if there is any doubt as to the patient's co-operation in oral dosage.

Premarin is a mixture of conjugated oestrogens derived from pregnant mare's urine and therefore relatively expensive. It is standardised as oestrone sulphate, and, taken at a dose of 2·5–5·0 mg tds it is almost free of side effects such as nausea or vomiting (Table 6.3). It can be given either orally or intravenously in the treatment of breast cancer.

Long-acting *depot injections* of oestrogen, such as the undecylate or valerianate esters should be used cautiously. If urgent complications such as heart failure or hypercalcaemia develop, their action cannot be swiftly terminated. The same objection applies to *implants* of oestrogens such as α-oestradiol 25 mg, or hexoestrol 500 mg, which are usually replaced at two-monthly intervals.

OESTROGEN DOSAGE

Diethyl stilboestrol is most commonly prescribed at a dose of 5 mg tds. A comparison of the clinical effectiveness of this dose with that of 0·5 mg tds, was carried out by the author (Stoll, 1950), and demonstrated a similar proportion of tumour growth remissions in breast cancer from either dose level. Nevertheless, the higher dose is generally recommended, as it was reported by Albert (1956) that diethyl stilboestrol dosage of more than 10 mg daily is required to inhibit gonadotropin secretion, and this is believed to be a major mechanism of its effect on breast cancer.

It was reported by Walpole and Paterson (1949) that 20 mg of dienoestrol daily was more efficacious in the treatment of breast cancer than was 1–2 mg daily. The lower dose is equivalent in its oestrogenic activity to approximately 0·25 mg diethyl stilboestrol and this may be an inadequate daily dose for the depression of breast cancer growth activity.

On the other hand, there is evidence that doses of diethyl stilboestrol higher than 15 mg daily, can achieve tumour control when the latter dose is found to be ineffective. The vaginal smear can be used in such cases as an indicator of the patient's oestrogen utilisation in the body. It has been shown by Liu (1957) and by the author (Stoll, 1967*b*), that there is a correlation between the degree of vaginal keratinisation and the likelihood of benefit from oestrogen therapy. If inadequate vaginal keratinisation follows prescription of stilboestrol 5 mg tds, it may be advisable to increase the dose, or even change from oral to parenteral prescription (*see* p. 108). A recent report (Veteran's Administration, 1967) of increase in deaths from cardiovascular complications following the prescription of even 5 mg diethyl stilboestrol daily in *males*, suggests caution in the

prescription of very high dosage also for females, until the possible dangers of such dosage are evaluated.

SIDE EFFECTS OF OESTROGEN THERAPY

The liver is known to inactivate oestrogens by conjugating them with glycuronides, and this ability may be impaired in some patients with liver cirrhosis according to Pincus *et al.* (1951). Thus the toxic side effects of oestrogens may be more manifest when the liver has been previously damaged. The following are the common side effects of therapeutic dosage:

1. *Nausea, vomiting, and anorexia.* Vomiting is complained of in 20 per cent of females taking 15 mg diethyl stilboestrol daily, and anorexia or nausea are even more common (Table 6.3). All these symptoms are usually transitory in nature, and they may be controlled by taking anti-emetics concurrently long enough for the patient to develop tolerance to diethyl stilboestrol. Chlorpromazine is better avoided for this purpose because, according to Khazan *et al.* (1962) it may stimulate prolactin secretion, and this hormone may play a part in the activation of breast cancer (*see* p. 109).

Alternatively, as suggested by Huseby (1958), a single dose of 5 mg diethyl stilboestrol taken before retiring at night is usually well tolerated, and further doses can be added gradually. In the author's experience (Stoll, 1950) tolerance is no greater to initial doses of 0·5 mg tds than to larger initial doses, and there is, therefore, little advantage in starting with low dosage.

In cases of persistent intolerance to diethyl stilboestrol, oral administration of ethinyl oestradiol or Premarin may be tried for a few weeks, after which it is usually found that the patient will tolerate stilboestrol without nausea. Alternatively oestradiol monobenzoate may be administered parenterally. In occasional cases, delayed intolerance may develop after several months of continuous diethyl stilboestrol therapy, and may even prevent further administration (*see* p. 64). Again, after oestrogen therapy is interrupted, its reintroduction may sometimes cause recurrence of vomiting.

2. *Sodium and water retention.* This is due to increased reabsorption of sodium salts and water by the kidney. Swelling of the ankles is seen to some extent in almost every patient taking oestrogens at the dose levels recommended. Less commonly, fullness of the breasts or gain in weight may result.

In elderly patients with a mild degree of heart failure, symptoms are usually increased after taking oestrogens at the dosage suggested. Diuretics and a restricted sodium diet may be useful in such cases.

In patients with severe heart failure, oestrogens are better avoided completely, although short intermittent courses of administration may control the tumour growth in patients with lesser degrees of heart failure (*see* p. 63).

3. *Urinary incontinence*. Dribbling of urine associated with cough or straining is often complained of by the older patient on oestrogen therapy. This is presumably due to the effect of oestrogen on the muscle tone of the bladder and is particularly marked in patients already suffering from cystocoel. The prescription of agents such as Tolazoline 100 mg daily (Priscol) has been found useful by the author in such cases.

4. *Uterine bleeding*. This occurs in the majority of postmenopausal females when oestrogen therapy is interrupted or withdrawn, and the patient should be forewarned of this to avoid anxiety. If severe, bleeding can be diminished by the administration of three or four doses of 100 mg testosterone propionate intramuscularly, at daily intervals.

Mucous discharge from the cervix uteri is not uncommon in patients receiving oestrogen therapy for breast cancer. 'Breakthrough' uterine bleeding occurs in a minority of patients even while taking 15 mg diethyl stilboestrol daily. It is not necessary to stop therapy or to curette the uterine lining if it occurs. By increasing the dose to 20 or even 30 mg daily, bleeding will nearly always cease, whereas stopping oestrogen administration will prolong the bleeding.

5. *Pigmentation of the skin*. Pigmentation of the nipples and areola occurs in almost all patients on diethyl stilboestrol therapy, and also in some on androgen therapy. Pigmentation varies from light brown to black, with scabbing on the surface of the nipple. Occasionally, pigmentation may occur also in the axillae or in old scars such as the striae gravidarum.

6. *Increase or decrease in libido, dizziness, irritability, excessive tiredness, breast tenderness or pelvic cramps* are occasional complaints in patients receiving oestrogen therapy at the dose suggested.

7. *Hepatotoxic effects*. Histological evidence of liver damage has been reported in postmenopausal breast cancer patients following therapy by a combination of the oestrogen Mestranol and the progestin Lynoestrenol (Stoll *et al.*, 1965) (*see* p. 71). No abnormality was found by the author in the liver function tests in a series of postmenopausal women receiving long-term diethyl stilboestrol therapy at the dosage recommended above.

TO SUMMARISE

Oestrogen therapy given as primary therapy will induce tumour regression in over 30 per cent of postmenopausal patients with advanced breast cancer. In such patients, undoubted prolongation of survival has been demonstrated. Objective evidence of tumour regression is seen most commonly in the presence of soft tissue metastases in older patients, and over 40 per cent of this group show remission of tumour growth. Lung and pleural metastases may also show objective evidence of regression in older patients, and survival is prolonged in such cases. A remarkable feature is that a second growth remission by the tumour is not uncommon on withdrawal of oestrogen therapy.

Diethyl stilboestrol is a suitable oestrogen for oral administration in the majority of patients. Dosage between 1·5 and 15 mg diethyl stilboestrol daily is recommended, but the adequacy of oestrogen intake is best assessed by serial examinations of the vaginal smear. Continuous or intermittent methods of dosage each has a place in management. Oestrogens may be poorly tolerated in a proportion of patients because of constant nausea or adverse effect upon cardiac failure. Exacerbation of the tumour growth by oestrogens is extremely rare in patients more than ten years postmenopausal.

Oestrogen Therapy

ILLUSTRATIVE CASE SUMMARIES

Patient A.D.E. Oestrogen-induced Regression of Soft Tissue Tumour on Three Occasions with an Additional Withdrawal Response. Hormonal Control Maintained over a Period of Six Years

A woman aged eighty-one presented in October 1953 with an inoperable breast cancer. It was fixed to the pectoralis muscles, and associated with overlying permeation nodules in the skin of the breast. Because of her advanced age primary treatment by oestrogen therapy was decided on, and a course of ethinyl oestradiol 0·5 mg tds was prescribed. It was maintained for a period of eleven months and resulted in almost complete disappearance of the breast tumour and of the infiltration of the skin for a total period of twenty-four months. When the tumour reactivated, a further eight months course of oestradiol therapy was given, and led to regression of the tumour for a further total period of eighteen months.

When the soft tissue tumour reactivated for the second time, the hormone was maintained uninterrupted for a period of twenty-two months—this time for as long as the tumour responded. When the tumour reactivated for the third time, *discontinuing* the hormone led to a withdrawal response with regression of the tumour lasting eight months. At the end of that time, a fourth attempt at oestradiol therapy was maintained for twelve months, but was unsuccessful in controlling the tumour. The patient died two months later, after tumour control by intermittent oestrogen therapy over a total period of six years.

Patient O.H.I. Control of Breast Tumour over a period of Five and a Half Years by Intermittent Administration of Oestrogen Therapy
A woman aged seventy-eight presented in July 1955 with a large inoperable carcinoma of the breast. It was invading all four quadrants and was associated with overlying peau d'orange of the skin of the breast. Because of her age and poor general condition, primary treatment by oestrogen therapy was decided on and a course of diethyl stilboestrol 5 mg tds was prescribed. Within six weeks there were early signs of regression in the tumour and this continued progressively.

Diethyl stilboestrol was continued by the patient for sixty-five months but only intermittently, because she disliked its side effects. During that time the breast tumour remained under control only as long as oestrogens were being taken, and reactivation occurred within two to three months of interrupting therapy. The patient's condition finally deteriorated suddenly after five and a half years of intermittent tumour control by oestrogen therapy.

Patient E.G.O. Oestrogen-induced Regression of Soft Tissue Tumour and an Additional Withdrawal Response. Hormonal Control Maintained over a period of Four Years
A woman aged seventy-one presented in October 1952, with an inoperable cancer of the breast. It was invading all four quadrants and associated with the presence of permeation nodules in the adjacent skin of the breast. Primary treatment was by a palliative course of X-ray therapy to the breast, adjacent areas of skin infiltration, axillary, and supraclavicular areas, to a minimum tumour dose of 4,000 roentgens in thirty days. Regression of the tumour followed the radiation therapy and was maintained for twenty months.

When tumour reactivation occurred, hormonal therapy was initiated with a course of ethinyl oestradiol 0·5 mg tds. Regression of tumour activity appeared after six weeks treatment, and, although oestradiol was discontinued after six months administration, tumour control was maintained for a total period of thirty-three months. At the end of that time, reactivation of growth again appeared. It did not respond to three months' administration of diethyl stilboestrol 5 mg tds, but, when stilboestrol was discontinued, a withdrawal response manifested with tumour regression lasting for thirteen months. In spite of further attempts at therapy, the patient died twelve months later, tumour control by oestrogen therapy having been achieved over a period of four years.

Patient A.R.I. Oestrogen-induced Recalcification of Bone Metastases, and Control of Pleural Effusion, for Twenty-three Months
A woman aged fifty-nine and seven years postmenopausal, presented in December 1953 with a Stage 2 carcinoma of the left breast. Primary treatment was by radical mastectomy followed by a prophylactic course of X-ray therapy to the mastectomy scar, axillary and supraclavicular draining node areas. After nineteen months she developed bone pain and radiographs showed the presence of multiple lytic areas of metastasis in bone, together with a malignant left pleural effusion.

Hormonal therapy was begun with the prescription of diethyl stilboestrol 5 mg tds but continuous nausea resulted. The prescription was changed to ethinyl oestradiol 0·5 mg tds, and this steroid relieved the bone pains within a month, followed later by radiographic evidence of recalcification in the previously lytic areas. No new evidence of bone destruction appeared, and for twenty-three months the patient remained on oestradiol treatment and maintained good activity, requiring no paracentesis for the pleural effusion or X-ray therapy for the bone metastases. She died suddenly one month later.

Patient F.H.O. Regression of Soft Tissue Tumour over a period of Four and a Half Years by Intermittent Administration of Oestrogens in a Patient with Cardiac Failure
A woman aged eighty presented in August 1954 with a Stage 2 cancer of the breast. Because of her poor cardiac condition, it was decided to initiate a trial of oestrogen therapy in preference to surgery or radiation therapy. A course of ethinyl oestradiol 0·5 mg tds was maintained for nine months, with some difficulty because of the fluid retention resulting from its use. Nevertheless it achieved regression of the tumour in the breast for a total period of eighteen months.

When the tumour reactivated at the end of that time a second course of ethinyl oestradiol was given for nine months, this time yielding a total period of twenty-six months of tumour control. A third and final nine months course of ethinyl oestradiol then controlled the tumour until the date of her death, which was four and a half years after coming under oestrogen treatment.

Patient E.F.E. Persistence In Spite of Oestrogen Intolerance Led to Control of Soft Tissue and Bone Metastases for Fourteen Months

A woman aged sixty-five presented in December 1954 with cancer of the breast complicated by the presence of multiple bone metastases. Radiographs showed these to be of a mixed lytic-sclerotic appearance. Because of the widespread metastases it was decided to begin treatment with oestrogen therapy.

A trial of diethyl stilboestrol 5 mg tds was prescribed but caused nausea and vomiting. A trial of ethinyl oestradiol was prescribed but again caused the same symptoms. A single dose of 2·5 mg of stilboestrol at night was then prescribed and found to be tolerated. The dosage was gradually increased till the patient was taking the full dosage of 5 mg tds. This dosage was continued for eight months without any further difficulty. During this time, the soft tissue tumour in the breast regressed in size and bone pains were almost completely relieved. The patient died as a result of bone marrow replacement by tumour, fourteen months after coming under treatment by oestrogens.

Patient F.W.H. Oestrogen-induced Regression of Soft Tissue Tumour for Two and a Half Years, but Intolerance to a Second Attempt at Oestrogen Therapy

A woman aged eighty-four presented in March 1955, with an inoperable scirrhous cancer of the breast. It was invading all four quadrants and was associated with overlying peau d'orange of the skin of the breast. Because of her advanced age, primary treatment by oestrogen therapy was decided on, and treatment with ethinyl oestradiol 0·5 mg tds was initiated. It was well tolerated and continued for sixteen months.

Regression in the size of the breast tumour was slow, appearing after two months but taking twelve months for shrinkage to occur from 7 to 3 cm diameter. Control of the tumour, once achieved, persisted for a period of twenty-nine months. When reactivation of tumour growth occurred at this stage, a further attempt at ethinyl oestradiol therapy was made, but this time it could not be tolerated because of nausea and vomiting. The patient died twenty-two months later, after further attempts at therapy by radiation.

Patient E.H.A. Oestrogen-induced Healing of Malignant Ulcer for Fifteen Months, but Treatment Curtailed by the Development of Late Drug Intolerance

A woman aged eighty-two presented in February 1956 with an inoperable ulcerated duct carcinoma invading all four quadrants of the breast. Because of her advanced age and poor general condition, hormone therapy was selected as the primary method of treatment. A course of diethyl stilboestrol 5 mg tds was prescribed, and within one month, early regression of the breast ulceration was apparent, and proceeded to complete healing.

Diethyl stilboestrol therapy was continued for ten months, but had to be discontinued at that stage because of the gradual development of intolerance as shown by nausea and vomiting. The soft tissue tumour remained healed for six months after stopping oestrogen therapy. Neoplastic growth then reactivated and the patient died eight months later.

Patient C.A.N. Oestrogen-withdrawal Response in Soft Tissue Tumour Without Prior Oestrogen Response

A woman aged sixty-seven, and sixteen years postmenopausal, presented in December 1953 with an inoperable cancer of the breast fixed to the underlying chest wall. Primary treatment was by a palliative course of X-ray therapy to the breast, axillary, and supraclavicular areas to a minimum tumour dose of 3,500 roentgens in twenty-six days. Regression of the tumour followed the X-ray therapy and was maintained for twenty-four months. When the tumour showed evidence of reactivation, hormonal therapy was initiated with a course of diethyl stilboestrol 5 mg tds. Regression of the soft tissue tumour was not obtained during the seven months that oestrogen was administered. However, when it was *withdrawn*, tumour regression occurred and persisted for six months.

Within twenty-four months the patient complained of bone pains and also of dyspnoea. Radiographs showed multiple areas of lytic bone metastases and also a malignant pleural effusion. A further attempt at hormonal therapy with ethinyl oestradiol 0·5 mg tds was instituted for a period of three months. This time, response was obtained neither during oestrogen administration nor after its withdrawal. The patient died one and a half years later, after further unsuccessful attempts at therapy.

Patient A.W.E.C. Oestrogen-induced Regression of Metastatic Axillary Nodes, but Not of the Primary Breast Tumour

A woman aged eighty-four presented in February 1956 with an inoperable cancer of the breast. It was invading all four quadrants of the breast, and associated with the presence of large fixed axillary nodes. Because of her advanced age, primary treatment by oestrogen therapy was decided on and a course of diethyl stilboestrol 5 mg tds prescribed. This resulted in rapid regression in size of the axillary nodes, but little change in size of the primary breast tumour. Because of this, oestrogen therapy was stopped after four months administration.

After an interval, a trial of prednisolone 5 mg qid was prescribed for one month. There was no change in size of the soft tissue tumour, and prednisolone had to be discontinued because of the embarrassment to the patient's cardiovascular condition. The patient died three months later.

Patient M.W.I. Oestrogen-induced Regression of Lung and Soft Tissue Metastases. Bone Metastases Progressed under Treatment
A woman aged sixty-seven, and twenty-one years post-menopausal, presented in May 1953 with a Stage 2 carcinoma of the breast. Primary treatment was by radical mastectomy followed by a prophylactic course of X-ray therapy to the mastectomy scar, axillary, and supraclavicular draining node areas. At twenty-six months following the operation she complained of cough and dyspnoea, and X-rays showed nodular opacities in the lung fields presumed to be metastatic in nature.

Hormonal therapy was begun with a course of diethyl stilboestrol 5 mg tds maintained for a period of three months. The pulmonary symptoms improved for a total period of twelve months and the lung opacities decreased considerably in size and density. At the end of twelve months, renewed activity appeared in the lung metastases, and at the same time, recurrent skin nodules appeared near the mastectomy scar. A second course of diethyl stilboestrol for two months was followed by regression in size of lung and soft tissue nodules, but at the end of four months there was radiographic evidence of bone metastases of a mixed lytic-sclerotic type.

After an interval, a course of testosterone propionate 100 mg intramuscularly three times a week was instituted for five months and led to relief of pain. Increasing bone marrow replacement by tumour caused death fifteen months later.

Patient I.J.O. Oestrogen-induced Regression of Soft Tissue Tumour on Two Occasions with an Additional Withdrawal Response. Mediastinal Node Metastases Progressed under Treatment
A woman aged sixty-three, and eighteen years post-menopausal, presented in July 1957 with a late Stage 2 carcinoma of the breast, fixing to the underlying pectoralis muscles. She received a pre-operative course of X-ray therapy to the breast and axillary

region to a minimum tumour dose of 4,000 roentgens in 30 days, and radical mastectomy was carried out three months later. Twelve months after mastectomy, recurrent skin nodules appeared in the region of the mastectomy scar, and, at the same time, multiple sclerotic areas of metastases in bone were visible in the radiographs.

Hormonal therapy was initiated with a course of diethyl stilboestrol 5 mg tds and was followed by flattening of the malignant skin nodules within five weeks. The nodules disappeared but, after only six months, reactivation occurred. When diethyl stilboestrol was stopped, a withdrawal response with regression of nodules occurred. The withdrawal response lasted for ten months—longer than the original remission. When the nodules reactivated for the second time, the patient also complained of cough and dyspnoea, and a radiograph of the chest showed enlargement of the mediastinal nodes. A further course of diethyl stilboestrol was prescribed, resulting in regression of the skin nodules for six months, but without change in the enlarged mediastinal nodes. The patient died seven months later.

Patient A.W.E. Oestrogen-induced Regression of Soft Tissue Tumour on Two Occasions. No Control from Attempted Androgen Therapy in the Interval
A woman aged eighty, presented in January 1953 with an inoperable cancer of the breast. It was invading the skin over the breast and fixed to the underlying pectoralis muscles. Primary treatment was by a palliative course of X-ray therapy to the breast, axillary, and supraclavicular node areas to a minimum tumour dose of 4,000 roentgens in twenty-eight days. Regression of the tumour followed the X-ray therapy and was maintained for thirteen months.

When reactivation of tumour occurred hormonal therapy was begun with a course of diethyl stilboestrol 5 mg tds, and was continued for fifteen months. Regression of the tumour resulted, but at the end of that period the tumour again showed signs of active growth. Oestrogen therapy was therefore discontinued and, after an interval, testosterone propionate intramuscularly 100 mg three times a week was prescribed. Although maintained for a period of six months, regression of tumour was not obtained. After an interval, a further course of diethyl stilboestrol 5 mg tds was instituted, and caused a further tumour regression for a period of six months. The patient died suddenly one month later.

Patient D.C.L. Oestrogen Stimulation of Calcium Excretion in the Presence of Bone Metastases, but No Benefit from Androgen Administration
A woman aged fifty-seven and fifteen years post-menopausal, presented in August 1957 with cancer

of the breast invading all four qudrants. She was complaining of bone pain, found to be associated with multiple lytic areas of metastasis in bone. The soft tissue tumour was primarily treated by a palliative course of X-ray therapy, delivering a minimum dose of 4,000 roentgens in twenty-seven days to the breast, axillary, and supraclavicular areas. Regression of the tumour followed the X-ray therapy, and it remained under control until death.

Serial estimations of urinary calcium excretion levels showed a rise on diethyl stilboestrol administration. Hormonal therapy was therefore begun with a course of testosterone propionate 100 mg intramuscularly three times a week, and continued for a period of three months. Although the calcium excretion level fell with androgen administration, relief of pain did not result, nor did recalcification of bone metastases occur. Within a further two months irregular metastatic enlargement of the liver was apparent, and the patient soon died.

Patient M.C.A. Oestrogen-induced Recalcification of Bone Metastases for Three Years, but Regression of Soft Tissue Tumour for only Twelve Months
A woman aged sixty-four, and twenty years postmenopausal, presented in June 1956 with a cancer of the breast. It was complicated by the presence of multiple lytic areas of metastasis in bone—mainly in the pelvis. Because of the widespread metastases, primary treatment by oestrogen therapy was decided on, and a course of ethinyl oestradiol 0·5 mg tds was prescribed for four months. As a result, pain was relieved for a total period of twelve months and radiographs showed recalcification in the bone metastases.

Pain recurred after twelve months, but once again responded rapidly to a course of ethinyl oestradiol. Thirteen months later the patient maintained her mobility free of pain but the breast tumour showed slow progression in size. Oestrogen therapy was therefore stopped, and after an eight-month interval, a three months' course of the corticosteroid dexamethasone 1·6 mg qid was prescribed. Corticosteroid therapy yielded no control of the soft tissue tumour growth, and the patient died five months later.

Patient B.R.O. Oestrogen-induced Regression of Soft Tissue Tumour on Two Occasions. No Control from Attempted Androgen Therapy in the Intervals
A woman aged sixty-three, and nineteen years postmenopausal, was treated in 1950 by a right radical mastectomy for breast carcinoma. After five years, tumour masses appeared in the opposite breast and axilla, and recurrent nodules appeared in the region of the mastectomy scar. She presented for treatment in January 1958, and because of the widespread

disease, primary treatment by oestrogen therapy was decided on and ethinyl oestradiol 0·5 mg tds was prescribed. Regression of soft tissue tumour was achieved, but the tumour showed signs of reactivation at the end of twelve months.

Oestrogens were discontinued and, after an interval, a course of fluoxymesterone 10 mg tds was prescribed for a period of three months. Tumour regression did not result. Diethyl stilboestrol 5 mg tds was tried after an interval but was not tolerated on account of nausea and vomiting. Premarin 5 mg tds was therefore substituted and a three months' course was well tolerated. Regression of the soft tissue tumour resulted from this oestrogen's administration for a total period of six months. At this stage the patient's condition deteriorated rapidly.

Patient G.B.E. Oestrogen-induced Regression of Soft Tissue Tumour on Two Occasions. Pleural Metastases Appeared under Treatment
A woman aged sixty-seven, with a history of a hysterectomy at the age of thirty-two, presented in April 1956 with an inoperable cancer of the breast. It was invading all four quadrants of the breast and associated with widespread permeation of the surrounding skin and also metastatic skin nodules. Because of the extensive nature of the disease it was decided to initiate treatment with a course of ethinyl oestradiol 0·5 mg tds. This was maintained for six months and led to regression of the breast tumour and metastatic nodules for a total period of thirteen months.

When the soft tissue tumour reactivated, it once again responded to a course of ethinyl oestradiol. At the end of four months, however, although the metastatic skin nodules had disappeared, a malignant effusion had appeared in the contralateral pleural cavity. The patient's condition deteriorated rapidly and she died soon after.

Patient E.B.O. Oestrogen-induced Regression of Soft Tissue Tumour on Two Occasions. No Control from Attempted Androgen Therapy in the Interval
A woman aged sixty-seven, and twenty years postmenopausal, presented in September 1954 with a large ulcerated cancer of the breast. Primary treatment was by a palliative course of X-ray therapy given to the breast, axillary, and supraclavicular areas, to a minimum tumour dose of 4,000 roentgens in thirty days. Although regression and healing of the tumour occurred following X-ray therapy, an enlarged metastatic node appeared in the opposite axilla seven months later. The breast tumour also showed evidence of reactivation at thirteen months after X-ray therapy.

Hormonal therapy was begun with a course of

ethinyl oestradiol 0·5 mg tds and was maintained for a period of eight months. This led to regression of the soft tissue tumours for a total period of twenty-two months. When the tumour reactivated, a course of fluoxymesterone 10 mg tds was given for five months, but did not result in tumour regression. After an interval, therefore, ethinyl oestradiol was reinstituted for a period of five months again resulting in objective regression of the tumour. The patient died suddenly at this stage from a cerebrovascular haemorrhage.

Patient S.W.I. Oestrogen-induced Healing of Ulceration on Two Occasions. No Subsequent Control from Androgen Therapy

A woman aged seventy-nine, presented in December 1952 with an ulcerated cancer of the breast, the ulcer measuring 7 × 5 cm in diameter. It was associated with a large parasternal tumour, presumably a metastasis originating in the internal mammary nodes, and also enlarged metastatic nodes in the opposite axilla. Because of her advanced age, primary treatment by oestrogen therapy was decided on, and ethinyl oestradiol 0·5 mg tds was prescribed for seven months. This resulted in complete healing of the ulceration and disappearance of the enlarged nodes.

Regression was maintained for a total period of thirteen months, and then recurrence of tumour activity occurred. This time treatment by stilboestrol 5 mg tds was given for five months, and again regression of tumour occurred for a total period of twelve months. When reactivation appeared for the second time, it did not respond to a trial of Sublings testosterone 10 mg qid for a period of two months. The patient died two and a half years later, after further attempts at therapy by radiation.

7

Progestin Therapy

EARLY REPORTS by Taylor and Morris (1951) and Gordon *et al.* (1952) described occasional cases of tumour regression following progesterone therapy in advanced breast cancer. Nevertheless, a later report by Volk *et al.* (1960) noted a complete absence of response in twenty-nine women given 2 G progesterone daily, although seven of the patients later showed favourable response to androgen or oestrogen therapy. There followed several trials in breast cancer of synthetic orally active progestins which have been developed more recently. (Since the major use of these agents has not been for assistance in the initiation of pregnancy, the author prefers to use the term 'progestin' rather than 'progestogen' or 'progestational agent').

FREQUENCY OF RESPONSE TO PROGESTINS

It was reported both by the author (Stoll, 1965*a*) and by Crowley and McDonald (1965) that the additional prescription of progestin led to tumour regression in

Various authors, using different progestins in the therapy of breast cancer, have reported a proportion with favourable response in limited series of patients and the results of the larger documented trials are summarised in Table 7.1. Briggs *et al.* (1967) have reviewed the literature of such progestin therapy and report tumour growth remission in 157 out of 634 patients with breast cancer—a 24·7 per cent tumour remission rate. This tumour remission rate is similar to the figure for androgen therapy (*see* p. 36).

From these observations it is obvious that there is a place for progestin therapy in the endocrine management of advanced breast cancer, but it is difficult to evaluate from the reports both the most efficacious group of agents, and the most suitable stage of the disease for their administration.

SELECTIVE ACTION OF PROGESTINS

By definition, a progestational agent is one which causes a secretory response in the uterine endometrium after oestrogen priming. Other criteria used

TABLE 7.1

Major Reports of Favourable Clinical Response in Patients with Breast Cancer Following Progestin Therapy

Author	Progestin	Regression in:
Jonsson *et al.*, 1959	Bromoketoprogesterone	7 of 34
Lewin *et al.*, 1959	Norethindrone	5 of 22
Curwen, 1963	Norethisterone acetate	21 of 55
Bucalossi *et al.*, 1963	Medroxyprogesterone	11 of 30
Stoll, 1967*a*	Lynoestrenol with Mestranol	9 of 42

breast cancer previously found unresponsive to oestrogen therapy. This suggested the possibility that a different mechanism of steroid activity was being utilised by these agents.

in the premenopausal female, are the postponement of menstruation, and the inhibition of ovulation, as shown by pregnanediol studies. The active progestins available have marked qualitative differences,

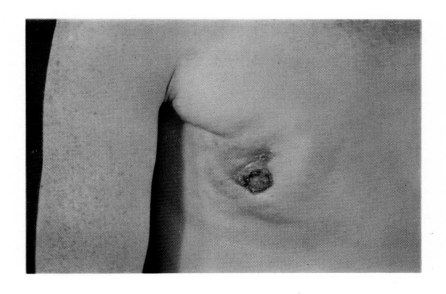

PLATE 1 Patient MM. Photographs to show healing of malignant ulceration of the breast within six months of surgical castration
Photographs taken 1 May and 4 November 1964

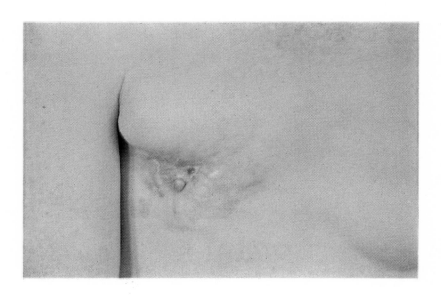

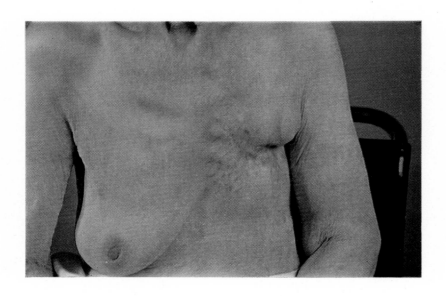

PLATE 2 Patient LM. Photographs to show healing of malignant ulceration of the chest wall within six months of instituting fluoxymesterone therapy 10 mg tds
Photographs taken 26 August 1957 and 8 February 1958

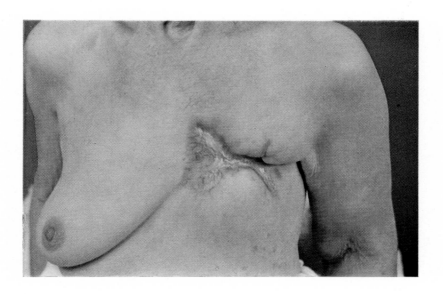

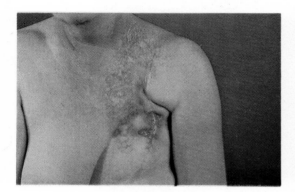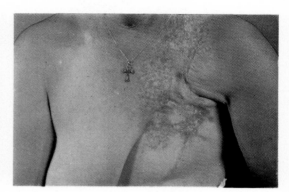

PLATE 3 (*a*) Patient DM. Photographs to show healing
of malignant ulceration of the chest wall within three months
of instituting fluoxymesterone therapy 10 mg tds
Photographs taken 4 November 1957 and 3 February 1958
Stoll, 1959 (courtesy Editor, *Medical Journal of Australia*)

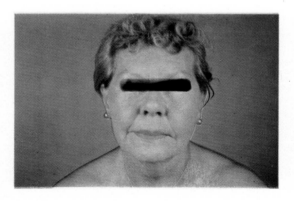

PLATE 3 (*b*) Patient DM. Facial appearance of patient to show
absence of virilisation after three months' therapy
with fluoxymesterone 10 mg tds, which has caused healing
of malignant ulceration of the chest wall
  Photographs taken 3 February 1958 (*see* Plate 3 (*a*))
  Stoll, 1959 (courtesy Editor, *Medical Journal of Australia*)

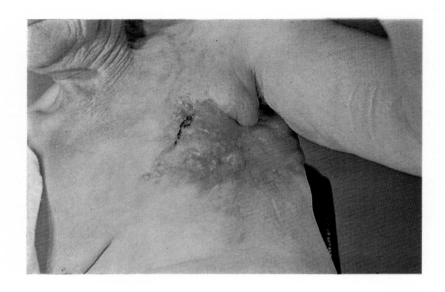

PLATE 4 Patient GB. Photographs to show regression of malignant infiltration of the breast within four months of ethinyl oestradiol therapy 0·5 mg tds
   Photographs taken 7 May and 24 September 1956

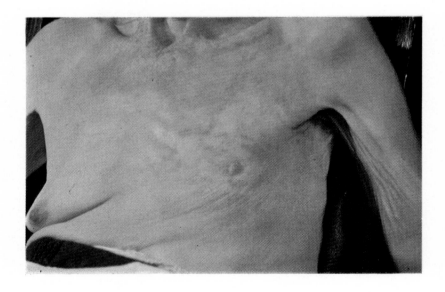

not only in respect to the above criteria, but also in their oestrogenicity, androgenicity, pituitary inhibiting properties, and metabolic activity. The importance of each of these properties in controlling breast cancer by progestins is unknown. Nevertheless, the androgenic and oestrogenic metabolites of each compound may be of considerable importance in deciding the choice of a progestin for breast cancer therapy, particularly in the case of the younger patient.

According to their parent chemical compound, progestins can be divided into three main groups of compounds—derivatives of 19-nortestosterone, of 17α-hydroxyprogesterone, and of testosterone respectively.

The 19-nortestosterone derivatives are probably metabolised to yield oestrogenic compounds, and, in addition, the group tends to be mildly anabolic and also androgenic in experimental animals. The 17α hydroxyprogesterone and the testosterone derivatives, on the other hand, are said to possess no inherent oestrogenicity, and no androgenic activity in the experimental animal according to Goldzieher (1964). In fact, some tend to have a pronounced anti-oestrogenic effect. Briggs et al. (1967) have suggested that all the progestins which give a good response in the treatment of breast cancer, have one thing in common—high pituitary inhibiting properties in animals. The possible mode of action of progestins in breast cancer is discussed later (see p. 71).

Since progesterone and many of its derivatives are fat soluble, they may have a very short life in the blood, and their rate of release from the fat deposits might have a very considerable bearing upon their efficacy in cancer control. This factor too could cause some selectivity of action in breast cancer, and the author (Stoll, 1966b, 1967c) has shown that patients failing to show favourable tumour reponse to one progestin may yet respond to another.

PROGESTIN-OESTROGEN COMBINATIONS

Lazarev (1960) on a theoretical basis, suggested that endogenous progesterone can counteract the benefit of oestrogen therapy in breast cancer (see p. 60). Nevertheless, Landau et al. (1962) noted tumour regression in two of seven previously hypophysectomised patients, following treatment by a combination of oestradiol and progesterone. Kennedy (1965b) noted a favourable response in two of four hypophysectomised patients from a stilboestrol, Delalutin combination. Crowley and MacDonald (1965) reported a favourable response in six of twenty-two breast cancer patients from the same

combination, after previous failure of oestrogen therapy.

A recent report by the author (Stoll, 1967a) described the results in breast cancer therapy of Lyndiol, a commercially available oral contraceptive containing Lynoestrenol (a progestin of the 19-nortestosterone group) combined with an oestrogen, Mestranol. Regression of soft tissue tumour in postmenopausal patients was noted in 22 per cent of sixty-five cases, the tumour remission rate being the same from the contraceptive dose as from a dose six times as high. Some of the patients showing tumour regression after Lyndiol had failed to respond to previous oestrogen therapy (Plate 5). As in the case of progestin therapy, there is no overall correlation between tumour response to Lyndiol administration, and previous response to either oestrogen or androgen administration.

SELECTION OF CASES FOR PROGESTIN THERAPY

In our present state of knowledge, the best results from progestin therapy in breast cancer appear to be in the treatment of soft tissue lesions (Jolles, 1962; Juret, 1966). The author (Stoll, 1966, 1967c) therefore compared agents belonging to the three groups of progestins in the management of soft tissue lesions from breast cancer. Tumour regression was noted in 16–22 per cent of seventy-two cases (Table 7.2). There was no significant difference in tumour remission rate between the three groups, although considerable differences in the nature and incidence of side effects were noted.

The palliative results of progestin therapy in the presence of bone metastases are disappointing according to Goldenberg and Hayes (1959) and Kaufman et al. (1964). The latter authors emphasise the appearance of hypercalcaemia in four out of seventeen patients treated with medroxyprogesterone acetate. In this connection it should again be noted that spontaneous hypercalcaemia occurs in 12 per cent of patients with bone metastases from breast cancer according to Kennedy et al. (1955).

According to Juret (1966) hydroxyprogesterone caproate is more effective in the older patient than in the younger age groups. Nevertheless, tumour regression in breast cancer was occasionally noted also in premenopausal women by Bucalossi et al. (1963) in a trial of medroxyprogesterone acetate.

Tumours responding favourably to progestin therapy do not necessarily belong to the same group as would respond favourably to conventional sex hormones. There is no correlation between tumour response to progestins and previous response of breast cancer either to castration or to androgen therapy (Jonsson *et al.*, 1959) or to oestrogen or androgen therapy (Stoll, 1967*c*). As noted above, the author (Stoll, 1965*a*) has shown that a proportion of patients with tumours failing to respond to oestrogen therapy, later show favourable response to progestin therapy.

Progestin therapy should be given a trial in the presence of breast cancer which is resistant to other forms of sex steroid therapy (*see* p. 125). In view of an apparently direct effect of a progestin oestrogen combination upon the tumour in hypophysectomised patients, as noted by Landau *et al.* (1962), and

PALLIATIVE EFFECTS OF PROGESTIN THERAPY

The earliest sign of tumour regression in soft tissue lesions from breast cancer is usually seen about six to eight weeks after starting progestin therapy. In some cases it is delayed for ten to twelve weeks. The average duration of tumour regression in the author's series was just over five months for the progestin treated cases, and over seven months for the Lyndiol treated cases. A further tumour regression on withdrawal of the hormones was noted in only one of sixty-five Lyndiol treated cases (Plate 5).

TABLE 7.2

Favourable Clinical Response to Progestin Therapy in Sixty-five Patients with Breast Cancer According to Agent Used (Stoll, 1967*c*). *By Permission of the Editor*, British Medical Journal

Therapy	Daily oral dose	Cases with regressing tumour	Group response in:
19 Nor-testosterone derivatives			
Norethisterone acetate	60 mg	2 of 12	} 3 of 19 = 16%
Lynoestrenol	30 mg	1 of 7	
17α Hydroxyprogesterone derivatives			
Medroxyprogesterone	200–400 mg	2 of 12	} 5 of 28 = 18%
Melengestrol	120 mg	1 of 5	
Megestrol	30 mg	2 of 11	
Testosterone derivatives			
Dimethisterone	300 mg	4 of 18	= 22%

Kennedy (1965*b*), such a combination is worth a trial also after failure of hypophyseal ablation therapy.

The author (Stoll, 1967*b*, 1967*c*) has reported that cytohormonal evaluation of the vaginal smear *before* steroid therapy can differentiate breast cancer patients with a 29 per cent likelihood of response to progestins, from those with only a 6 per cent likelihood of such response (Table 7.3). The former show an intermediate pattern, the latter an atrophic pattern, in the vaginal smear. The pattern of the vaginal smear before steroid therapy has a similar predictive value in the case of treatment with the progestin oestrogen combination, Lyndiol, according to a report by the author (Stoll, 1967*a*).

In the author's series regression of metastatic skin nodules or nodes did not occur in areas which had previously been the site of X-ray therapy, but was confined to adjacent unirradiated areas. This suggests that an undamaged blood supply is necessary for endocrine factors to affect the tumour. Regression of soft tissue lesions from breast cancer was often found to be associated with slow progression of metastases in other systems such as pleura or bone. Excerbation of tumour growth by progestin administration has not been noted by the author, but the relatively higher incidence of hypercalcaemia in the series of Kaufman *et al.* (1964) has been ascribed to this cause (*see* p. 69).

Subjective benefit is common, and many patients

experience a gain in weight and improvement in appetite, while on progestin therapy. Some patients note a marked feeling of euphoria while on such therapy, the effect being most pronounced in the author's experience from dimethisterone (Secrosteron) administration.

SIDE EFFECTS OF PROGESTIN THERAPY

The use of 17α hydroxyprogesterone caproate in the treatment of breast cancer is associated with almost complete absence of side effects according to Jolles (1962) and Juret (1966). Nevertheless, other types of

The possible modes of action of progestins in controlling breast cancer include
(i) Direct inhibition of tumour growth.
(ii) Suppression of pituitary hormone secretion.
(iii) Sensitisation of the tumour to the effect of oestrogens.
(iv) Conversion of progestins to another steroid.

1. DIRECT INHIBITION OF TUMOUR GROWTH
A direct effect of progestins upon breast cancer is suggested by observations on organ cultures *in vitro*. These observations were discussed previously together with similar effects of oestrogens and androgens (*see* p. 16).

TABLE 7.3

Favourable Clinical Response to Different Groups of Steroids in Relation to Cytohormonal Assessment of Pretreatment Vaginal Smear (Stoll 1967a). *By Permission of the Editor*, British Medical Journal

Form of hormonal therapy	Patients showing tumour regression if smear:		Significance
	Atrophic	Intermediate	
Lyndiol	1 of 16 (6%)	8 of 20 (40%)	Sig. $p < 0.03$
Progestin	2 of 32 (6%)	14 of 48 (29%)	Sig. $p < 0.03$
Androgen	11 of 36 (31%)	7 of 20 (35%)	Not sig.
Oestrogen	21 of 57 (37%)	14 of 45 (31%)	Not sig.

progestin therapy, in the dosage used by the author for the treatment of breast cancer, may be associated with varying degrees of backache, headache, breast tension, and leg or abdominal cramps (Stoll, 1967c). Severe nausea or vomiting may occasionally be sufficient to stop treatment, and is seen mainly with members of the 19-nortestosterone group. Severe mental depression or minor degrees of irritability have been noted in some patients, but euphoria in others. 'Break-through' uterine bleeding is only rarely noted at the dosage prescribed. Gain in weight, and increase in appetite have already been referred to.

Biochemical and histological evidence of liver damage following the administration of oral contraceptives has been reported by Eisalo *et al.* (1964) and by the author and colleagues (Stoll, 1965b, 1966a). Only with members of the 19-nortestosterone group of progestins were such changes recorded.

MODE OF ACTION OF PROGESTINS IN BREAST CANCER

It is established that progestins may inhibit the secretion of gonadotropin, may yield oestrogenic or androgenic metabolites and can behave either as anti-androgens or as anti-oestrogens.

A direct effect is also suggested by the observation of Landau *et al.* (1962) and Kennedy (1965b) of a beneficial response from a progestin oestrogen combination upon advanced breast cancer in hypophysectomised patients. Kim (1965) has observed in hypophysectomised rats an effect from such a combination on the growth of hormone sensitive mammary carcinoma.

2. SUPPRESSION OF PITUITARY HORMONES
Brown *et al.* (1964) reviewed the conflicting evidence concerning the effect of progestins on total gonadotropin excretion. It has been suggested by Diczfalusy (1965) that a decrease in the luteotropin secretion may be the only effect common to such agents. (Luteotropin is thought to be merely one function of prolactin.)

High pituitary inhibiting properties are said to be shared by all progestins effective in breast cancer therapy (Briggs *et al.*, 1967). It is of interest in this respect that Curwen (1963) reported a favourable response to progestin therapy to be associated with a high likelihood of similar response to subsequent hypophysectomy.

3. SENSITISATION OF TUMOUR TO THE EFFECT OF OESTROGEN

In the case of the uterine endometrium, oestrogen priming is necessary before achieving a progestin secretory response. A similar observation has been made by Sherman and Woolf (1959), on the need for oestrogen priming before neoplastic response in the uterine endometrium to progestins. In the case of hormone sensitive mammary carcinoma in rats, Huggins *et al.* (1962) have shown that the effect of progesterone upon the tumour varies according to the presence and concentration of oestrogen.

If such a mechanism also applies to the progestin treatment of human breast cancer, significant beneficial response to progestin therapy may depend on the presence of an adequate oestrogen concentration. This may account for the very poor tumour remission rate reported by the author (Stoll, 1967*b*, 1967*c*) in postmenopausal patients with an atrophic vaginal smear, as such a smear indicates an almost complete absence of oestrogen stimulation.

Whereas oestrogen therapy alone causes no tumour regression in human breast cancer after hypophysectomy (*see* p. 59), it was noted above that a combination with progesterone, has been reported by Landau *et al.* (1962), to yield objective evidence of tumour regression in some cases.

4. CONVERSION TO ANOTHER ACTIVE STEROID

It is generally agreed that many of the 19-nortestosterone derivatives have both oestrogenic and androgenic metabolites. The author's observation on breast cancer patients suggest that this may also be true of some 17α-hydroxyprogesterone derivatives (Stoll, 1967*c*). Difference in metabolic breakdown products may explain favourable response to one progestin after failure of response to another, which has been noted by the author in breast cancer therapy (Stoll, 1967*c*).

TO SUMMARISE

A palliative effect upon advanced breast cancer has been shown for progestin therapy in over 20 per cent of women so treated. Clinical benefit has been seen in patients with tumours previously not responding to oestrogen or androgen therapy, suggesting that tumours responding favourably to progestin therapy do not necessarily belong to the same group as would respond favourably to conventional sex hormones. Progestin therapy is therefore worth a trial in the case of patients with breast cancer failing to show tumour remission from androgen or oestrogen therapy. In combination with oestrogens, progestins are also worth a trial in patients failing to show tumour remission from hypophyseal ablation.

The progestins form a heterogeneous group of steroids with differing biological effects and metabolites in the body. A direct effect upon breast cancer tissue may be an important mode of action in their controlling effect, at least in the case of some members of the group.

Progestin Therapy

ILLUSTRATIVE CASE SUMMARIES

Patient A.G.R. Lyndiol-induced Regression of Soft Tissue Tumour for Twenty-one Months, both from Therapy and from Withdrawal Response. Previous Oestrogen Therapy Ineffective

A woman aged seventy-nine presented in February 1960 with a carcinoma of the breast. Primary treatment was by simple mastectomy. At forty-five months after operation, recurrent skin nodules appeared in the mastectomy scar, associated with the presence of enlarged metastatic nodes in the axilla. Hormonal therapy was initiated with a course of stilboestrol 5 mg tds, prescribed for three months, but without clinical signs of response.

Within five months, the skin nodules were ulcerated, new supraclavicular node metastases had appeared, and ulcerated tumour was present on the under surface of the opposite breast. Lyndiol 6 tablets daily, was prescribed for ten months. Within three months of instituting treatment, the enlarged nodes had regressed and the ulcerated areas healed. When new skin nodules appeared at the end of ten months Lyndiol administration was ceased. Withdrawal regression of the nodules then occurred and persisted for a further eleven months (Plate 5).

Patient D.H.A. Short-term Regression of Soft Tissue Tumour following Lyndiol Previous Regression for Five Years following Castration

A premenopausal woman aged forty-eight, presented in 1956 with a carcinoma of the breast. Primary treatment was by radical mastectomy, but at twenty-one months after operation, recurrent skin nodules appeared in the mastectomy scar. Endocrine therapy was begun with X-ray castration and, as a result, the nodules regressed, and remained under control for a period of five years.

At the end of this period, a localised area of recurrence of nodules was treated by a palliative course of X-ray therapy, and such treatment was repeated at approximately annual intervals for the next three years. At this stage, intracutaneous metastatic nodules appeared also in the scalp. A course of Lyndiol 6 tablets daily, was prescribed for six months, with almost complete regression of all nodules. When they reactivated at the end of this time, Lyndiol was stopped, but a withdrawal response did not occur.

Patient L.M.I.E. Short-term Regression of Soft Tissue Tumour following Norethisterone Acetate Therapy. Previous Oestrogen- and Androgen-induced Regressions

A woman of seventy-eight presented in November 1954 with an advanced inoperable cancer of the breast, invading all four quadrants and ulcerating through the skin. Hormonal therapy was initiated with a course of ethinyl oestradiol 0·5 mg qid and was continued for seven months. Complete healing of the ulceration resulted for a total period of twenty-seven months. When the tumour recurred, a further course of ethinyl oestradiol was attempted for five months but found ineffective. After an interval, a course of fluoxymesterone 10 mg tds was prescribed for three months, and this caused further healing of the ulceration and regression of the tumour for a period of fifteen months.

When recurrence occurred at the end of this time, a two month's course of fluoxymesterone, and a three month's course of stilboestrol were attempted but found ineffective. However, when norethisterone acetate 20 mg tds was prescribed for three months after an interval, it caused tumour regression for a total period of seven months. The patient died four months later, after tumour control over a period of five years by various methods of hormonal therapy.

Patient G.C.O. Short-term Regression of Soft Tissue Tumour following Norethisterone Acetate Therapy. Previous Androgen Therapy Ineffective

A premenopausal woman aged forty-six presented in 1957 with a carcinoma of the breast. Primary treatment was by radical mastectomy, and prophylactic surgical castration was carried out at the same time. At two years after mastectomy, recurrent skin nodules appeared in the mastectomy scar and also over the upper abdomen. At the same time, enlarged metastatic nodes were palpable in the axilla and in the inguinal region.

Hormonal therapy was initiated with a course of methyl testosterone 25 mg qid and continued for a period of six months, but without clinical signs of response. This was followed after an interval by a course of norethisterone acetate 20 mg tds for three months and as a result, the nodules and metastatic nodes completely disappeared for a period of eight months, and then slowly recurred.

Patient L.M.I.T. Short-term Regression of Soft Tissue Tumour following Medroxyprogesterone Therapy

A woman aged forty-five and four years postmenopausal, presented in November 1956 with a Stage 2 carcinoma of the right breast. Primary treatment was by radical mastectomy, followed by a prophylactic course of X-ray therapy to the axillary, supraclavicular, and internal mammary draining node areas. At twenty-seven months after mastectomy, metastatic enlargement of the right supraclavicular nodes was palpable, and was found to be associated with a malignant pleural effusion.

Hormonal therapy was begun with a course of medroxyprogesterone acetate 50 mg qid continued for a period of four months. During this time, the enlarged nodes regressed almost completely, although there was no decrease in the size of the pleural effusion. The patient's general condition deteriorated subsequently and she died six months after stopping steroid therapy.

8

Corticosteroid Therapy

THE PLACE of corticosteroids in the hormonal therapy of advanced breast cancer needs clarification. The results in the literature do not agree on the stage of the disease suitable for this form of therapy, nor on the proportion of patients likely to show objective evidence of tumour regression. There is also uncertainty as to the most effective agents and their optimal dose levels.

'MEDICAL' ADRENALECTOMY

It was shown by Wilkins et al. (1952) that cortisone administration leads to diminished oestrogen secretion by the adrenal glands. Since its long continued administration can finally lead to atrophy of the adrenal cortex, cortisone therapy in breast cancer has been described as a 'medical' adrenalectomy. This term is often applied when corticosteroid therapy is the sole method of treatment. Since *ovarian* oestrogen production is not inhibited by cortisone administration (Segaloff et al., 1954a), most authorities insist on ovarian ablation in addition, in order to make it comparable with the surgical procedure.

Ovarian ablation would certainly be a major factor in the clinical benefit reported in breast cancer patients, from a combination of castration and corticosteroid therapy by Nissen Meyer and Vogt (1959) and by Brinkley and Kingsley Pillars (1960). This has been discussed previously (*see* p. 28). On the other hand, varying degrees of clinical benefit have been claimed from corticosteroid therapy given alone in this disease, the major reports being by Segaloff et al. (1954a), West et al. (1954), Read (1957), Taylor et al. (1958), Kolodziejska (1959), Kennedy (1957b), Kofman et al. (1957), Lemon (1959), Gilse (1962), Gardner et al. (1962), and the author (Stoll, 1960c, 1963b). The last two reports confirm that objective evidence of tumour regression is sometimes obtained in premenopausal patients also.

PALLIATION BY CORTICOSTEROID THERAPY

The subjective benefit from corticosteroid therapy on the clinical status of seriously ill patients with advanced breast cancer, is often dramatic. Pain arising from metastases in bone or in the liver is usually markedly reduced, the appetite is improved, and the patient may return to near normal activity. Nevertheless in the majority of cases where such subjective benefit results, there is little or no associated objective evidence of tumour regression.

In only approximately 15 per cent of patients with local soft tissue metastases, is there also objective evidence of regression in the size of metastatic nodes or nodules, mainly affecting the smaller lesions (Plate 6). The peau d'orange, redness and pain of an 'inflammatory' breast cancer are often reduced, and lymphoedema of the arm, from whatever cause, is usually rapidly relieved. Objective evidence of control, when it does occur after corticosteroid therapy, rarely lasts longer than nine months in the author's experience (Stoll, 1963b).

Partial reduction in the size of pleural, peritoneal or even pericardial fluid accumulation is often achieved rapidly but lasts only for a few months in the great majority of cases (Fig. 8.1). Recalcification of lytic bone metastases is very rarely seen, but corticosteroid therapy may be useful in the presence of severe leuco-erythroblastic anaemia, as it may counteract the bleeding tendency. The relief of coma from brain metastasis, decrease in pain from liver metastasis, or of gross dyspnoea from lung metastasis are very gratifying although short-lived in most cases.

In Fig. 8.2 the progress is graphically shown of a patient with androgen induced hypercalcuria. It was successfully controlled by corticosteroid therapy after other ancillary therapy had failed (*see* p. 43). As soon as the serum calcium level is brought down to normal by this means, an attempt is made to replace prednisone therapy (Fig. 8.3). Major endocrine

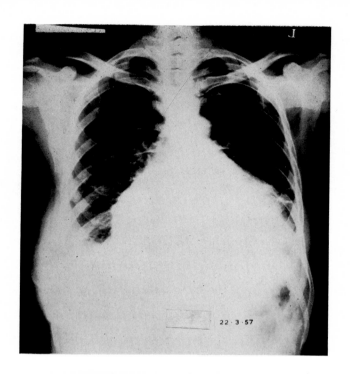

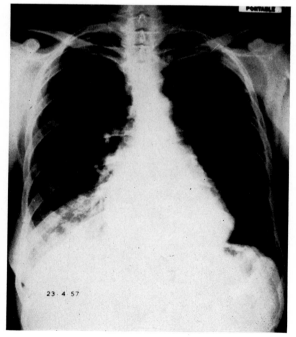

FIGURE 8.1 Patient B.H. Radiographs to show regression of
malignant pericardial effusion, secondary to breast cancer, after
four weeks of prednisolone therapy 20 mg tds

Radiographs taken 22 March and 23 April 1957

ablation may finally be necessary to control the hypercalcaemia in such cases.

In view of the dramatic controlling effect of corticosteroid administration in hypercalcaemia, it is remarkable that Hall *et al.* (1963*a*) have noted hypercalcaemia to develop in five out of fifty-eight patients while receiving corticosteroid for the treatment of bone metastases in breast cancer.

and psychosis, puffiness of the face, ankle oedema, and hirsutism. In addition, for months after such corticosteroid therapy, the adrenal insufficiency induced may lead to 'crises' in cases of severe infection or surgical operation, unless corticosteroids are administered prophylactically.

Therefore it is of interest to compare with the earlier results from high dosage, the benefit re-

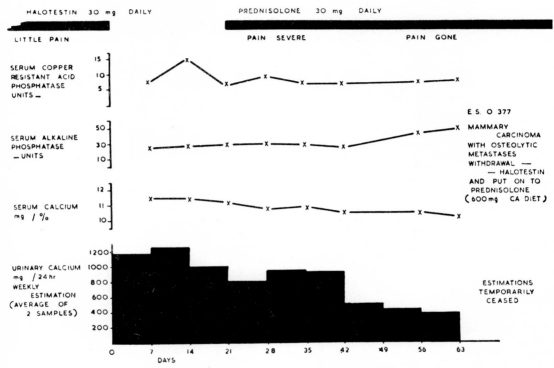

FIGURE 8.2 Patient E.S. The effect of prednisolone therapy on the urinary calcium excretion and on the serum calcium and enzyme levels, in a patient with bone metastases from breast cancer

Stoll, 1959 (courtesy, Editor, *Medical Journal of Australia*)

CORTICOSTEROID DOSE CONSIDERATIONS

Early reviews (*see* p. 74) reported that treatment by cortisone at a dose of 100–400 mg daily, or prednisolone at a dose of 50–200 mg daily, was followed by objective evidence of tumour regression in 20–30 per cent of treated cases of breast cancer. However, it is well established that prolonged dosage of 100–200 mg prednisone (or prednisolone) daily may give rise to serious complications such as peptic ulceration, hypertension, osteoporosis, diabetes or hyperglycaemia. Even 50–100 mg daily can give rise to glycosuria and diabetes, dyspepsia and peptic ulceration, increased susceptibility to infection, insomnia

ported from only 30 mg prednisone daily in advanced breast cancer. Because of the depressing effect of prednisolone on thyroid function, Lemon (1957) combined this with the administration of tri-iodothyronine, and Gardner *et al.* (1962) with liothyronine, and noted 48 per cent and 24 per cent respectively, of patients to show objective evidence of tumour regression. The author's series (Stoll, 1963*b*), treated only with 30 mg prednisolone daily, yielded objective evidence of tumour regression in 11 per cent of eighty cases. The relatively lower percentage response in the author's series is probably explained by a difference in the criteria of tumour remission, as an additional 11 per cent in the series showed 'arrested

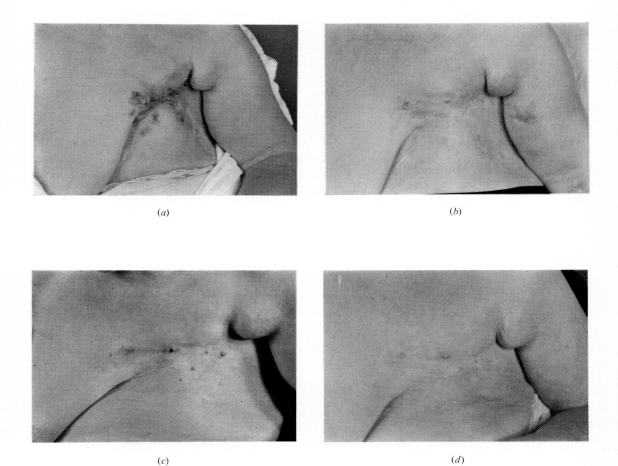

(*a*)   (*b*)

(*c*)   (*d*)

PLATE 5 Patient AG. Photographs to show (*a*) malignant ulceration of the breast and chest wall,
              (*b*) healing four months following the institution of Lyndiol therapy,
              (*c*) recurrence of activity after fifteen months hormonal therapy,
              (*d*) second regression within six months of hormone withdrawal

Photographs taken 9 August 1964, 21 December 1964, 17 November 1965, and 19 May 1966
Stoll, 1966 (*a* and *b* courtesy Editor, *Medical Journal of Australia*)
Stoll, 1967 (*c* and *d* courtesy Editor, *British Medical Journal*)

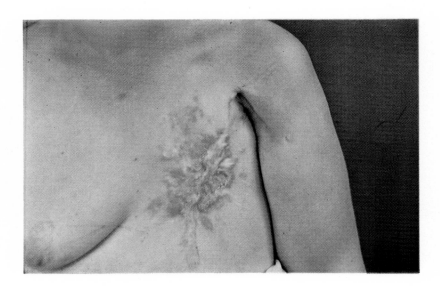

Plate 6 Patient EM. Photographs to show partial regression of malignant ulceration of the chest wall secondary to breast cancer within four months of dexamethasone therapy 1·6 mg qid

Photographs taken 23 March and 6 July 1959

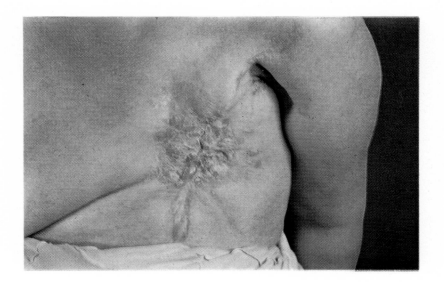

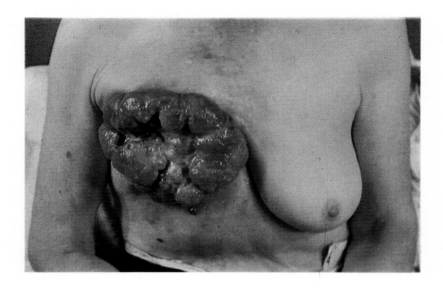

PLATE 7 Patient FH. Photographs to show partial regression of massive breast carcinoma following a course of 345 mg of thioTEPA in seventeen weeks
Photographs taken 29 January and 7 May 1963

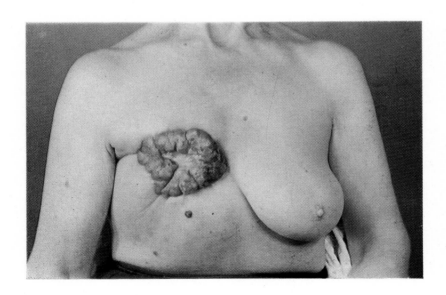

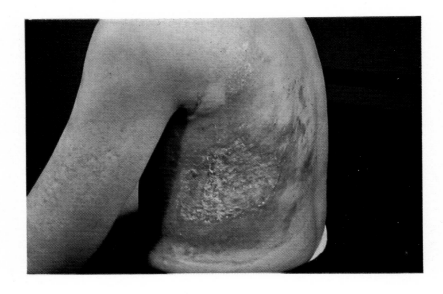

PLATE 8 Patient EE. Photographs to show partial regression of ulcerating breast cancer following a course of 285 mg of thioTEPA in twenty-two weeks
Photographs taken 27 September 1961 and 5 April 1962

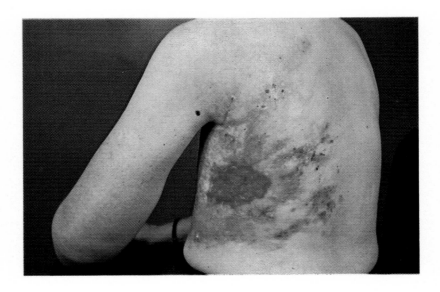

disease' which is accepted by some authors as evidence of tumour control.

The side effects resulting from three to six months administration of prednisolone at this dosage include mild puffiness of the face and ankles and slight increase of hirsuties in most patients, and only occasionally, mild dyspepsia or euphoria. In only one out of eighty patients was a more serious symptom seen by the author, and this took the form of temporary hypomania.

Taylor *et al.* (1958) suggested that larger doses of corticosteroids give better control of symptoms in

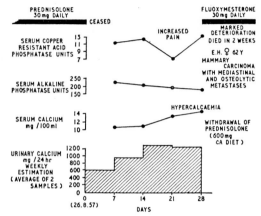

FIGURE 8.3 Patient E.H. The effect of ceasing prednisolone therapy on the urinary calcium excretion and on the serum calcium and enzyme levels, in a patient with bone metastases from breast cancer

Stoll, 1963 (courtesy, Editor, *British Medical Journal*)

breast cancer. This is possible, but there would appear to be no concrete advantage, yet a considerable increase in side effects, in using in *all* cases of breast cancer a dosage of prednisolone or prednisone higher than 30 mg daily. Elderly patients with cardiac disease may not tolerate even 20 mg prednisolone daily. On the other hand, according to Dao *et al.* (1961) and the author (Stoll, 1963*b*), dosage less than 50 mg cortisone or 15 mg prednisolone daily does not cause objective evidence of tumour regression in breast cancer. The author regards the commonly prescribed dose of prednisolone 5 mg tds as being marginal in its effects on breast cancer, except as part of a 'tapering off' procedure.

High dosage levels of 60–100 mg prednisolone daily may nevertheless be attempted in patients not responding to the lower dosage recommended above. The stage in the disease at which they are prescribed depends on the severity of the disease symptoms, and this is weighed against the dangers of severe side

effects from the steroids. High dose levels are always used in emergencies, such as hypercalcaemia (Connor *et al.*, 1956), acute dyspnoea due to pulmonary or mediastinal metastases, and coma due to cerebral metastases from breast cancer. In all cases, dosage should be reduced to 60 mg daily as soon as control of symptoms is achieved, and to 30 mg daily as soon as the patient is ambulatory. Reduction of the dosage to 20 mg daily may be attempted, but as the disease progresses, it is more often found necessary to increase the dose of corticosteroid in order to maintain control over the symptoms over a prolonged period. The risk of increased side effects is justified if no other method of treatment remains for the patient.

A higher proportion of visceral metastases has been found at autopsy in corticosteroid treated patients, compared to a group treated by major endocrine ablation therapy (Sherlock and Hartmann, 1962). The significance of this finding is uncertain, as patients with visceral metastases are likely to be selected for corticosteroid therapy, and rejected for major endocrine ablation.

Prednisone and prednisolone are of equal effectiveness in the treatment of breast cancer. Attempts by the author to replace prednisolone with dexamethasone, betmaethasone, or paramethasone in pharmacologically equivalent dosage were no more successful (Stoll, 1960*c*). Nevertheless dexamethasone 1–2 mg tds has been suggested as an alternative to prednisone. Dosage of corticosteroids must be tailed off slowly if they have been used for long periods, because of the adrenocortical atrophy induced. In such cases, a course of slow acting ACTH (80 units tapered on successive days to 20 units) may be necessary to counteract the depressant effects of corticosteroids on the secretory capacity of the adrenal cortex.

FACTORS INFLUENCING CORTICOSTEROID RESPONSE

It has been suggested by Lemon (1959) that surgical castration is an essential prerequisite to successful corticosteroid treatment in breast cancer. Nevertheless, objective evidence of tumour regression in premenopausal patients has been confirmed by Gardner *et al.* (1962) and by the author (Stoll, 1963*b*). These same reports noted that no correlation could be established between the likelihood of tumour regression from corticosteroid therapy and the patient's age group (Table 8.1).

In two series of patients (Gardner *et al.*, 1962; Stoll, 1963*b*), it was found that tumour response to corticosteroids cannot be correlated with previous response to sex hormone therapy (Table 8.2). Nevertheless, cortisone suppression of urinary calcium excretion has been suggested by Emerson and Jessiman (1956) as a method of identifying sex hormone sensitivity in breast cancer. This appears unlikely in view of the observation by Plimpton and Gellhorn (1956) that hypercalciuria associated with

TABLE 8.1

Favourable Clinical Response to Corticosteroid Therapy in Relation to Menopausal Age Group (Stoll, 1963*b*)

Age group	Cases with regressing tumour	Percentage with regressing tumour	Significance
Premenopausal or within 5 years of menopause	21 of 79	27%	Difference not sig.
Over 5 years post-menopausal	16 of 75	21%	

TABLE 8.2

Favourable Clinical Response to Corticosteroid Therapy in Relation to Previous Sex Hormonal Therapy Response (Stoll, 1963*b*)

	Now regress after corticosteroids in:		Significance
	Cases	Percentage	
Previous tumour regression after sex hormones	9 of 24	37%	Difference not sig.
Previous failure of sex hormones	13 of 59	22%	

malignant disease of types *not* generally regarded as under gonadal influence, can be controlled by corticosteroid administration. This is presumably because of its non-specific calcium retaining effects.

CORTICOSTEROID THERAPY AND ADRENALECTOMY

It has been suggested by Nissen Meyer and Vogt (1959) and Lemon (1961) that the beneficial results of corticosteroid therapy are as good as those from either hypophysectomy, or from bilateral adrenalectomy and oophorectomy, in the treatment of advanced breast cancer. In fact, it has even been suggested by some that the beneficial effects of bilateral adrenalectomy may be due to the cortisone replacement therapy used after the operation. Nevertheless, Dao *et al.* (1961) have shown that this dose level is ineffective in causing objective evidence of tumour regression in breast cancer. Disagreement

on benefit from corticosteroid therapy may be due to different criteria of response (*see* p. 112).

Fracchia *et al.* (1959) suggested that a favourable clinical response in breast cancer to corticosteroid therapy predicts a similar response to adrenalectomy. The author (Stoll, 1963*b*) has shown that this is not always true. According to Dao *et al.* (1961) too, adrenalectomy may be followed by a favourable clinical response even if previous corticosteroid therapy has been unsuccessful.

Objective evidence of tumour regression following corticosteroid administration is not usually as prolonged or as complete as that following adrenalectomy. In the series of Lemon (1959) the average length of remission from corticosteroid therapy is 8·5 months, and in the author's series (Stoll, 1963*b*) only 6·5 months, while that for adrenalectomy is over 12 months (*see* p. 91). Corticosteroids, however, have the advantage of causing marked subjective benefit in seriously ill patients, and they may even improve their condition sufficiently to face later major ablative surgery (Hellstrom and Franksson, 1958). If so used, the corticosteroid therapy does not appear to prejudice the result of the operation or the subsequent postoperative management of the patient.

MODE OF ACTION OF CORTICOSTEROID THERAPY

It has been mentioned at the beginning of this section that the administration of corticosteroids, like the operation of adrenalectomy, causes suppression of adrenal oestrogen secretion. It has, therefore, been suggested that this may be its mechanism in controlling the growth of breast cancer. It should be noted that, according to Wilson *et al.* (1960) hypophysectomy causes a far more profound adrenal atrophy than does corticosteroid administration. Furthermore, it has been shown that the success of endocrine ablation therapy is not dependent on decrease in oestrogen secretion (*see* p. 14). Segaloff *et al.* (1954*a*) have observed that although corticosteroid administration depressed ACTH secretion, it may cause *increase* in gonadotropin secretion by the pituitary. This may result from the fall in oestrogen and androgen levels which follows corticosteroid therapy (Lemon *et al.*, 1958).

The absence of a correlation between the nature of the response to corticosteroids and that to sex hormone therapy in breast cancer, has led to the suggestion by Taylor *et al.* (1958) that the effect of corticosteroids in this disease is a local one upon the tumour or upon the tumour bed. The katabolic effect of the hormone may decrease protein synthesis by the tumour. An anti-inflammatory action would decrease vascular permeability and oedema around the tumour or its metastases, and thus relieve symptoms of pressure by the tumour.

Such an action would explain the author's observation of rapid but transitory reduction in size (but rarely disappearance) of pulmonary opacities, metastatic skin nodules and nodes following corticosteroid therapy. Such an action would explain the rapid but temporary improvement noted in the coma of cerebral metastases from breast cancer by Kofman *et al.* (1957). According to Kofman *et al.* (1957) and Galicich *et al.* (1961), similar relief has been noted also in patients with *primary* brain tumours treated with corticosteroids, suggesting that the action is not a specific one.

Gerbrandy and Hellendorn (1957) and Taylor *et al.* (1958) suggest that in the case of hypercalcaemia, the effect of corticosteroids is probably by a specific action on calcium metabolism, and the relief of pain from bone metastases is by an action on the tumour bed. As stated above, recalcification of bone metastases is rarely seen to follow corticosteroid therapy.

CORTICOSTEROIDS COMBINED WITH ALKYLATING AGENTS

A combination of corticosteroid therapy with that of alkylating agents has been reported in the treatment of advanced breast cancer by McCarthy (1955), Curreri and McIver (1956), the author (Stoll, 1960*d*), and by Freckman *et al.* (1964).

The last authors noted tumour regression in 34 per cent of seventy-one of a series of patients with breast

TABLE 8.3

Favourable Clinical Response of Intrathoracic Metastases to Prednisolone, With or Without Added Nitromin (Stoll, 1963*b*)

Therapy	Cases with regressing tumour	Percentage with regressing tumour	Significance
Prednisolone	2 of 33	6%	Difference sig.
Prednisolone with Nitromin	17 of 31	55%	$p < 0.05$

cancer treated by Chlorambucil and prednisolone. The effect of prednisolone combined with Nitromin in a large series of patients with cancer of all types, was reported by the author (Stoll, 1960*d*), but it was only in the case of breast cancer that an additive effect appeared. This is most marked in the regression of intrathoracic metastases (Table 8.3). Alkylating agents given alone in breast cancer yield only poor results in the treatment of lung metastases (Hurley *et al.*, 1961).

In the presence of lung or brain metastases from breast cancer the author advises (Stoll, 1963*b*) that treatment should be initiated with prednisolone and an alkylating agent (Figs. 8.4, 8.5, 8.6). Sex hormone therapy is introduced later, when an attempt is made to taper off the therapy with prednisolone and alkylating agent. The combination of corticosteroids and alkylating agents yields early but transient clinical improvement in the majority of patients, while subsequent therapy by sex hormones may induce a delayed but prolonged control in the hormone sensitive minority.

A combination of prednisolone and an alkylating agent is useful also in the management of metastatic serous effusions—either pleural or peritoneal. A 'loading' dose of thioTEPA or cyclophosphamide is injected into the serous cavity and followed by a maintenance course of the alkylating agent combined with prednisolone. This is continued until satisfactory control of the effusion is obtained or until evidence of haemopoietic toxicity develops. Sex hormone therapy is then instituted. Control of the effusion is often achieved for one to three years in many such cases.

TO SUMMARISE

Corticosteroid therapy is indicated especially for patients who are too ill for major endocrine ablation therapy, and for those whose tumours are not sensitive to sex hormone administration. It yields objective signs of tumour regression in the presence of visceral metastases, such as those of the liver, pleura and peritoneum. It is indicated as emergency treatment especially in the presence of hypercalcaemia, lung, and brain metastases. Apart from these emergencies, there appears to be no proven clinical advantage, but considerable disadvantages in exceeding a dose of 30 mg prednisone or prednisolone daily.

The patient's age group, and previous response to sex hormone therapy, are not correlated with the likelihood of favourable response of breast cancer to corticosteroid therapy. The effect of corticosteroids on breast cancer is probably a local one upon the tumour bed. Objective evidence of tumour regression is in general not as prolonged or as complete from corticosteroid therapy as it is following bilateral adrenalectomy, but subjective benefit is more common. Combination with an alkylating agent gives remarkable if short lived, palliation of symptoms

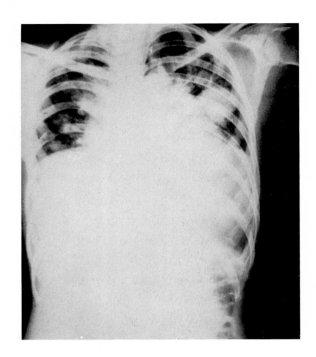

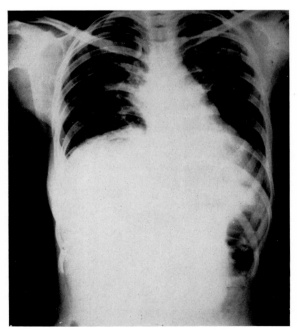

FIGURE 8.4 Patient J.R. Radiographs to show regression of pulmonary metastases from breast cancer within three weeks of instituting therapy with prednisolone combined with Nitrogen mustard oxide. Radiographs taken 23 May and 12 June 1956

Stoll, 1960 (courtesy, Editor, *Acta Unio Int. Contra Cancer*)

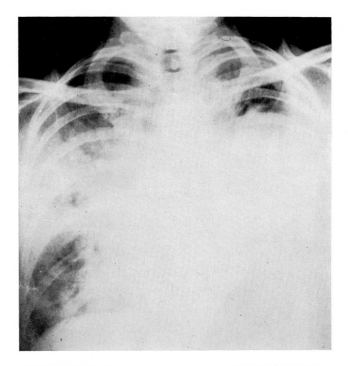

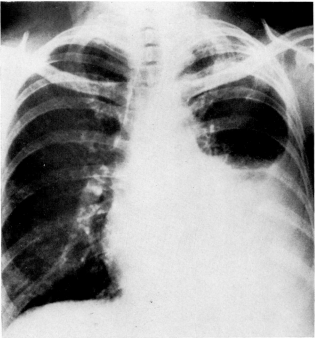

FIGURE 8.5 Patient J.G. Radiographs to show regression of pulmonary metastases from breast cancer with two weeks of initiating therapy with prednisolone combined with thioTEPA

Radiographs taken 16 June and 29 June 1956

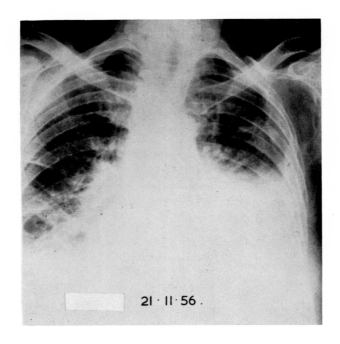

21 · II · 56 .

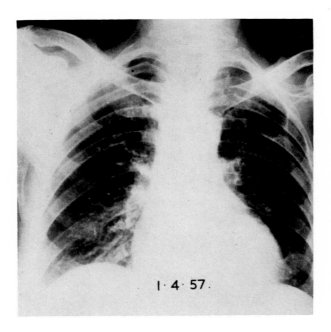

I · 4 · 57 .

FIGURE 8.6 Patient E.C. Radiographs to show regression of lung infiltration from breast cancer within four months of initiating therapy with prednisolone combined with thioTEPA

Radiographs taken 21 November 1956 and 1 April 1957

from intrathoracic metastases, and prolonged control of serous effusions. Disagreement on the benefit to be expected from corticosteroid therapy is probably a result of different criteria of favourable response.

Corticosteroid Therapy

ILLUSTRATIVE CASE SUMMARIES

Patient E.O.R. Corticosteroid-induced
Recalcification of Bone Metastases for Twenty-three
Months after Androgen-induced Control of Pain
A woman aged sixty-four and twelve years post-menopausal, presented in March 1956 with an advanced cancer infiltrating all four quadrants of the breast, and associated with palpable metastatic enlargement of the supraclavicular nodes. She also complained of bone pains, and radiographs showed multiple lytic areas of metastasis in bone. A palliative course of X-ray therapy was given to the breast, axillary, and supraclavicular areas to a minimum tumour dose of 3,500 roentgens in twenty-eight days. At the same time, hormonal therapy was initiated with a course of Primoteston depot 250 mg weekly intramuscularly and continued for thirty-four months.

Regression of the soft tissue tumour followed the X-ray therapy and was maintained until death. The androgen therapy resulted in relief of pain from the bone metastases, but no radiographic evidence of recalcification in the metastases. Multiple nodular opacities suggestive of metastases, had appeared in the lung fields during androgen therapy, and it was therefore stopped after almost three years administration, when new supraclavicular node enlargement also appeared.

The urinary calcium excretion was estimated before and during prednisolone therapy. As a fall in the level resulted from corticosteroid administration, prednisolone 10 mg tds was prescribed for the next twenty-three months. Recalcification of bone metastases occurred after three months of this therapy but control of soft tissue tumour did not occur and the patient died six months after stopping corticosteroid treatment.

Patient B.H.U. Short-term Regression of Soft
Tissue Tumour following Corticosteroid Therapy
but No Control of Bone Metastases
A woman aged sixty-three and eleven years post-menopausal, presented in January 1957 with a carcinoma of the right breast. Primary treatment was by radical mastectomy followed by a prophylactic course of X-ray therapy to the mastectomy scar, supraclavicular, and axillary draining node areas. Within nineteen months of the operation, the patient complained of bone pains. Multiple lytic areas of metastasis were visible in skeletal radiographs and soon afterwards, recurrent skin nodules appeared in the vicinity of the mastectomy scar.

Hormonal therapy was initiated with a course of prednisolone 5–10 mg tds and was maintained for seven months. As a result, the skin nodules regressed in size during that time, and bone pain was partly relieved. In spite of this, the radiographs showed no evidence of recalcification in the metastases. The patient died two months after stopping corticosteroid therapy.

Patient L.S.Y. Corticosteroid-induced Regression
of Soft Tissue and Bone Metastases for Eleven
Months, after Failure of Androgen Therapy
A premenopausal woman aged forty presented in July 1957 with a Stage 2 carcinoma of the left breast. Primary treatment was by radical mastectomy followed by a prophylactic course of X-ray therapy to the mastectomy scar, axillary, and supraclavicular draining node areas. At forty-one months after the operation, the patient developed bone pains associated with multiple lytic areas of skeletal metastasis.

Hormonal therapy was initiated with a course of testosterone propionate 100 mg intramuscularly three times a week. After four months therapy there was no relief of pain or evidence of recalcification in the radiographs of the bone metastases. The steroid was discontinued when the patient developed multiple nodular opacities of metastasis in the lung fields, and also a malignant pleural effusion. Soon afterwards, nodular recurrence appeared in the skin near the mastectomy scar, and metastatic enlargement of the left supraclavicular nodes was palpable.

A course of prednisolone 10 mg tds was prescribed, and continued for a period of fifteen months. As a result, the skin nodules regressed in size for eleven months of that time, and the previously lytic areas of bone metastasis showed evidence of recalcification. However, the patient's general condition slowly deteriorated and she died soon after stopping corticosteroid therapy.

Patient D.M.A. Short-term Regression of Soft Tissue Tumour Following Corticosteroid Therapy, after Androgen-induced Regression

A woman aged fifty-four, with a history of hysterectomy nine years previously, presented in July 1957 with a Stage 2 carcinoma of the left breast. Primary treatment was by radical mastectomy, followed by a prophylactic course of X-ray therapy to the mastectomy scar, axillary, and supraclavicular draining node areas. Within twenty-three months of the operation, recurrent skin nodules appeared in the vicinity of the mastectomy scar.

Hormonal therapy was begun with a course of stilboestrol 5 mg tds, and was continued for ten months, but without clinical evidence of benefit. After an interval, a four month's course of fluoxymesterone 10 mg was prescribed, and this resulted in complete healing of the skin nodules for a period of seventeen months. When the nodules again reactivated, a course of the corticosteroid dexamethasone 1·6 mg qid was prescribed for four months, and this also resulted in regression of the skin nodules. At the end of four months, however, bilateral malignant pleural effusions developed, and treatment was continued by the use of cytotoxic agents, viz. nitrogen mustard, Mitomycin, and cyclophosphamide. These were all without clinical benefit, and the patient soon died.

Patient J.M.A. Short-term Control of Symptoms from Cerebral Metastases following Corticosteroid Therapy

A premenopausal woman aged forty-one, presented in June 1956 with a carcinoma of the breast considered inoperable because of its fixation to the underlying pectoralis muscles. Primary treatment was by a course of X-ray therapy to the breast, axillary, and supraclavicular draining node areas, completing a tumour dose of 4,000 roentgens in twenty-seven days. At the same time, prophylactic radiation castration was added, delivering a dose of 1,000 roentgens in fourteen days to the region of the ovaries. At the end of six months, radical mastectomy was carried out.

At forty-nine months after the operation, the patient complained of cough and dyspnoea, and multiple nodular opacities of metastasis were visible in radiographs of the lung fields. One month later, she developed papilloedema, and localising signs of cerebral metastases. An attempt at stilboestrol therapy was made but not tolerated on account of vomiting. A course of prednisolone 10–20 mg tds was prescribed, and this abolished the signs of raised intracranial pressure and cerebral symptoms for a total period of four months. The patient died three months later.

Patient R.C.O. Short-term Regression of Soft Tissue Tumour following Corticosteroid Therapy after Failure of Oestrogen Therapy

A woman aged forty-nine, with a history of a hysterectomy four years previously, presented in March 1955 with a carcinoma of the breast. It was considered inoperable because of fixation to the underlying pectoralis muscles, and primary treatment was by a palliative course of X-ray therapy. A dose of 3,500 roentgens was delivered in thirty-four days to the breast, axillary, and supraclavicular areas. Regression of the breast tumour followed the X-ray therapy, and was maintained for a period of six months, after which nodular infiltration appeared in the skin.

Hormonal treatment was begun with a course of stilboestrol 5 mg tds, but after three months' treatment, no regression of the soft tissue tumour was visible. After an interval, a course of prednisolone 10 mg tds was prescribed for four months, and this led to temporary regression of the nodules. Within three months of discontinuing prednisolone, a malignant pleural effusion appeared which increased in size despite an oral course of 750 mg of the alkylating agent Nitromin. The patient's condition deteriorated and she died three months later.

Patient L.M.U. Short-term Regression of Liver Metastases following Corticosteroid Therapy, after Soft Tissue and Bone Metastases Failed to Regress after Castration and Androgen Therapy

A woman aged forty-four, with a history of hysterectomy two years previously, presented in June 1954 with a carcinoma of the left breast. Primary treatment was by radical mastectomy followed by a prophylactic course of X-ray therapy to the mastectomy scar, axillary, and supraclavicular draining node areas. The tumour was reported to be of an anaplastic grade. Within twenty months of mastectomy, subcutaneous nodular metastases appeared in the scalp, and bone metastases of a mixed lytic-sclerotic type were visible in the radiographs.

Hormonal therapy was initiated with a course of X-ray therapy to the ovaries in order to ablate any residual secretory activity, giving 500 roentgens in a single dose. At the same time, a course of testosterone propionate 100 mg intramuscularly three times a week was instituted for three months. Regression of tumour activity did not result from the combined treatment, and at the end of three months the liver showed irregular enlargement due to metastatic involvement. A course of prednisolone 10 mg tds was prescribed for a period of three months. The liver enlargement decreased as a result, and the associated pain was much improved for two months, although the patient's general condition deteriorated and she died soon after.

Patient J.R.I. Regression of Lung Metastases following a Combination of Prednisolone and Nitromin, after Previous Failure of Response to Castration and Androgen Therapy

A premenopausal woman aged thirty-five, presented in August 1954 with breast carcinoma. Primary treatment was by radical mastectomy followed by a prophylactic course of X-ray therapy to the mastectomy scar, axillary and supraclavicular draining node areas. Within twenty months of the operation, metastatic enlargement of supraclavicular nodes was palpable on both sides. The patient also complained of cough and dyspnoea found to be associated with the presence of multiple nodular opacities of metastasis in the lung fields.

Endocrine therapy was begun by carrying out X-ray castration, delivering a dose of 1,000 roentgens to the region of the ovaries. At the same time, a course of testosterone propionate 100 mg intramuscularly every week was begun and maintained for a period of three months. Regression of soft tissue and lung metastases did not follow the combined treatment. After an interval, a course of prednisolone 10 mg tds was prescribed and with this was associated a cytotoxic agent—a course of Nitromin 750 mg orally. Within a few days of starting treatment there was a dramatic relief of the pulmonary symptoms, and within two weeks, radiographic evidence of marked regression in the lung opacities. Because of this response to therapy, the patient was referred for bilateral adrenalectomy and oophorectomy, but she died postoperatively.

Patient M.V.A. Short-term Regression of Soft Tissue Tumour following a Combination of Prednisolone and Nitromin after Failure of Androgen Therapy

A premenopausal patient aged forty-one, presented in November 1953 with a Stage 2 carcinoma of the left breast. Primary treatment was by radical mastectomy, but within one month of operation, multiple lytic areas of metastasis appeared in bone. Endocrine therapy was initiated by carrying out X-ray castration, delivering a dose of 1,000 roentgens in sixteen days to the region of the ovaries. At the same time, a course of testosterone propionate 100 mg intramuscularly, three times a week was initiated and continued for three months. Relief of the patient's bone pain resulted within a month and persisted for twenty months, but recalcification of bone metastases did not occur.

At the end of twenty months recurrent skin nodules appeared near the mastectomy scar. A further course of testosterone propionate for eight months failed to control further growth of the nodules. After an interval, a course of prednisolone 10 mg tds was prescribed for three months, and with this was associated a cytotoxic agent—a course of Nitromin 750 mg orally. This combined treatment was followed by regression of soft tissue tumour for a period of four months. Because of this response, bilateral adrenalectomy and oophorectomy were advised and carried out. The operation relieved the patient's bone pain for four months, but achieved no objective regression of either the bone or the soft tissue metastases. She died five months after the operation.

Patient D.T.R. Response of Cerebral and Soft Tissue Metastases following a Combination of Prednisolone and Nitromin

A premenopausal woman aged forty-nine, presented in April 1956 with a carcinoma of the left breast which was treated primarily by radical mastectomy. Within sixteen months of the operation a left parasternal tumour appeared, presumably a metastasis arising in the internal mammary nodes. In addition, enlarged metastatic nodes were palpable above the left clavicle.

Endocrine therapy was initiated by carrying out X-ray castration, delivering a dose of 800 roentgens in five days to the region of the ovaries. Within two months of castration, symptoms and signs of cerebral metastasis developed. A course of treatment with prednisolone 10 mg tds was prescribed and with this was associated a cytotoxic agent—a course of Nitromin 750 mg orally. The cerebral symptoms improved remarkably, and the supraclavicular node enlargement regressed. Because of this response to therapy, bilateral adrenalectomy and oophorectomy were carried out but the patient died postoperatively.

Patient E.H.I. Recalcification of Bone Metastases following a Combination of Prednisolone and Nitromin

A woman aged fifty-five and three years postmenopausal, presented in March 1957 with a carcinoma of the right breast. Primary treatment was by radical mastectomy, followed by a prophylactic course of X-ray therapy to the mastectomy scar, axillary and supraclavicular draining node areas. At fifty-seven months after operation she complained of difficulty in swallowing, and Barium examination showed pressure on the oesophagus from grossly enlarged mediastinal nodes. A course of palliative X-ray therapy given to the mediastinum resulted in relief of symptoms. However, within seventeen months she developed bone pains found to be associated with multiple lytic areas of skeletal metastasis.

Hormonal therapy was started with a course of prednisolone 10 mg tds maintained for three months, and with this was associated a cytotoxic agent—a course of Nitromin 750 mg orally. This combination therapy resulted in relief of the patient's bone pain and, later, recalcification of the previously lytic areas in bone. Nevertheless, recurrent skin nodules appeared near the mastectomy scar two months after stopping prednisolone therapy, and the patient died soon afterwards.

Patient B.M.O. Short-term Regression of Soft Tissue and Pleural Metastases following a Combination of Prednisolone and ThioTEPA, after Oestrogen-induced Regression

A woman aged forty-four, with a history of a hysterectomy six years previously, presented in September 1956 with a Stage 2 carcinoma of the right breast, which was treated primarily by radical mastectomy. At seventy-five months after the operation, recurrent skin nodules appeared near the mastectomy scar and examination showed enlarged mestastatic nodes palpable above the clavicle. The soft tissue tumour was treated by a palliative course of X-ray therapy.

Endocrine therapy was initiated by giving a course of X-ray therapy to the ovaries, to a dose of 1,000 roentgens in five days, in order to ablate any residual secretory activity. In spite of this, the nodules spread progessively, and there was no clinical response to a course of dexamethasone therapy 1·6 mg qid which was prescribed for three months. Nor was there response to a course of fluoxymesterone 10 mg tds prescribed subsequently for a period of six months. After an interval, a course of Premarin 5 mg tds was prescribed, and this natural oestrogen preparation resulted in regression of soft tissue tumour. Treatment was, however, stopped after seven months when the patient developed bilateral malignant pleural effusion.

After an interval, a course of prednisolone 10 mg tds was given for three months, and with this was associated a course of the cytotoxic agent thioTEPA intramuscularly to haemopoietic tolerance. This combination controlled both the pleural effusion and the soft tissue tumour for a period of four months. The patient died two months later.

Patient E.N.I. Short-term Regression of Soft Tissue Tumour following a Combination of Prednisolone and Nitromin, after Failure of Androgen Therapy

A woman aged seventy-five presented in January 1955 with a Stage 2 breast carcinoma. Because of her age and poor general condition, it was decided on primary treatment by radon needle implant to the region of the tumour. The implant was followed by regression of the growth that was maintained for eighteen months. At the end of that time, an area of permeation nodules appeared in the skin of the breast.

Hormonal therapy was initiated with a trial of fluoxymesterone 10 mg tds. It was maintained for a period of three months but without evidence of clinical response. After an interval, a course of prednisolone 10 mg tds was prescribed for three months, and with this was associated a cytotoxic agent—a course of Nitromin 750 mg orally. This combination therapy led to regression of the soft tissue tumour for a period of four months. Reactivation then occurred and the patient died three months later.

Patient C.S.M. Short-term Regression of Pleural and Soft Tissue Metastases following a Combination of Prednisolone and Nitromin, and Later following Androgen Therapy

A woman aged sixty-six and eleven years postmenopausal, gave a history of right radical mastectomy ten years previously for breast carcinoma. She presented in March 1956 with a right parasternal tumour presumably a metastasis arising in the internal mammary nodes, and with this was associated a malignant right pleural effusion. A palliative course of X-ray therapy was given to the parasternal tumour, and hormonal therapy was initiated with a course of Sublings testosterone 10 mg qid. In spite of androgen therapy for five months, new recurrent skin nodules appeared near the mastectomy scar.

After an interval, a course of prednisolone 10 mg qid was prescribed for five months, and with this was associated a cytotoxic agent—a course of Nitromin 750 mg orally. Regression resulted for five months in the soft tissue tumour and in the pleural effusion following this combined treatment. When reactivation occurred, a course of fluoxymesterone 10 mg qid was prescribed, and yielded similar regression, but this time only for a period of three months. In spite of the androgen therapy, lytic areas of metastasis then appeared in bone, and the patient died two months later.

Patient M.R.E. Short-term Regression of Liver Metastases following a Combination of Prednisolone and Nitromin, after Androgen-induced Recalcification of bone Metastases

A premenopausal patient aged thirty-four, presented in March 1953 with a Stage 2 carcinoma of the left breast. Primary treatment was by radical mastectomy followed by a prophylactic course of X-ray therapy to the mastectomy scar, axillary and supraclavicular draining node areas. Within eleven months of the operation, a new tumour appeared in the opposite breast, and this too was treated by radical mastectomy. Endocrine therapy was initiated by carrying out X-ray castration, delivering 1,000 roentgens in eleven days to the region of the ovaries.

Within twenty-seven months, the patient complained of bone pains, found to be associated with multiple lytic areas of skeletal metastasis. A course of fluoxymesterone 10 mg tds was prescribed for a period of six months, and resulted in relief of pain and evidence of recalcification in the radiographs. Nevertheless, at the end of six months, the liver showed irregular enlargement due to metastatic involvement. A course of prednisolone 10 mg tds was prescribed for five months, and with this was associated a cytotoxic agent—a course of Nitromin 750 mg orally. The liver enlargement decreased and the associated pain was much improved. Nevertheless, the patient's general condition deteriorated, and she died one month after stopping prednisolone therapy.

Patient E.M.A. Short-term Regression of Soft Tissue and Lung Metastases following Corticosteroid Therapy, but Failure of Subsequent Androgen Therapy

A premenopausal woman aged thirty-nine, presented in February 1957 with a very large carcinoma of the left breast. Primary treatment was by a 'toilet' mastectomy. Within two months of the operation, enlarged metastatic nodes were palpable in the left supraclavicular region and in the right axilla. Endocrine therapy was begun by carrying out X-ray castration, delivering a dose of 1,000 roentgens in twelve days to the region of the ovaries. At the same time a palliative course of X-ray therapy was given to the metastatic nodes.

Within eleven months of the castration recurrent skin nodules had appeared in the vicinity of the mastectomy scar. The patient also complained of a cough and dyspnoea, and the radiographs showed multiple nodular opacities of metastases in the lung fields. A course of prednisolone 10 mg tds was prescribed, and with this was associated a course of Nitromin 750 mg orally. Regression in the size of the skin and lung nodules for a period of six months followed this combined treatment.

When reactivation occurred, a course of fluoxymesterone 10 mg tds was prescribed for four months, but resulted in no obvious clinical benefit. In addition, multiple lytic areas of metastasis in bone appeared while the patient was under androgen therapy, and it was therefore stopped. After an interval, a course of the corticosteroid dexamethasone 1·6 mg qid was prescribed for four months. During that time the cutaneous nodules, but not the metastatic nodes, showed regression in size. Nevertheless, the patient's general condition deteriorated progessively, and she died two months after ceasing cortocosteroid therapy.

Patient L.C.R. Short-term Regression of Pleural Metastases following a Combination of Prednisolone and Nitromin, after Oestrogen-induced Regression of Soft Tissue Tumour

A woman aged seventy-one presented in September 1953 with a Stage 2 carcinoma of the left breast. Primary treatment was by radical mastectomy followed by a prophylactic course of X-ray therapy to the mastectomy scar, axillary and supraclavicular draining node areas. Within seven months of the operation, recurrent skin nodules appeared near the mastectomy scar.

Hormonal therapy was initiated with a course of ethinyl oestradiol 0·5 mg tds for a period of fifteen months. This led to regression in the size of the skin nodules that was maintained for a total of twenty-nine months but at the end of that period, a malignant pleural effusion appeared. A course of prednisolone 10 mg tds was prescribed for three months, and with this was associated a cytotoxic agent—a course of 750 mg of Nitromin orally. The pleural effusion regressed, and remained under control for a period of six months. Control was then lost, and the patient died two months later.

Patient K.M.O. Short-term Regression of Soft Tissue Tumour following a Combination of Prednisolone and Nitromin, but Subsequent Failure of Oestrogen and Androgen Therapy

A woman aged sixty-three and thirteen years postmenopausal, presented in June 1956 with a carcinoma of the right breast which was treated primarily by radical mastectomy. At twenty-eight months after the operation, she developed a malignant right pleural effusion, and, in addition, enlarged metastatic nodes were palpable above the right clavicle. Hormonal therapy was begun with a course of Sublings testosterone 10 mg qid that was prescribed for a period of four months, but tumour regression did not result. At the end of four months, recurrent skin nodules appeared near the mastectomy scar, and the patient complained of bone pains that were found to be associated with multiple lytic areas of metastasis in bone.

A course of prednisolone 10 mg tds was prescribed for three months, and with this was associated a cytotoxic agent—a course of Nitromin 750 mg orally. This combination therapy led to regression in the size of the recurrent skin nodules and the enlarged nodes for a period of four months, but there was no relief of pain or recalcification in the bone metastases. Therefore, after an interval, a course of fluoxymesterone 10 mg tds was prescribed for three months. This failed to control either the pain or the tumour growth. A subsequent trial of stilboestrol 5 mg tds for two months was equally unsuccessful. The patient died of widespread disease nine months later.

9

Major Endocrine Ablation Therapy

WITH THE advent of cortisone replacement therapy, Huggins and Bergenstal (1952) were able to report tumour regression following bilateral adrenalectomy in the treatment of advanced breast cancer, and Perrault *et al.* (1952) reported similar benefit from the practice of hypophysectomy.

The nature of this book precludes a discussion of the technical aspects of adrenalectomy or of the different methods of hypophyseal ablation. For these, the major references quoted can be consulted, or the excellent review by Juret (1966). Nevertheless, the selection of patients for major endocrine ablation, and the selection of the most suitable method of treatment, need to be considered in a review of the hormonal management of advanced breast cancer.

EARLY MAJOR ENDOCRINE ABLATION THERAPY

If hormonal control in breast cancer is based upon oestrogen dependence, the benefit to breast cancer patients from hypophysectomy should summate, in theory, those of all lesser procedures. This has not been demonstrated in practice. The author, like Randall (1960), Hortling *et al.* (1961), Dobson (1962), Juret (1966), Donegan (1967), and many others, believes that planned sequential therapy (*see* p. 118) in hormone-sensitive breast cancer leads to an average total survival longer than that from hypophyseal ablation alone, or from bilateral adrenalectomy alone. This question is more fully discussed in Chapter Thirteen.

Apart from the likelihood of longer survival from sequential therapy, the author believes that operations which 'transform patients into veritable artificial satellites of their endocrinosurgical clinic' (Gennes, 1960) should be postponed as long as is possible. The Joint Committee of the AMA (1961) reported that the results of major endocrine ablation therapy in breast cancer are best if operation is

carried out early in the progress of the disease—especially within six months of recurrence appearing. If early endocrine ablation is advantageous, it is surprising that Patey (1960) in evaluating the benefit of 'prophylactic' bilateral adrenalectomy carried out at the time of mastectomy, was unable to demonstrate any improvement in prognosis from its practice.

SELECTION OF PATIENTS FOR MAJOR ENDOCRINE ABLATION THERAPY

It is now generally agreed that castration should be given a trial in all premenopausal women before considering major endocrine ablation therapy, whether in the form of bilateral adrenalectomy or of hypophyseal ablation (*see* p. 25). Of those patients showing favourable response to oophorectomy, 52 per cent gave a further response to hypophysectomy and 40 per cent to bilateral adrenalectomy, according to MacDonald (1962). Of those not responding to oophorectomy, only 14 per cent and 10 per cent respectively showed a tumour remission from the more major procedures. A more marked difference was noted by Pearson and Ray (1960) in their hypophysectomy series. Whereas 100 per cent of patients showing a tumour remission from castration, showed a subsequent favourable response to hypophysectomy, only 25 per cent of castration non-responders did so.

It seems that the more stringent the criteria of regression fulfilled by the response to castration, the greater is the likelihood of subsequent favourable response to major endocrine ablation. Thus, an extreme experience is that of Escher (1958) who states that castration non-responders never respond favourably to subsequent bilateral adrenalectomy, and can thus be spared needless major surgery.

In addition to castration, the response to other forms of hormone therapy may possibly aid in the selection of patients for major endocrine ablation. According to Jessiman et al. (1959), Pearson and Ray (1960), and Kennedy and French (1965), there is a positive correlation between favourable response to oestrogen or androgen therapy and subsequent favourable response to hypophysectomy, but this is not confirmed by Atkins et al. (1966). Again, Douglas (1957) and Hellstrom and Franksson (1958) suggest positive correlation between favourable response to oestrogen or androgen therapy and subsequent favourable response to bilateral adrenalectomy, but this is not confirmed by Byron et al. (1962) and Dao and Nemoto (1965). Edelstyn et al. (1968) suggest, on the other hand, that failure to respond to oestrogen therapy predicts a favourable response to hypophysectomy.

With regard to radiation ablation of pituitary function, Ahlquist et al. (1968) found no correlation between response to X-ray castration or hormone therapy, on the one hand, and subsequent response to radioactive Yttrium implantation of the hypophysis, on the other. Therefore, even in the absence of a favourable response to castration in the younger patient or to sex steroid therapy in a postmenopausal woman, a favourable response to hypophyseal ablation is still a possibility. Because of the low likelihood of success, transphenoidal surgery or radioactive Yttrium implant will probably be preferred to the more extensive transfrontal operation in patients who have failed to respond to castration or sex steroids.

Apart from the effect of previous hormonal manipulation, the length of the free interval between mastectomy and recurrence, is also of value in selecting patients for major endocrine ablation therapy. Hellstrom and Franksson (1958) and Cade (1966) have noted that the longer the free interval, the more likely a remission following bilateral adrenalectomy. In the case of hypophysectomy, a similar correlation has been noted by Luft et al. (1958), Pearson and Ray (1960), and Boesen et al. (1961). The remission rate from hypophysectomy is 33 per cent for patients with a free interval of less than one year, but is 66 per cent if the free interval since mastectomy is over four years (Pearson and Ray, 1960).

The effect of the patient's age group, and the site and size of metastasis on the likelihood of favourable response to bilateral adrenalectomy or hypophyseal ablation is discussed later under the heading of each technique. The suggested use of pre-operative oestrogen excretion levels or of the 'discriminant function' or of other biochemical criteria, for selecting breast cancer patients more likely to respond favourably to major endocrine ablation therapy is discussed in Chapter Ten.

SELECTION OF METHOD FOR MAJOR ABLATION THERAPY

The percentage of patients showing tumour regression in breast cancer, as measured by objective criteria, is listed for the larger adrenalectomy series in Table 9.1. The remission rate varies from 28 to 51

TABLE 9.1

Major Reports of Favourable Clinical Response to Bilateral Adrenalectomy in Patients with Breast Cancer

Author	Cases with regressing tumour	Percentage with regressing tumour
Dao and Huggins, 1955	95	41%
Cade, 1958	137	39%
Hellstrom and Franksson, 1958	150	51%
Fracchia et al., 1959	155	35%
Daicoff et al., 1962	455	28%
Byron et al., 1962	248	38%

TABLE 9.2

Major Reports of Favourable Clinical Response to Hypophyseal Ablation in Patients with Breast Cancer

Author	Cases with regressing tumour	Percentage with regressing tumour	Method of ablation
Luft et al., 1958	59	46%	Surgery
Pearson and Ray, 1960	333	42%	Surgery
Boesen et al., 1961	111	42%	Surgery
Greening et al., 1960	100	12%	[198]Au
Juret et al., 1964	150	37%	[90]Y
Forrest et al., 1965	138	28%	[90]Y

per cent of operated cases. Objective tumour remission rates for hypophysectomy and for pituitary ablation by radioactive isotopes are listed similarly on Table 9.2. The remission rate varies from 12 to 46 per cent of operated cases. Figures of up to 60 per cent of remissions have been claimed in smaller series, but these high rates are either in selected series of patients previously responding to castration, or tend to include non-progressing disease among their criteria of benefit.

The Joint Committee of the AMA (1961) pooled the results of bilateral adrenalectomy or hypophysectomy in the treatment of the patients from twelve North American clinics, and showed virtually no difference between the results of the two procedures (Table 9.3). Their overall tumour remission rate of 31–32 per cent is more realistic than some quoted above. The postoperative mortality rates for the two procedures are also similar to each other—13–15 per cent. The average survival of patients responding favourably following the operations is between twenty-one and twenty-two months as compared to only seven to eight months for non-responders (Table 9.3).

The difficulty of completely ablating the pituitary

Some results of the radioactive Yttrium method are given in Table 9.2. Recently the use of ultrasonic waves to ablate hypophyseal function in breast cancer has been reported by Arslan (1966), with a total absence of postoperative complications. The use of cryogenic therapy for the same purpose has been reported by Bleasel and Lazarus (1965) and Wilson et al. (1966). The results of these newer techniques have not, so far, been sufficiently evaluated.

In our present state of knowledge, therefore, radioactive Yttrium implantation of the pituitary is recommended in the very ill patient where the more drastic ablative procedures are contraindicated. The proportion of patients palliated justifies this rela-

TABLE 9.3

Reports of Tumour Remission from Bilateral Adrenalectomy Compared to that from Hypophysectomy in Advanced Breast Cancer. (MCV = Mean Clinical Value)

Author		Bilateral adrenalectomy	Hypophysectomy
Joint Committee, 1961	Total cases	404	467
	% tumour remissions	31·7%	31·3%
	Mean survival	22 months	20·6 months
Atkins *et al.*, 1960	Total cases	79	70
	MCV improvement	5·48	6·57
	Mean survival	14·2 months	20·3 months

tissue has caused various modifications in technique to be proposed. The comparative results of different methods of hypophyseal ablation depend, in the main, on the experience and skill of the operators. The transfrontal approach, with curettage of the fossa, is the method which has been used in the majority of reported series. Postoperative cauterisation of the fossa with Zenker's solution, or the sealing of the cavity to prevent revascularisation of any residual pituitary tissue, have been suggested.

The transethmoidal, trans-sphenoidal approach does not permit as good access, although reported results of palliation in breast cancer appear to be encouraging in some series. Section of the pituitary stalk and interposition of an inert disc between the two cut ends causes necrosis of the pituitary gland, and has also yielded remission of tumour growth in the treatment of breast cancer. The results of this technique have not yet been sufficiently evaluated.

Interstitial irradiation of the pituitary by radioactive sources—radon, radioactive gold, or radioactive Yttrium—has also been used with success. The two former methods have been largely abandoned due to the high incidence of damage to the optic tracts and to the motor cranial nerves of the eyes.

tively minor procedure even in patients with a poor prognosis.

The difference in results to be expected between bilateral adrenalectomy and hypophyseal ablation in one of its forms depends, in the main, on the experience of available specialists. One practical advantage of hypophyseal ablation over adrenalectomy, according to Juret (1966), is that postoperative electrolyte management problems are less common in the former group. This is probably due to the fact that aldosterone secretion is relatively unaffected after hypophyseal ablation.

Although the Joint Committee of the AMA (1961) showed no significant difference between the overall results of the two operations, Atkins *et al.* (1960) conclude that hypophysectomy is marginally the better operation *in their institution*, in the quality of the remission (Table 9.3).

SELECTION OF METHOD FOR THE INDIVIDUAL

As mentioned in the discussion on androgen therapy (*see* p. 39), similarity in *overall* results by two methods does not necessarily imply that the methods are equally applicable to individual patients. The selection of a method of major endocrine ablation may depend on individual factors such as general condition, age, site of metastasis, size of metastasis, or other criteria as yet undertermined.

A recent symposium opened by Greenberg (1962) illustrates one aspect of this problem in the selection of major endocrine ablation therapy. The overall opinion of the participants (although some disagreed) was that, whereas hypophysectomy yields objective evidence of tumour regression in about 30 per cent of patients with liver metastases, the results of adrenalectomy are considerably inferior in such cases. It is possible that such differences in experience may reflect, apart from differences in criteria of response, a different selection of clinical material. Cade (1966) has pointed out that, whereas small metastatic nodules in the liver may regress completely after bilateral adrenalectomy, large metastases are not usually affected. He suggests that a similar differential sensitivity of smaller nodules applies also to cerebral metastases from breast cancer. It is now generally agreed that adrenalectomy should be advised only if metastases are small, in the case of involvement of the brain or the liver.

In a similar way the circumstances of age, general health, site of metastases, and biochemical criteria in each individual patient may determine the advisability and selection of a method of major endocrine ablation. The influence of such factors is discussed in the following paragraphs, keeping in mind that the results of a technique in a large series represents merely an average of all responses, and the selection of the suitable patient is more important than the selection of a technique.

PALLIATION FROM BILATERAL ADRENALECTOMY

The relief of pain from bone metastases which occurs within two to three days of adrenalectomy is often dramatic, but also often very transient in nature. Although pain relief occurs in the majority of such patients after bilateral adrenalectomy, in the individual patient it bears no relationship to the likelihood of objective evidence of tumour regression.

The likelihood of objective remission from adrenalectomy in breast cancer varies according to the site of metastasis. According to Hellstrom and Franksson (1958) and to Fracchia et al. (1959), it is highest in the case of local soft tissue and bone metastases, occurring in 40–50 per cent of such cases. It is slightly less in the case of lung and pleural metastasis—30–40 per cent of cases, and it is lowest in the case of brain, liver, and peritoneal metastases —10–20 per cent of cases.

As mentioned previously, it is now generally agreed that in the presence of large brain, liver, or peritoneal metastases, adrenalectomy is contra-indicated. Whereas Cade (1958) noted that all sites of metastasis respond or fail to respond equally to adrenalectomy, Jessiman (1958) has noted healing of bone lesions associated with progression of soft tissue metastases, as is commonly seen with oestrogen therapy (see p. 55).

The average duration of objective tumour remission from bilateral adrenalectomy is between twelve and eighteen months, although occasional examples of survival over five years are recorded. Prolongation of survival in operated over non-operated patients was shown by Daicoff et al. (1962) in 455 adrenalectomised patients. The five-year survival of the former group was 12·5 per cent compared to 3·7 per cent for the latter group.

The correlation between response to adrenalectomy and other factors such as previous response to castration or hormonal therapy, or the length of the 'free interval', has been discussed earlier in the chapter. The correlation between response to adrenalectomy and biochemical criteria such as preoperative oestrogen excretion levels or the 'discriminant ratio', is discussed in Chapter Ten. Although Dao and Huggins (1955) suggested that well differentiated breast carcinoma is more likely to respond favourably to adrenalectomy than is an anaplastic tumour, most reports fail to confirm this correlation.

The age of the patient has been suggested as an indicator of the likelihood of response to adrenalectomy, in that older patients are said to be more likely to respond favourably than younger patients. Hellstrom and Franksson (1958) noted a favourable response in 52 per cent of patients over fifty, but in 48 per cent under forty-nine years of age, and the corresponding figures noted by Fracchia et al. (1959) are 39 per cent and 29 per cent respectively. However, Dao and Huggins (1955) and Galante et al. (1957) showed no difference in tumour remission rates between these age groups. If the older patient is more likely to respond favourably to bilateral adrenalectomy and oophorectomy, this is difficult to explain on the oestrogen-dependence hypothesis of breast cancer control (see p. 13).

ADRENALECTOMY AND CORTISTEROID THERAPY

A comparison of bilateral adrenalectomy with cortisone therapy in the palliation of breast cancer has been reported by Dao et al. (1961) and is discussed on p. 78. It may be noted here that cortisone maintenance therapy after major endocrine ablation usually involves dosage of 12·5 mg two or three times a day. When dosage of cortisone replacement is as high as 75 mg a day, or of prednisolone 15 mg a day, there is a possibility that any tumour regression observed, or relief of pain experienced, may be due, at least in part, to corticosteroid effects upon the tumour (*see* p. 77).

In this connection too, it may be mentioned that Lipsett *et al.* (1957) have reported survival of two adrenalectomised cases without cortisone maintenance therapy, and such survival has been ascribed to cortisone secretion by accessory adrenal tissue.

ADRENALECTOMY AND CASTRATION

The relative places of castration and of bilateral adrenalectomy in the treatment of advanced breast cancer are discussed later (*see* p. 108).

In the premenopausal patient, bilateral adrenalectomy is never carried out as the sole ablative procedure—ovariectomy is carried out at the same time if it has not been done previously. This is now generally extended to patients of all age groups, as it is believed (*see* p. 8) that postmenopausal secretion of oestrogens by the ovary may continue for many years. Several authors have compared the tumour remission rate from bilateral adrenalectomy alone with that from ovario-adrenalectomy. Comparative figures are 40 per cent and 52 per cent respectively, by Hellstrom and Franksson (1958) and 27·4 per cent and 41·5 per cent by Fracchia *et al.* (1959). Added castration thus increases the proportion responding, and also the duration of tumour growth remission.

PALLIATION FROM HYPOPHYSECTOMY

The likelihood of objective evidence of tumour regression from hypophysectomy in breast cancer varies according to the site of metastasis. According to Pearson and Ray (1960) it is greatest for bone metastases—46–55 per cent of cases. It is somewhat less for lung and pleural metastases—42–55 per cent of cases—and local soft tissue metastases—38–48 per cent of cases. It is least for liver metastases—35 per cent of cases. The range of site sensitivity does not appear to be as wide as that for adrenalectomy (*see* p. 91). With regard to size of metastasis, some authorities suggest that hypophysectomy be advised only if liver or brain metastases are small in size.

The age of the patient also appears to influence the likelihood of tumour growth remission from hypophysectomy, but in a direction different to that suggested by Hellstrom and Franksson (1958) and by Fracchia *et al.* (1959) for adrenalectomy. Older postmenopausal patients are more likely to benefit from hypophysectomy than are recently postmenopausal patients, according to Pearson and Ray (1960). They noted a favourable tumour response in 40 per cent of patients under fifty-four, but in 56 per cent of patients over sixty years of age. Nevertheless, premenopausal patients show favourable tumour response in 60 per cent of cases, compared to a 46 per cent response overall for postmenopausal patients. The two age peaks for favourable response are, therefore, in the premenopausal age group and in patients aged over sixty.

Prolongation of survival following hypophysectomy has also been shown. The average survival of hypophysectomised cases was twelve months longer than that of non-hypophysectomised cases in a series of patients with a free interval of more than two years studied by Taylor and Perlia (1960). The correlation between response to hypophysectomy and other factors such as the nature of the previous response to castration or to hormone therapy, and the length of the free interval has been discussed earlier in the chapter. The correlation between response to hypophysectomy and biochemical criteria, such as hormonal excretion, is discussed in Chapter Ten.

It is important to note that a favourable response to hypophysectomy is achieved in 20 per cent of patients who have not responded to bilateral adrenalectomy, according to Pearson and Ray (1960). The mean duration of such response is twelve to eighteen months. Benefit from hypophysectomy in such cases is not necessarily associated with a further reduction in the oestrogen excretion levels. Hypophyseal ablation, possibly by trans-sphenoidal surgery or radioactive Yttrium implant, is therefore worth a trial in some cases after unsuccessful adrenalectomy.

COMPLETENESS OF HYPOPHYSEAL ABLATION

The likelihood of tumour growth remission following hypophyseal ablation in breast cancer does not appear to be related to the completeness of ablation, as measured by presently accepted criteria of pituitary function. The development of hypopituitarism after ablation therapy is usually assessed by measuring the radioactive iodine uptake, the protein bound Iodine and urinary 17 ketosteroid excretion levels before and after the operation. The failure of metyrapone to elevate the 17 oxogenic steroid levels is a reliable sign of ACTH disappearance after ablation, but the disappearance of urinary gonadotropin excretion is said to be the most sensitive indicator of all according to McCullagh *et al.* (1965). Biochemical evidence suggesting incomplete ablation of pituitary function may be due in some cases to subtotal removal of the hypophysis or to compensatory hyperplasia of pituitary tissue cells in the wall of the pharynx (Muller, 1958). According to Greenwood and Bulbrook (1957) the majority of patients continue to excrete oestrogens after hypophysectomy, but their source is uncertain (*see* p. 8).

It has been suggested from the experience of Bateman (1962) that the development of diabetes insipidus after hypophysectomy (presumably associated with damage to the pituitary stalk) is more likely to be associated with a favourable therapeutic response. Other authors do not agree. An early report by Boyland *et al.* (1958) suggested that patients with tumour regression after hypophyseal irradiation included a higher proportion with a marked fall in gonadotropin excretion than did the non-responding patients. Overall, according to Beck *et al.* (1966) there is no correlation between the likelihood of tumour growth remission and the completeness of ablation as judged by either pituitary-adrenal-thyroid function tests or by autopsy examination.

PAIN RELIEF FOLLOWING HYPOPHYSEAL ABLATION

It is commonly observed that relief of pain from bone metastases occurs within two or three days of hypophyseal ablation in the majority of cases treated. Such relief usually lasts from three to twenty-four months. Relief of bone pain is not related to the likelihood of objective evidence of tumour regression or the healing of bone metastases in such cases. Juret *et al.* (1962) has suggested that the analgesic effect obtained from hypophyseal implantation of radioactive gold or Yttrium sources cannot always be ascribed to the endocrine effect of the procedure. Although relief of pain was obtained in the majority of patients with bone metastases from breast cancer treated by these methods, only a small proportion showed endocrinological evidence of complete hypophyseal destruction.

It is reported, too, that hypophyseal implantation of radioactive Yttrium is able to relieve the pain of bone metastases secondary to cancers of the rectum or cervix, which are at present not regarded as hormone dependent tumours. It is therefore suggested by Juret (1966) that the analgesic effect of radioactive implants into the pituitary may be due to trauma to the diencephalon (*see* p. 9) or to the adjacent sympathetic plexus. A similar mechanism may explain the relief of pain, although of shorter duration, which follows pituitary stalk section.

TO SUMMARISE

Both bilateral adrenalectomy and hypophyseal ablation yield objective evidence of tumour regression in over 30 per cent of patients with advanced breast cancer for an average duration of just less than two years. Such procedures should be preceded by less drastic attempts at endocrine therapy such as castration or sex hormone therapy. The difference in results to be expected from different methods of major endocrine ablative surgery depends in the main, on the experience of the available specialists. Nevertheless, trans-sphenoidal hypophysectomy or radioactive implantation of the hypophysis are preferred in very ill patients.

Patient factors such as age, general condition, site and size of metastasis, length of 'free interval', response to previous hormonal manipulation, and biochemical criteria of hormone excretion, will determine the advisability, and selection of a method of ablation therapy.

Major Endocrine Ablation

ILLUSTRATIVE CASE SUMMARIES
Patient T.N.O. Hypophysectomy-induced Regression of Bone and Soft Tissue Metastases for Twenty-four Months. Previous Adrenalectomy and Androgen Therapy Resulted only in Subjective Benefit
A premenopausal woman aged forty presented in March 1953 with a carcinoma of the left breast. Primary treatment was by radical mastectomy. At twenty-four months after the operation she developed recurrent skin nodules in the region of the mastectomy scar, and these were treated by a palliative course of X-ray therapy. Within eighteen months, she developed bone pains, found to be associated with multiple lytic areas of skeletal metastases.

The patient was not castrated, but instead, a course of Primoteston depot 250 mg a week was administered intramuscularly for ten months. Although pain was relieved, there was no objective evidence of response in the bone metastasis. When, eight months later, enlarged metastatic nodes appeared in the left supraclavicular and right axillary regions, the patient was referred for bilateral adrenalectomy and oophorectomy. The operation resulted in relief of pain for only two months, but no regression of soft tissue tumour, and again there was no evidence of recalcification in the bone metastases.

At eight months after adrenalectomy, it was decided to proceed to transfrontal hypophysectomy. As a result of the operation, bone pain was relieved for twenty-four months, the soft tissue tumours regressed in size, and the previously lytic bone lesions showed recalcification in the radiographs. The patient died twenty-seven months after hypophysectomy.

Patient M.S.H. Adrenalectomy-induced Recalcification of Bone Metastases for Three Years
A woman aged fifty presented in December 1953 with bone pains which were found to be associated with widespread lytic areas of skeletal metastasis. About ten years previously, a Stage 1 carcinoma of the left breast had been treated by radical mastectomy, and seven years previously, hysterectomy had been performed for non-malignant uterine disease.

Bilateral adrenalectomy and oophorectomy were advised as the initial method of hormonal therapy. Within a few days of the operation, the patient was almost completely relieved of her pain, and she later regained near-normal activity. After approximately three months, the radiographs showed the first evidence of recalcification in previously lytic areas. She remained fairly free of pain for a total period of three years, after which new bone metastases appeared, and the patient eventually died as a result of bone marrow replacement.

Patient M.H.O. Hypophysectomy-induced Regression of Soft Tissue Tumour but Malignant Serous Effusions Developed within Twelve Months of Treatment
A premenopausal woman aged forty-two, presented in September 1956 with a Stage 2 carcinoma of the breast. Primary treatment was by radical mastectomy, followed by a prophylactic course of X-ray therapy to the axillary, supraclavicular, and internal mammary draining node areas. At the same time, prophylactic X-ray castration was carried, delivering a dose of 800 roentgens in four days to the region of the ovaries.

At twenty months after the operation, recurrent skin nodules appeared in the region of the mastectomy scar, and soon afterwards, new tumour appeared in the opposite breast and axillary nodes. Transfrontal hypophysectomy was advised as the initial method of hormonal therapy. Following the operation, the soft tissue tumour regressed, but after a period of twelve months the patient manifested a malignant pleural effusion and malignant ascites.

Her condition gradually deteriorated and she died four months later.

Patient U.T.Y. Adrenalectomy-induced Control of Bone and Lung Metastases for Three and a Half Years. Previous Recalcification of Bone Metastases from Castration and Androgen Therapy
A premenopausal woman aged forty-six, presented in January 1953 with an advanced cancer involving all four quadrants of the breast, and with overlying permeation nodules in the skin. She complained of bone pains, and radiographs showed multiple lytic areas of skeletal metastasis. Treatment was begun with a palliative course of X-ray therapy to the breast, axillary, and supraclavicular node areas to a minimum tumour dose of 4,300 roentgens in twenty-nine days. Regression of the breast tumour followed X-ray therapy and was maintained for five years.

Endocrine therapy was initiated by carrying out X-ray castration, delivering a dose of 2,000 roentgens in twenty-two days to the region of the ovaries. At the same time a course of testosterone propionate 100 mg intramuscularly three times a week was begun, and maintained for fifteen months. Following this combined treatment, the patient's bone pains were partly relieved, and evidence of recalcification was seen in previously lytic areas in bone. However, at the end of fifteen months, multiple nodular opacities of metastasis were visible in radiographs of the lung fields.

Bilateral adrenalectomy and oophorectomy were now carried out. As a result, the bone metastases remained under control for a period of three and a half years following the operation, and during that time there was no visible change in the lung opacities. At the end of three and a half years, renewed activity occurred in the bone metastases, and the patient died five and a half years after first coming under treatment.

Patient M.G.O. Hypophysectomy-induced Recalcification in Bone Metastases for Thirteen Months. Further Remission from Subsequent Castration and Androgen Therapy
A premenopausal woman aged fifty, presented in January 1958 with a Stage 1 carcinoma of the right breast which was treated primarily by radical mastectomy. At eleven months after operation, the patient complained of back pain and multiple lytic areas of bone metastasis were noted in the radiographs. Soon after, the patient's menses ceased spontaneously.

Transfrontal hypophysectomy was advised as the initial method of hormonal therapy. Relief of pain rapidly resulted after the operation, and was maintained for thirteen months. The radiographs showed recalcification in previously lytic areas of bone metastasis. When pain recurred, surgical castration was carried out and, at the same time, a course of fluoxymesterone 10 mg tds was prescribed for a period of four months. As a result of this combined treatment, pain was controlled and the sclerotic appearance in the radiographs was maintained, until the patient's death ten months later as a result of bone marrow replacement.

Patient J.M.C. Adrenalectomy-induced Regression of Soft Tissue Metastases, after Previous Failure of Androgen Therapy

A premenopausal woman aged thirty-one, presented in May 1956 with a Stage 2 carcinoma of the right breast. Primary treatment was by radical mastectomy, followed by a prophylactic course of X-ray therapy to the mastectomy scar, axillary and supraclavicular draining node areas. At eighteen months after the operation, widespread tumour recurrence appeared in the soft tissues, including recurrent skin nodules in the scar, metastatic enlargement of the axillary and supraclavicular nodes, and also tumour in the opposite breast and axillary nodes.

The patient was not castrated, but instead, hormonal therapy was initiated with a course of testosterone propionate 100 mg intramuscularly three times a week, and continued for six months. Regression of soft tissue tumour did not result, and at the end of six months, the patient complained of bone pains found to be associated with multiple skeletal metastases of a mixed lytic-sclerotic appearance. Bilateral adrenalectomy and oophorectomy were carried out, and led to relief of pain, and regression in the soft tissue tumour manifestations. Control lasted for a period of twelve months, after which new bone metastases appeared. The patient died two months later.

Patient J.F.A. Regression of Bone and Soft Tissue Metastases following Adrenalectomy Associated with Androgen and ThioTEPA Therapy

A premenopausal woman aged thirty-four, presented in July 1959 with an advanced cancer of the breast, associated with nodular skin infiltrational lytic bone metastases, pleural effusion, and malignant ascites. Bilateral adrenalectomy and oophorectomy were advised as the initial method of hormonal therapy. This was immediately followed by a course of Primoteston depot 250 mg intramuscularly weekly, and a course of thioTEPA to haemopoietic tolerance levels. As a result, the pleural effusion and ascites regressed in size, and did not require further paracentesis, and the previously lytic bone metastases showed recalcification, with relief of pain.

At twelve months after the operation, recurrence of bone pain appeared. Because of the success of the

previous hormonal manipulation, the patient was referred for transfrontal hypophysectomy. Unfortunately, she died postoperatively, without relief of pain. The excised pituitary gland was found to be extensively replaced by metastasis.

Patient R.H.A. Regression of Bone and Soft Tissue Metastases following Hypophysectomy after Previous Failure of Androgen Therapy

A woman aged forty-six and one year postmenopausal, presented in October 1955 with a Stage 1 carcinoma of the right breast which was treated primarily by radical mastectomy. At sixty-nine months after the operation, recurrent skin nodules appeared in the region of the mastectomy scar. The patient also complained of bone pains and radiographs showed multiple lytic areas of skeletal metastasis.

Hormonal therapy was initiated with a course of testosterone propionate 100 mg intramuscularly three times a week and continued for five months. This did not result in relief of the patient's pain or healing in the bone metastases. The patient was therefore referred for transfrontal hypophysectomy. The operation was followed by regression of skin nodules, relief of pain, and recalcification in previously lytic areas of bone metastases. Control lasted for seven months, at which juncture the patient died suddenly.

Patient L.S.I. Short-term Regression of Bone Metastases follows Adrenalectomy, after Previous Failure of Combined Castration and Androgen Therapy

A premenopausal woman aged forty-nine, presented in October 1954 with a Stage 1 carcinoma of the left breast. Primary treatment was by radical mastectomy, followed by a prophylactic course of X-ray therapy to the mastectomy scar, axillary and supraclavicular draining node areas. At twenty-six months after operation, she developed bone pains, found to be associated with multiple lytic areas of skeletal metastases.

Endocrine therapy was initiated by carrying out X-ray castration, delivering a dose of 1,500 roentgens in eighteen days to the region of the ovaries. At the same time, a course of testosterone propionate 100 mg intramuscularly three times a week was prescribed. In spite of treatment, the patient's pain continued with no evidence of healing in bone metastases, except those treated by X-ray therapy. After eleven months of androgen therapy, the patient was referred for bilateral adrenalectomy and oophorectomy. The operation was followed by dramatic relief in the pain which persisted for seven months. Partial recalcification of previously lytic bone deposits was observed in the radiographs, but the patient's condition gradually deteriorated, and she died ten months after the operation.

Patient M.A.L. Subjective Benefit from Hypophysectomy in the Presence of Bone Metastases. Subsequent Androgen and Cyclophosphamide Therapy Ineffective

A woman aged forty-two with a history of a hysterectomy five years previously, presented in October 1959 with a carcinoma of the left breast which was treated primarily by radical mastectomy. At eleven months following operation, the patient complained of bone pains and these were associated with multiple lytic areas of skeletal metastasis. Transfrontal hypophysectomy was advised as the initial method of hormonal therapy. This resulted in relief of bone pain for four months, but no evidence of sclerosis in the bone metastases.

At seven months after the operation, recurrent skin nodules appeared near the mastectomy scar. A trial of testosterone propionate 100 mg intramuscularly three times a week was instituted, followed by a single intravenous dose of the cytotoxic agent cyclophosphamide 50 mg/kilo body weight. Neither method of treatment was followed by clinical evidence of response. The patient died eleven months after hypophysectomy.

Patient J.A.N. Subjective Benefit from Adrenalectomy in the Presence of Bone Metastases, after Previous Similar Result from Combined Castration and Androgen Therapy

A premenopausal woman aged thirty-two, presented in July 1955 with an advanced breast cancer, associated with the presence of bone pain and multiple areas of lytic bone metastases. Endocrine therapy was initiated by carrying out X-ray castration delivering a dose of 1,200 roentgens in ten days to the region of the ovaries. At the same time, a course of testosterone propionate 100 mg intramuscularly three times a week was prescribed and continued for twelve months.

As a result of the combined treatment, there was relief of pain for a period of six months. Nevertheless, the breast tumour showed no evidence of regression, nor did the lytic bone metastases show evidence of sclerosis in the radiographs. At the end of twelve months, therefore, the patient was referred for bilateral adrenalectomy and oophorectomy. This resulted in dramatic relief of pain shortly after the operation, but it persisted only for about four weeks. The patient died two months later of increasing bone marrow replacement.

Patient M.A.D. Absence of Response to Hypophysectomy after Oestrogen-induced Regression of Soft Tissue Tumour

A woman aged fifty-five and three years postmenopausal, presented in December 1955 with a Stage 2 carcinoma of the left breast. Primary treatment was by radical mastectomy, followed by a prophylactic course of X-ray therapy to the mastectomy scar, axillary and supraclavicular draining node areas. Within ten months of the operation recurrent skin nodules appeared in the region of the mastectomy scar.

Hormonal therapy was initiated with a course of stilboestrol 5 mg tds and maintained for eleven months. As a result, almost complete regression of the skin nodules occurred. When reactivation occurred, the patient was referred for transfrontal hypophysectomy. The operation achieved no control of the tissue tumour activity, and the patient died sixteen months later, after further attempts at local therapy.

Patient E.E.D. Adrenalectomy Ineffective for Intrathoracic Metastases, after Androgen-induced Recalcification of Bone Metastases

A woman aged fifty-six and eight years postmenopausal, presented in May 1957 with cancer of the breast. She complained of bone pains found to be associated with multiple lytic areas of skeletal metastasis. The urinary calcium excretion was estimated before and during androgen therapy. As a fall in level resulted from androgen administration, a course of fluoxymesterone therapy 10 mg tds was prescribed for three months. This led to relief of pain and partial recalcification of the bone metastases.

At the end of three months, the patient complained of increasing cough and dyspnoea, and demonstrated multiple nodular opacities of metastasis in both lung fields, and also a malignant pleural effusion. She was referred for bilateral adrenalectomy and oophorectomy. Following the operation, there was no subjective benefit or change in the appearance of the intrathoracic metastases, and the patient died four months later.

Patient M.S.T. Adrenalectomy Death, after Androgen and Oestrogen-induced Regression of Soft Tissue Tumour

A woman aged forty-nine and six years postmenopausal, presented in February 1957 with a history of carcinoma of the left breast nine years previously. It had been treated by radical mastectomy, followed by a prophylactic course of X-ray therapy to the chest wall and draining node areas. She now presented with a left parasternal tumour presumed to be a metastasis arising in the internal mammary nodes. Shortly afterwards, metastatic nodes were palpable in the supraclavicular area.

Hormonal therapy was initiated with a trial of prednisolone 10 mg tds for three months, and with this was associated an oral course of 750 mg of the cytotoxic agent Nitromin. Regression of the tumours did not result. After an interval, a course of fluoxymesterone 10 mg tds was instituted for four months and led to partial regression of the soft tissue tumour. After a further interval, a course of stil-boestrol 5 mg tds was prescribed for three months and this led to a similar short-term regression of tumour. Hormonal sensitivity of the tumour was therefore assumed, and the patient referred for bilateral adrenalectomy and oophorectomy. Unfortunately she died postoperatively.

Patient R.W.E. Hypophysectomy Death, after Control of Bone Metastases by Castration and Androgen Therapy for Two Years
A premenopausal woman aged forty-eight, presented in November 1956 with a carcinoma of the left breast, which was treated primarily by radical mastectomy. At nineteen months after the operation, she complained of bone pains which were found to be associated with multiple lytic areas of skeletal metastasis. Endocrine therapy was initiated by carrying out X-ray castration, delivering a dose of 1,000 roentgens in twelve days to the region of the ovaries. Recalcification in the bone metastases resulted and persisted for fifteen months. Together with a subsequent course of fluoxymesterone 10 mg tds, pain was kept under control for a total period of two years.

The patient at this juncture developed hypercalcaemia, which failed to respond to massive doses of hydrocortisone and prednisolone. She was referred for transfrontal hypophysectomy, and, although there was an immediate fall in the serum calcium level after the operation, the patient died in the immediate postoperative period.

Part Three

INDIVIDUALISED HORMONAL MANAGEMENT IN BREAST CANCER

10

Laboratory Criteria of Hormonal Responsiveness

As STATED in Chapter One (*see* p. 4) an essential prerequisite for the practice of individualised hormonal therapy in breast cancer, is to be able to determine in a scientific manner, the 'hormonal responsiveness' of the individual's tumour. This term is used to designate the activity of a breast cancer in relation to its hormonal environment in a particular individual.

Our knowledge is still undeveloped, but the laboratory criteria that have been suggested to determine hormonal responsiveness, include the following groups of indices:

Group (*a*)—indices reflecting the tumour's activity.
Group (*b*)—indices reflecting the tumour's sensitivity to hormones.
Group (*c*)—indices reflecting the hormonal environment of the tumour.

It is difficult to draw a sharp dividing line between indices of tumour activity and those of tumour sensitivity to hormones. Members of the former group can be included in a test system and used to assess the response to hormonal therapy. Nevertheless, for convenience, such a division is made, and the indices considered in this chapter are the following:

Group (a)
Urinary calcium excretion.
Serum calcium level.
Serum alkaline phosphatase.
Serum phosphohexose isomerase.
Serum lactic dehydrogenase.
Serum glycoproteins.

Group (b)
Serial tumour biopsies.
Radioactive phosphorus uptake of the tumour.
Radioactively labelled oestrogen uptake by the tumour.
Effect of steroids on the tumour *in vitro*.

Group (c)
Urinary oestrogen excretion.
Cytohormonal assay of the vaginal or urethral smear.
Urinary gonadotropin excretion.
Urinary prolactin excretion.
Urinary 'discriminant function'.
Tumour sex chromatin determination.

URINARY CALCIUM EXCRETION

It was suggested by Pearson *et al.* (1952) and by Emerson and Jessiman (1956), that in the presence of osteolytic bone metastases, serial assays of the urinary calcium excretion could be used to predict sensitivity to castration in breast cancer. A 'baseline' urinary calcium excretion is measured daily for a period of five to seven days, the patient being on a 200 mg calcium diet intake. A provocative course of diethyl stilboestrol, 5–10 mg daily, is then given for three days, and a rise in the urinary calcium excretion is watched for within the next few days.

Correlation is said to exist, between the rapidity of onset, extent, and duration of the *rise* in the calcium excretion which may ensue, and the hormone dependency of the breast cancer. The test is limited in its application, because of the danger that tumour provocation may cause dangerous symptoms to arise, and as a result, an emergency castration or adrenalectomy may be called for. For this reason, Emerson and Jessiman (1956) suggested a suppression test by cortisone (no dose being specified) instead of provocation by diethyl stilboestrol, in the presence of tumour symptoms which might be aggravated.

It should be noted that the provocation test is of little value when bone metastases are few, as provocation of the limited bone destruction would have little effect upon the urinary calcium levels. Furthermore, change in calcium excretion bears no relation to the clinical benefit from bilateral adrenalectomy

(Dao and Huggins, 1955). With regard to the significance of the cortisone suppression test in breast cancer, control of hypercalciuria by corticosteroid therapy has been noted by Plimpton and Gellhorn (1956) in various other tumours not regarded as sex hormone dependent. In the experience of the author (Stoll, 1963*b*), cortisone suppression of hypercalciuria is not a sign of sex hormone sensitivity in breast cancer.

It should be mentioned that in the case of sex hormone administration, correlation between a *fall* in the level of urinary calcium excretion, and tumour growth remission in breast cancer is not clearly established. In postmenopausal women *without* breast cancer, either oestrogen or androgen administration may lead to a decrease in the urinary excretion of calcium, as a result of the specific calcium retaining effect of these steroids. Thus, it is not surprising that Gerbrandy and Hellendoorn (1957) have found that a fall in calciuria following oestrogen or androgen therapy in postmenopausal patients with bone metastases from breast cancer, does not necessarily predict tumour growth remission in the disease. Examples of the effects of steroids on urinary calcium excretion in breast cancer patients are shown in Figs 5.1, 5.4, and 8.2.

SERUM CALCIUM LEVEL

A raised serum calcium level is not uncommonly seen in the presence of bone metastases from breast cancer. It may also be seen occasionally in the absence of bone metastases. Gerbrandy and Hellendoorn (1957) suggest that there is a positive correlation between the level of serum calcium, and that of the calciuria, in practically all cases of this type. A difference of 1 mg per cent in the serum calcium level reflects a difference of approximately 100 mg calcium in the daily urinary excretion. Although not quite as sensitive, similar prediction of hormonal sensitivity after steroid administration is often possible from assessing changes in serum calcium levels, as from the laborious investigation of urinary calcium excretion in patients placed on a rigid diet at rest in bed. This index has the fallibility mentioned above for the urinary calcium index, in the presence of limited bone metastases.

Hall *et al.* (1963*a*) have pointed out that a *rise* in the serum calcium to hypercalcaemic levels after androgen or oestrogen administration, indicates sensitivity of the tumour to steroids, but does not always predict increased tumour activity. In some patients, it was followed by regression of tumour deposits when hormonal therapy was persisted with (*see* p. 60).

An example of the effect of androgen therapy in causing a fall in serum calcium levels in a patient with breast cancer is shown in Fig. 10.1. It demonstrates the correlation with pain relief from bone metastases which often exists in such cases. It is

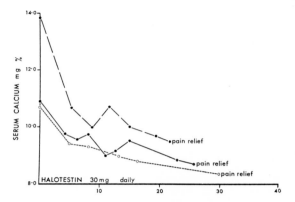

FIGURE 10.1 Serial fall in serum calcium associated with pain relief in three patients with bone metastases from breast cancer, receiving fluoxymesterone (Halotestin) therapy

essential in any case, that serial serum calcium estimations be carried out once or twice monthly, in every patient with bone metastases from breast cancer whether or not she is receiving steroid therapy. Apart from their value in reflecting sensitivity to steroid therapy (Fig. 10.2) they are an essential precaution, because of the danger of hypercalcaemia developing at any stage in the disease.

SERUM ALKALINE PHOSPHATASE

A raised serum alkaline phosphatase level is often seen in the presence of bone metastases from breast cancer. It is thought to reflect an increased osteoblastic activity in the normal bone surrounding the destroyed areas, which, if successful, will lead to bone repair in the metastases (Woodard *et al.*, 1954). It is, of course, understood that the presence of liver metastases must be excluded in such cases as the cause of the raised enzyme level.

Kennedy (1965*a*) noted that in patients with bone metastases, an initially high alkaline phosphatase level tended to be associated with a better remission from hormonal therapy. A high enzyme level in such cases presumably reflects an effective stromal response to the presence of tumour. Kennedy's observation may be correlated with the observation that breast cancer with a slower rate of growth (permitting better stromal response), is more likely to respond to most forms of endocrine therapy (*see* p. 116). It may be noted here, that a sclerotic appearance of bone metastases in untreated cases of breast cancer, is manifested most frequently in patients whose disease spans the natural menopause. Such a picture may reflect the slower rate of tumour growth at times of hormonal change (*see* p. 12), which permits an attempt at bone repair.

When endocrine therapy by castration or by steroids is instituted in the presence of bone metastases from breast cancer, it is often followed within a month, by an initial 'flare' in the alkaline phosphatase level. The 'flare' is independent of whether the patient derives benefit from treatment or not, and often occurs again when steroid treatment is

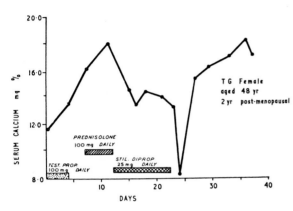

FIGURE 10.2 Patient T.G. Serial serum calcium estimations in a patient with bone metastases from breast cancer associated with hypercalcaemia; to show effect of consecutive courses of therapy with androgen, corticosteroid, and oestrogen on the serum calcium level

discontinued. It reflects an attempt at bone repair, which tends to occur during any period of hormonal imbalance, according to Woodward *et al.* (1954). Both oestrogens and androgens are known to stimulate osteoblastic activity.

If clinical benefit follows endocrine therapy, the serum alkaline phosphatase level will tend to fall, but only after an interval of about two to three months. Even if no clinical benefit ensues, there is often a fall in the enzyme level, and it therefore has little practical value for *early* prediction of response in the endocrine therapy of breast cancer. The significance of the serum alkaline phosphatase level is best assessed in conjunction with other enzyme levels such as the serum phosphohexose isomerase level or with the serum calcium level. When recalcification of bone metastases finally occurs after successful endocrine therapy, the alkaline phosphatase level usually returns to normal.

SERUM PHOSPHOHEXOSE ISOMERASE

This enzyme is involved in the conversion of glucose-6-phosphate to fructose-6-phosphate. A rise in serum glycolytic enzyme levels tends to occur whenever there is extensive tissue necrosis, whether it is due to malignant or to non-malignant causes. The serum phosphohexose isomerase level was suggested by Bodansky (1954) as a valuable index of breast cancer activity, after the diagnosis has been made. Levels are found to be raised in 85 per cent of patients with disseminate breast cancer (Joplin and Jegatheesen, 1962), the highest levels being in the presence of large osseous or hepatic metastases. In the author's experience, raised levels are much less common in the presence of a small volume of localised tumour. The excess enzyme is thought to be liberated from tissues compressed by the growing tumour.

A reduction in the serum phosphohexose isomerase level after pituitary ablation is correlated with favourable clinical response of breast cancer, according to Joplin and Jegatheesan (1962) and to Beck *et al.* (1966). According to Griffith and Beck (1963), raised enzyme levels are present in over 80 per cent of breast cancer patients, and a change in the enzyme level correlates well with the clinical response to oestrogen or androgen therapy. A decrease in the enzyme level is associated with objective evidence of tumour regression, while an increase is associated with evidence of tumour activation.

A change in the enzyme level, whether in the form of increase or decrease, usually occurs within a few days of endocrine therapy, and always antedates clinical evidence of change in the tumour by days or even by weeks according to Myers and Bodansky (1957) and Griffith and Beck (1963). The former authors report that the serum level of phosphohexose isomerase is more reliable in demonstrating changes in the activity of bone metastases than is the urinary calcium excretion level.

A rise in the phosphohexose isomerase level is the basis of a provocation test for assessing steroid sensitivity in breast cancer, as suggested from the experience of Beck *et al.* (1966). They noted a rise in the enzyme level in some patients within only four to five days of beginning the administration of oestrogens or androgens. This suggested provocation of tumour activity, as the level fell again when hormone therapy was stopped. The test appears to be independent of the type of metastasis present, unlike the sensitivity test of Emerson and Jessiman (1956) (*see* p. 101), which is restricted to cases of bone metastases. Nevertheless, the phosphohexose isomerase provocation test can be used to supplement evidence from serum calcium and alkaline phosphatase estimations, if bone metastases are present.

To assess the presence of hormone sensitivity in metastatic breast cancer, the enzyme level is measured before, and four days after, a three day course of injections of oestradiol monobenzoate, 1 mg daily intramuscularly. If the serum enzyme level is already considerably raised, it is safer to try the effect of an androgen such as testosterone propionate 100 mg intramuscularly daily for three days or fluoxymesterone 10 mg tds for a period of seven days. Depression of the raised enzyme level within seven days indicates hormone sensitivity in these cases.

It should be stressed that ingestion of food may cause temporary changes in the serum phosphohexose isomerase level, and it is therefore essential that all serial blood specimens be taken in the morning with the patient in a fasting state. Major surgery and the presence of liver damage are also said to affect the enzyme level.

SERUM LACTIC DEHYDROGENASE

Lactic dehydrogenase is found in relatively higher concentration in malignant tissue than in adjacent normal tissue. According to Hill and Levi (1954), this may reflect the higher rate of anaerobic glycolysis in tumours. The excess enzyme may overflow into the blood stream as shown by Wroblewski and La Due (1955).

Brindley and Francis (1963) examined a group of patients with advanced cancer of various types, and attempted to correlate increase in the serum enzyme level, with observed increase in size of the tumour. The correlation was generally good except in terminal cases. Furthermore, according to Hall et al. (1963b), changes in serum lactic dehydrogenase levels can be correlated with shrinkage of the tumour occurring after treatment by radiotherapy or by cytotoxic agents.

Joplin and Jegatheesan (1962) and Beck et al. (1966) consider that, as an index of tumour activity in breast cancer, the lactic dehydrogenase level in the blood is less reliable than the phosphohexose isomerase level.

SERUM GLYCOPROTEINS

It has been suggested by Burnett et al. (1963) that the serum glycoprotein level could be used to select patients with breast cancer who are likely to respond favourably to major endocrine ablation. The mean pre-operative level in cases showing favourable response is said to be appreciably higher than in non-responding cases. It has recently been suggested that to simplify the test, only the seromucoid bound carbohydrate and seromucoid bound tyrosine levels need be considered.

It is claimed that such an estimation might avoid subjecting patients to an unnecessary operation, and unlike Bulbrook's 'discriminant function' (see p. 109), the significance of the serum glycoprotein assay is not affected by recent oophorectomy or by steroid administration.

SERIAL TUMOUR BIOPSIES

Examination of serial tumour biopsies has been suggested as a means of establishing a response to hormonal therapy before clinical evidence of response becomes obvious. Wolff (1957) showed a decrease in the percentage of mitotic cells in the specimen, in the majority of patients responding favourably to oestrogen therapy. The change in radioactive phosphorus uptake noted in serial biopsies was investigated by Nevinny and Hall (1963) (see below).

Emerson et al. (1953; 1960) attempted to correlate changes in lysosomal enzyme activity with the effect of steroid administration. The heterogenous histology of breast cancer has so far prevented an effective biochemical assessment of this nature, as areas of spontaneous degeneration are common in the tumour.

MEASUREMENT OF RADIOACTIVE PHOSPHORUS UPTAKE BY THE TUMOUR

Certain malignant tumours including breast cancer, show a selectively high uptake of radioactive phosphorus. Noting this, Low-Beer and Green (1952) suggested that a change in the surface measurement of radioactive phosphorus uptake of advanced breast cancer might be useful as an indicator of tumour response to hormonal therapy. A report by Ellis et al. (1961) noted a fall in the radioactive phosphorus uptake of advanced breast cancer after a palliative course of X-ray therapy.

Nevinny and Hall (1963) attempted to apply the method to evaluation of hormonal response in advanced breast cancer. They measured the difference in radioactive phosphorus uptake before and after hormonal therapy, at first in biopsy specimens of the breast tumour, and later by surface counting measurement. Hale (1961), on the other hand, used continuous recording by implanted Geiger counters, and noted that those breast cancers showing a cyclical fluctuation in the radioactive phosphorus uptake, had a higher likelihood of favourable response to subsequent steroid therapy.

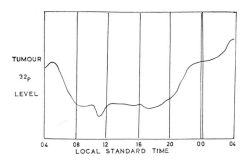

FIGURE 10.3 Diurnal periodicity in the radioactive phosphorus uptake of breast cancer. A composite curve derived by additive superposition of the individual curves from five patients

Stoll and Burch, 1968 (courtesy, Editor, *Cancer*, Philadelphia)

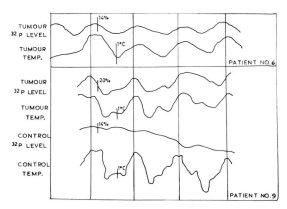

FIGURE 10.4 Recordings from two patients with breast cancer showing the relationship between the uptake of radioactive phosphorus and the adjacent skin temperature. The tumorous breast shows coincident diurnal periodicity in both, while the lower tracings show periodicity in the temperature over the normal breast, but no periodicity in the radioactive phosphorus uptake

Stoll and Burch, 1968 (courtesy, Editor, *Cancer*, Philadelphia)

The presence of cyclical fluctuations in the radioactive phosphorous uptake of some breast cancers has recently been confirmed by Bleehan and

Bryant (1967), Taylor *et al.* (1968), Wooley-Hart *et al.* (1968), and Stoll and Burch (1968). The last authors preferred the use of surface counting techniques and showed that the cycling frequency when present, was actually circadian—of a 24-hour periodicity (Fig. 10.3). This pattern presumably indicates that the metabolism of the tumour continues to respond to endogenous circadian hormonal stimulation (Fig. 10.4). Bleehan and Bryant (1967) reported that administration of oestrogens or androgens caused changes in the cycle in some patients and, in such cases, a favourable response by the tumour was always associated. Taylor *et al.* (1968) showed a correlation between clinical response to oestrogen therapy and a change in the radioactive phosphorus uptake of the tumour during therapy, but this method of predicting hormone sensitivity is still too complex for routine use.

RADIOACTIVELY LABELLED OESTROGEN UPTAKE BY THE TUMOUR

It has been suggested that the oestrogen sensitivity of a breast cancer is a measure of the tumour's capacity to fix circulating oestrogen. A selectively higher uptake of radioactively labelled oestrogen in some cases of human breast cancer was shown by Folca *et al.* (1961) and Crowley *et al.* (1962). The radioactively labelled oestrogen was administered to patients before bilateral adrenalectomy, and a relatively greater uptake of the isotope in breast cancer tissue was shown by Folca *et al.* (1961) in patients responding favourably to the adrenalectomy. Selectively higher uptake of androgen also, has been shown in some cases by Deshpande *et al.* (1963) in human breast cancer compared to normal tissue. Nevertheless, high uptake of a steroid by a tumour is significant of hormone sensitivity only if the concentration can be shown to be higher in hormone responsive than in hormone unresponsive tumours.

Assessment of oestrogen uptake by breast cancer maintained in organ culture *in vitro* has been suggested (Jensen *et al.*, 1967). It has the advantage that it is possible to correlate the quantitative uptake of an oestrogen with demonstrable metabolic effects in the target tissue. It also avoids the injection of radioactive materials into the patient. Jensen *et al.* (1967) suggested the possibility of measuring the blocking power of a steroid with anti-oestrogenic properties by incubating it *in vitro* together with tumour tissue and radioactively labelled oestrogen. The presence of these properties in a steroid does not necessarily indicate the clinical usefulness of such an agent in hormonal therapy.

EFFECT OF STEROIDS ON THE TUMOUR *IN VITRO*

The methods described in the previous section may suggest a likelihood of hormone sensitivity by breast cancer, *if this term is equated with higher oestrogen uptake*. However, as explained in Chapter Three, the oestrogen dependent theory of hormonal control in breast cancer does not apply to all therapy and, in fact, in postmenopausal women, high therapeutic oestrogen levels in the blood are associated with regression and not stimulation of breast cancer growth. It is possible that for every breast cancer there is an optimal level of oestrogen requirement for stimulation of its growth, so that either higher or lower concentrations may depress its activity (Segaloff, 1967a).

The observation of growth inhibition or stimulation in an organ culture of the patient's tumour incubated with different concentration of a steroid, can provide an individualised bio-assay of steroid response. It must be taken into account that such a method will not necessarily predict the effect of the steroid clinically, as it eliminates the influence on the tumour of the steroid metabolites, or of other endogenous hormones present in the body. It also ignores any indirect action that the steroid might have on endogenous hormone secretion. Nevertheless, to support the use of such a method, there is now considerable evidence that steroid hormones exert a direct effect upon breast cancer tissue *in vitro*, at concentrations comparable to the pharmacological concentrations existing at the target organ.

Hollander *et al.* (1958; 1959) have demonstrated an oestrogen sensitive dehydrogenase in some human breast cancer specimens and in the adjacent normal breast tissue. An attempt was made to correlate in a very small series of patients the enzymatic activity of the specimen with the clinical response to subsequent endocrine ablation. Rienits (1959) reported the effect of androgen or oestrogen on the respiration of incubated tissue slices of breast cancer, while Heuson and Legros (1963) reported the effect of these hormones in inhibiting protein synthesis in breast cancer maintained *in vitro*.

Morphological signs of growth inhibition, by androgen, oestrogen, and progesterone incubated with monolayer or organ cultures of mammary carcinoma, have been reported by Kellner and Turcic (1962), Rivera *et al.* (1963), and Flaxel and Wellings (1963). The development of an individualised bio-assay method in the past, has been frustrated by difficulties in the maintenance of organ culture of human breast cancer, and these problems have been fully described by Foley and Aftonomos (1965). Recent improvements in technique have, however, led to encouraging reports such as those of Altmann and Chayen (1967) and Tchao *et al.* (1968).

URINARY OESTROGEN EXCRETION

If the hormonal sensitivity of breast cancer was equated with its oestrogen dependence, one would expect that a favourable tumour response to endocrine therapy in an individual with breast cancer would be associated with a fall in the oestrogen excretion level. An accurate method for the measurement of urinary oestrone, oestradiol 17β, and oestriol excretion was reported by Brown (1955) and Bauld (1956). It enabled Strong *et al.* (1956), Bulbrook *et al.* (1958), Gordon and Segaloff (1958), Scowen (1958), Hiisi Brummer *et al.* (1960), McAllister *et al.* (1960), Irvine *et al.* (1961), Swyer *et al.* (1961), Hortling *et al.* (1962), Palmer and Helstrom (1962), and Jull *et al.* (1963) to report that after oophorectomy, bilateral adrenalectomy or hypophysectomy, oestrogens may continue to be secreted, and their persistence in some patients bore no relationship to the likelihood of favourable clinical response in their breast cancer.

Again, it could be expected that a very low preoperative oestrogen excretion level, might indicate a lesser likelihood of oestrogen dependence in breast cancer. Dao and Huggins (1955) and Block *et al.* (1959) did indeed note that if oestrogen excretion levels are very low before bilateral adrenalectomy, the operation is less likely to be successful. However, Birke *et al.* (1958) and Irvine *et al.* (1961) could not confirm this observation.

In spite of such reports, the problem may have to be reinvestigated. It had been suggested by Bulbrook *et al.* (1960b) that the older chemical methods of oestrogen assay may yield unreliable results, at the low levels being measured after castration and major endocrine ablation therapy. This applies particularly in the presence of the metabolites of hormone replacement therapy.

A more sensitive method of oestrogen determination has been developed by Brown (1967). By its use, it is possible to distinguish persistent oestrogen secretion by the ovary, from that of the adrenal cortex, in postmenopausal women. The former shows a cyclical variation in oestrogen level through the month (Brown, 1967). An alternative method of distinction is the dexamethasone suppression test, which suppresses only adrenocortical oestrogen in the postmenopausal patient, but not the ovarian fraction (Schweppe *et al.*, 1967). Such information should clarify the endocrine management of post-menopausal breast cancer patients, with signs of persistent oestrogen secretion. Castration would be recommended only for those patients in whom the secretion can be shown to be ovarian in origin.

The persistence of small quantities of oestrogen, pregnanediol, androsterone, and aetiocholanolone excretion after combined bilateral adrenalectomy and oophorectomy for breast cancer, is thought by Bulbrook *et al.* (1960b), to indicate residual secretion arising in aberrant adrenal tissue overlooked at operation. The findings of Strong *et al.* (1956) and Sim *et al.* (1961) do not agree with this assumption as the levels do not rise with ACTH stimulation. An alternative explanation which has been suggested is that breast cancer is capable of synthesising oestrogens from other steroids (Adams and Wong, 1968).

Bonser *et al.* (1961) examined biopsies from the remaining breast in patients who had had a mastectomy for breast cancer. They looked for evidence of prolactin stimulation, and also estimated the urinary oestrogen excretion in these patients. They claim that from these two criteria they could recommend a choice between bilateral adrenalectomy, hypophysectomy, and no endocrine ablation surgery in the presence of advanced disease. They were able to predict correctly the response in fourteen of eighteen patients subjected to major endocrine ablation therapy, but the series was uncontrolled. Furthermore, the histological interpretation of prolactin stimulation of the normal breast tissue is difficult.

CYTOHORMONAL ASSAY OF URETHRAL OR VAGINAL CYTOLOGY

Castellanos and Sturgis (1958) suggested that examination of the cytological sediment of an early morning urine specimen, yields a more accurate indication of endogenous oestrogen activity in the body than does the vaginal smear as it will differentiate ovarian from adrenal oestrogens. ACTH administration is said to increase the oestrogen effect on the urethra, if the oestrogens originate in the adrenal cortex. The urethral smear is also said to reflect accurately the effect of steroid administration. In a later report, Castellanos *et al.* (1963) suggest that examination of the urethral smear after dexamethasone administration, can be used to demonstrate the persistence of ovarian activity in the postmenopausal patient with an oestrogenised smear showing a karyo-pyknotic index of over 20 per cent.

The vaginal smear in the normal postmenopausal woman reflects the concentration of circulating endogenous steroid hormones. Atrophic, intermediate and oestrogenic (cornified or keratinised) patterns

are recognised. According to Rubinstein and Duncan (1941) and Young *et al.* (1957) there is a close correlation between the level of oestrogen excretion, measured biologically or biochemically, and the vaginal smear pattern. The distribution of such patterns in a group of postmenopausal patients with breast cancer, is no different from that of a control group of the same age distribution, according to Struthers (1956) and Liu (1957).

According to Green (1961), the pretreatment vaginal smear can be used to indicate the most suitable method of hormonal therapy in breast cancer. In his view, an oestrogenised smear requires oestrogen suppressive therapy, and an atrophic smear requires oestrogen therapy. Nevertheless, Liu (1957) and the author (Stoll, 1967b) have shown that in a series of patients treated by oestrogen therapy (and in the case of androgen therapy too), the pretreatment vaginal smear pattern cannot be correlated in this way with the likelihood of tumour growth remission (*see* Table 7.3).

In the case of progestin therapy of breast cancer, however, there is a suggestion of such a correlation in the author's series (Stoll, 1967c). The presence of an atrophic vaginal smear before treatment (signifying the complete absence of hormonal stimulation)

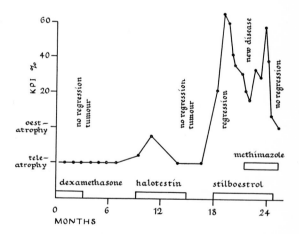

FIGURE 10.5 Patient B.M. Record of tumour regression in breast cancer in relation to the vaginal smear pattern, following the successive administration of dexamethasone 6·4 mg daily, fluoxymesterone (Halotestin) 40 mg daily, stilboestrol 15 mg daily, and added methimazole 30 mg daily

Stoll, 1967 (courtesy, Editor, *Cancer*, Philadelphia)

appears to be associated with a significantly lower tumour remission rate, than is the presence of an intermediate or oestrogenised smear (*see* p. 70).

Moreover, during the course of steroid therapy of

breast cancer, the vaginal smear can be used as a bio-assay of the patient's hormone utilisation in the body, and the degree of absorption from the bowel (Fig. 10.5). According to Liu (1957) and the author (Stoll, 1967b), there is a correlation between the *degree* of vaginal smear cornification, and the likelihood of clinical benefit in breast cancer from oestrogen

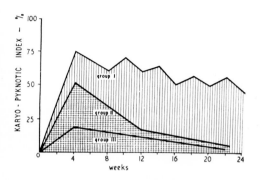

FIGURE 10.6 Diagrammatic representation of the vaginal smear response to oestrogens. Categorised into three group patterns—

Group 1 A rise in the karyopknotic index above 60 per cent, followed by a gradual fall over a period of six months or longer

Group 2 A rise in the KPI to 50 per cent (approx.), followed by a rapid fall after two months

Group 3 No rise in the KPI above 25 per cent throughout treatment

Stoll, 1967 (courtesy, Editor, *Cancer*, Philadelphia)

therapy. The degree of oestrogen-induced cornification of the smear in some patients may be interfered with by androgen activity in the body or other metabolic factors. It may be possible to increase the cornification of the vaginal smear in such patients, according to Pundel (1958), either by using a higher dose of oestrogen, or by changing from oral to parenteral administration.

The author has observed a tendency in the individual patient, for a progressive decrease with time in the cornification response to continuous oestrogen administration (Fig. 10.6). To maintain a highly cornified vaginal smear in the treatment of breast cancer, it may be necessary to progressively increase the oestrogen dose at intervals (*see* p. 61).

URINARY GONADOTROPIN EXCRETION

It has been noted previously (*see* p. 106) that there is no correlation between the likelihood of tumour

regression in breast cancer after oophorectomy, bilateral adrenalectomy, or hypophysectomy, on the one hand, and the degree of postoperative persistence in urinary oestrogen excretion, on the other. It suggests that oestrogen withdrawal may not be a major factor in the favourable response noted in some patients after hormonal ablation therapy. On the other hand, it was shown by Douglas *et al.* (1961) and Pommatau (1963) that gonadotropin levels tend to rise to especially high levels in breast cancer patients achieving remission of tumour growth after oophorectomy and adrenalectomy. The author has therefore suggested (Stoll, 1964b) on a theoretical basis, that the tumour growth remission usually ascribed to oestrogen withdrawal in the younger patient, might be associated with an increased gonadotropin secretion released by removal of inhibiting oestrogen. Lazarev (1960), on the other hand, incriminates gonadotropin as a stimulator of breast cancer. The difference of opinion would be resolved by a clinical trial of human gonadotropin therapy in advanced breast cancer in young women.

In the case of postmenopausal patients with little or no circulating oestrogens, the position appears to be different. According to Loraine *et al.* (1957) a high gonadotropin level before stilboestrol therapy in postmenopausal breast cancer suggests a poor prognosis, as does also a high gonadotropin level persisting after high dose diethyl stilboestrol therapy according to Stewart *et al.* (1965). To account for the different hormonal response of the postmenopausal patient to oestrogen administration it has been postulated (*see* p. 14) that breast cancer manifesting in the postmenopausal female has developed in a different hormonal background from that in premenopausal females.

It is possible that estimation of gonadotropin levels before and after endocrine therapy in breast cancer may be useful to predict clinical response, if premenopausal and postmenopausal cases were considered separately. A change in the level may be more important than the actual height of the level. According to Segaloff (1967a), chronic debilitating illness may lead to low gonadotropin excretion levels. This factor, or a mixture of clinical material, may account for the inconclusive results of Segaloff *et al.* (1954b) and Martin (1964) connecting gonadotropin levels, and the likelihood of favourable response in breast cancer to endocrine therapy. Androgen therapy by fluoxymesterone is not correlated with a specific trend in the subsequent level of gonadotropin excretion (Segaloff *et al.*, 1958).

With regard to hypophyseal ablation, it was noted by Boyland *et al.* (1958) that breast cancer patients showing tumour regression following the operation, included a higher proportion with a marked fall in gonadotropin excretion than did non-responders. In such cases, the fall in level is a measure of the completeness of ablation, yet most other authorities have failed to correlate the likelihood of tumour regression after hypophyseal ablation with the completeness of ablation (*see* p. 92).

URINARY PROLACTIN EXCRETION

The problems of separating human growth hormone from prolactin are complex and there are considerable doubts as to their assay methods as described by Ferguson and Wallace (1961) and Barrett *et al.* (1961). The evidence linking human growth hormone with the stimulation of breast cancer is based on pain and calcium excretion as indices of response (Pearson and Ray, 1959), and is not confirmed by Lipsett and Bergenstal (1960).

With regard to prolactin, the evidence is somewhat more conclusive. Castration decreases prolactin secretion (Meites and Nicoll, 1966). Tumour regression in breast cancer patients after oestrogen administration was early reported by Segaloff *et al.* (1954*b*) to be associated with a fall in the urinary prolactin level. Hadfield (1957) reported that clinical response to hypophysectomy was associated with abolition of urinary prolactin excretion. Furthermore, Pearson (1957) reported that administration of prolactin to patients after hypophysectomy may cause reactivation of controlled breast cancer. Finally, McCalister and Welbourn (1962) have reported that an increase in calcium excretion, following provocative injections of ovine prolactin in patients with bone metastases, predicts a likelihood of tumour regression after hypophysectomy.

All these findings can be interpreted to suggest that decrease of prolactin secretion may be a factor involved in the benefit from oestrogen therapy or from hypophysectomy in human breast cancer (*see* p. 16). If a reliable method of assay can be established it may be useful to predict changes in tumour activity. Surprisingly, Segaloff *et al.* (1958) have reported that favourable response of breast cancer to the androgen, fluoxymesterone, is associated with a *rise* in the prolactin level (*see* p. 18).

URINARY 'DISCRIMINANT FUNCTION'

It was reported by Bulbrook *et al.* (1960*a*) that the clinical response of breast cancer patients to bilateral adrenalectomy or to hypophysectomy, can be correlated with the proportion of androgen and corticosteroid metabolites in the urine before operation. The 'discriminant function' is regarded as negative in patients excreting abnormally low quantities of aetiocholanolone relative to the quantity of 17 hydroxycorticosteroids. According to Thomas *et al.* (1967), patients with a negative discriminant showed tumour growth remission from major ablation therapy in only 11·5 per cent of cases, whereas those with a positive discriminant showed such remission in 38·7 per cent of cases.

The likelihood of remission from major ablation therapy was almost negligible in negative discriminant cases, if they had a short free-period between mastectomy and recurrence or if they were within six years of the menopause.

Similar correlation with the discriminant function has been obtained by Juret *et al.* (1964) for the results of hypophyseal destruction by radioactive Yttrium implant and by Wilson *et al.* (1967) for bilateral adrenalectomy. More recently, it has been suggested by Miller *et al.* (1967) and Ahlquist *et al.* (1968) that instead of aetiocholanolone, the total 11 deoxy 17 oxosteroids may be more simply measured. Although the discriminant function using this latter criterion was shown by Thomas *et al.* (1967) to be related to the results of major endocrine ablation therapy, Ahlquist *et al.* (1968) showed that it did not apply to other forms of hormonal therapy. The urinary discriminant function cannot be related to the likelihood of clinical response to major endocrine ablation, either in elderly patients, or in those who have recently been subjected to castration or to steroid therapy.

So far, the value of the discriminant function has not been proven significantly in a prospective series, to select patients for major endocrine ablation.

A negative discriminant is associated with a relatively subnormal level of androgen excretion in the urine, and is increasingly common with advancing age of the patient. A report by Bulbrook and Hayward (1962) has shown that negative discriminants are considerably more common in patients with breast cancer than in the normal population. Such a steroidal abnormality may, therefore, precede or even predispose to the development of breast cancer. In addition, according to Bulbrook *et al.* (1964*a*) a negative discriminant at the time of mastectomy carries a poor prognosis, with a likelihood of early recurrence and death from the disease.

Some of the conclusions of Bulbrook *et al.* (1960*a*) have been criticised by Nabarro (1960) on the grounds that the discriminant ratio can be affected by various constitutional factors such as anxiety, stress or surgical operation. Adrenal androgen excretion is reduced during chronic illness. Thyroid function may also be involved, as Hellman *et al.* (1961) have shown that the total amount of circulating corticosteroids, and the proportion of their constituents, is related to the level of thyroid hormone in the circulation. A wide variation has been observed in the thyroid function of patients with recurrent breast cancer according to Strong (1963) and the author (Stoll, 1965b). There is also a possibility that the tumour itself may be responsible for causing the steroid abnormality found in patients with negative discriminants.

TUMOUR SEX CHROMATIN DETERMINATION

A nuclear chromatin body peculiar to female somatic cells is believed to represent the second 'X' chromosome. It is referred to as the sex chromatin and various authors have suggested that the presence or absence of the sex chromatin in the breast cancer cells can be used as a guide to the selection of patients for hormonal therapy. Reports include those of Kimel (1957), Moore and Barr (1957), Regele et al. (1964), Bohle (1965), and Shirley (1967).

The presence of sex chromatin in less than 5 per cent of cell nuclei is generally regarded as abnormally low (male karyotype), while its presence in over 15 per cent of nuclei is regarded as normal (female karyotype). If the proportion is between 5–15 per cent, the morphology is categorised as intermediate in type. It is claimed by Regele and Vagacs (1962) that an abnormally low sex chromatin count is associated with a below normal oestrogen excretion, and the normal karyotype with a normal oestrogen excretion.

Between 60–70 per cent of patients with breast cancer appear to have tumours with normal sex chromatin counts, and about 20–25 per cent have tumours with abnormally low sex chromatin counts, the rest being intermediate in character. According to Kimel (1957), Regele et al. (1964), and Bohle (1965) tumours with low sex chromatin counts respond poorly to prophylactic oophorectomy or androgen therapy. According to Regele et al. (1964) 76 per cent of such cases died after mastectomy and prophylactic androgen therapy, compared to 40 per cent of those with normal sex chromatin counts. The relationship between karyotype and response to oestrogen therapy is difficult to classify because Kimel (1957) regards a clinical remission from oestrogen therapy as representing an 'oestrogen independent' tumour, but no clinical response to the same steroid as representing an 'oestrogen dependent' tumour.

Sex chromatin bodies are said to be more easily recognised in well-differentiated tumour cells. Although Kimel (1957) does not agree, Bohle (1965) notes a worse prognosis and a greater likelihood of metastasis in patients whose breast cancer shows a low sex chromatin content. This may reflect the fact that these are likely to represent poorly differentiated tumours, according to Moore and Barr (1957). However, Atkin (1967) doubts the existence of a correlation between sex chromatin count and histological grading.

Shirley (1967) considers the presence of sex chromatin in over 45 per cent of all tumour cells—an unusually *high* proportion—also to be associated with a poor response to hormonal therapy in younger women. More information is needed before sex chromatin counts can be used to predict the outcome of hormonal therapy.

11

Clinical Criteria of Hormonal Response

IN DISCUSSING the selection of individualised hormonal therapy in patients with late breast cancer, the previous chapter considered the guidelines provided by laboratory criteria of hormonal responsiveness. When we come to assess benefit from such treatment, we require agreement on significant clinical criteria of hormonal response.

For a radical form of treatment in cancer, the length of survival is the logical choice of index for assessing the results of therapy. (Although this index is widely used for comparing results from different centres, care should be taken to distinguish between recurrence-free survival rates, crude survival rates, net survival rates, and corrected survival rates.) However, in the case of a palliative form of treatment, such as endocrine therapy in breast cancer, the survival rate may not be a valid index for comparing benefit from different forms of therapy. It is possible that patients with slowly growing tumours may, as a group, show a greater likelihood of favourable response to one type of endocrine therapy than to another. Prolonged survival of the responding members of such a group need not necessarily indicate the beneficial results of treatment.

CRITERIA OF RESPONSE AND OF PALLIATION

In assessing the results of endocrine therapy in late breast cancer, the difficulties of agreement on criteria of response are considerable. Some of the problems have been recently discussed in a symposium edited by Hayward and Bulbrook (1966).

The criteria of response and of palliation may be classified and subdivided as follows:

1. Subjective response as judged by:
   (a) Improvement in appetite, well-being, or performance.
   (b) Relief of pain or of other symptoms, e.g. cough or dyspnoea.

2. Objective response as shown by a change in the tumour:
   (a) Histology
   (b) Size of lesion
   (c) Laboratory criteria
       e.g. enzyme levels
   (d) Indirect effect of lesion
       e.g. neurological signs
   Change should be qualified according to:

   (i) Overall incidence
   (ii) Extent of response
   (iii) Duration of response
   (iv) Site sensitivity

   } SPECIFIC CRITERIA OF RESPONSE

   (a) Improvement in exercise tolerance or return to work
   (b) Increase in weight
   (c) Laboratory criteria returned to normal, e.g. ESR, blood urea, serum calcium, or haemoglobin level.

   } NON-SPECIFIC CRITERIA OF PALLIATION

The essential point of contention is as to whether evidence of *response* to endocrine therapy, or evidence of *palliation* from endocrine therapy is being assessed. Evidence of response is important to the observer for assessing the hormonal sensitivity of breast cancer, although in some cases it may not even be apparent to the patient. Visible evidence of hormonal sensitivity implies a possible controlling effect upon occult metastases also. As an example, we may consider decrease in size of metastatic skin nodules, probably our most accurately measured criterion of response. A limited inhibiting effect on the growth of such lesions does not in all cases, lead to appreciable physical benefit to the patient. In other words, a short-term limited shrinkage in size of skin nodules, although significant of hormone sensitivity, does not necessarily qualify as clinical hormonal palliation.

111

Therefore, when clinical response to endocrine therapy is being specified for comparative purposes, such a statement needs to describe the average *extent*, *duration*, and *site selectivity* of the response, in addition to its *incidence*. The sum of the three former qualifying factors will define also the degree of palliation, while the latter defines only the hormonal response.

CONFUSION IN CLINICAL CRITERIA OF RESPONSE

The following factors have been described by the author (Stoll, 1964*a*) as the more obvious causes of conflicting reports in the literature by observers of endocrine therapy in breast cancer.

INCLUSION OF NON-PROGRESSIVE OR QUIESCENT DISEASE

It is not uncommon to see in late breast cancer, manifestations such as metastatic nodules or nodes which barely change in size over a period of several months. Most observers (but by no means all), therefore, insist that the disease must show recorded signs of measurable progression over a period of two months at least, before instituting a trial of endocrine therapy. This should avoid claims of endocrine control of what is actually quiescent disease (Segaloff, 1960).

The growth rate of an individual metastasis declines progressively with increasing size of the lesion, and a tendency to necrosis is common in large lesions. For this reason it is suggested by Brennan (1966) that it is more accurate to judge advancing growth on the basis of new lesions appearing, rather than by a change in existing lesions.

ACCEPTANCE OF RESTRICTED OBJECTIVE BENEFIT

Some observers will accept as a tumour growth remission the shrinkage of existing lesions under endocrine therapy even if lesions in other systems are meanwhile developing. Thus it is not uncommon (especially with corticosteroid therapy or cytotoxic chemotherapy), to see soft tissue metastases from breast cancer regressing under treatment, yet two to three months later a malignant pleural effusion is clinically obvious. Most observers will recognise tumour growth remission only if *all* systems show measurable signs of tumour control for a specified minimum time period.

The estimation of the 'mean clinical value' has been devised by Walpole and Paterson (1949) for the assessment of response in such cases. Each existing lesion is measured separately at each attendance and given a rating according to its progress. The mean value of all ratings is calculated and used as an index. Such an index measures hormonal response but not palliation, because regression of isolated skin nodules is given the same 'weighting' as regression of lung or bone metastases.

Again, there is no unanimity on the percentage decrease in size of a lesion which must be attained to justify the term 'remission'. In a recent assessment by Rimm *et al.* (1966) of tumour response to cytotoxic chemotherapy in 253 patients, he found that he could quote a 7 per cent tumour remission rate or a 48 per cent tumour remission rate, according to whether a 50 per cent decrease or a 10 per cent decrease in size was demanded.

There is no unanimity as to the minimum duration of tumour growth remission following endocrine therapy for it to be considered valid. Most authorities insist on a minimum period of three months, some insist on at least six months regression, while others accept lesser periods as long as tumour regression is useful, and objectively established. Again, the difference in criteria is basically one between palliation and objective evidence of hormonal response.

There is also disagreement as to whether a patient with lesions remaining unchanged in size during endocrine treatment (while previously advancing), should be regarded as being in growth remission or non-responding, or classified in a separate group. This applies particularly to bone metastases from breast cancer, where associated with relief of pain, it is common for the radiographic appearance barely to change over months of therapy, whereas it was showing progression before treatment.

FAILURE TO ALLOW ADEQUATE INTERVAL BETWEEN TREATMENTS

Unless there are urgent manifestations of advancing disease, six months should be allowed after radiation endocrine ablation, and at least two months after surgical endocrine ablation, before considering such therapy to have failed. After oestrogen or androgen therapy have lost control, one should wait at least two months in order to observe a withdrawal response. The latter is seen after stopping oestrogen therapy in about 30 per cent of all cases of breast cancer where favourable response has been achieved and then lost (*see* p. 59). If the existence of a withdrawal response is not appreciated, the observed remission may in such cases be credited to the newly administered form of treatment.

EXCLUSION OF CASES FROM ASSESSMENT

Many reports exclude from calculation of the tumour remission rate all patients who die, or who discontinue medication, within one month of beginning any course of steroid treatment for breast cancer.

Exclusion is justified on the basis that the drug has had insufficient time to demonstrate its effect. These patients are indeed failures of palliation, but not necessarily of hormonal response, because clinical trial has not been adequate. Other observers would insist on regarding these patients as a failure also of hormonal response.

A similar problem applies to cases of early post-operative death after surgical or radiation endocrine ablation. They are failures of treatment, but whether of palliation or of hormonal response is a matter of contention. Different interpretation of these patients' category will lead to differences in tumour remission rates. The presence of a high proportion of terminal patients in a clinical trial of a new modality can affect results considerably for this reason.

CONFUSION BETWEEN CRITERIA OF
HORMONAL 'RESPONSE' AND NON SPECIFIC
'PALLIATION'

Some reports of endocrine therapy in breast cancer are based purely upon macroscopic change in every measurable lesion. Others include among the criteria of benefit—increase in weight, increase in exercise tolerance or increase in 'performance status' (Karnosfsky and Burchenal, 1958). These criteria are evidence of non-specific palliation, but do not necessarily indicate a hormonal cancer restraining influence. Nor, necessarily, do changes in erythrocyte sedimentation rate, blood urea, or haemoglobin levels during endocrine management.

Changes in serum calcium level or urinary calcium excretion need not necessarily signify inhibition of tumour activity (see p. 102). Systemic upset with pyrexia at the onset of steroid treatment is not uncommon but has not been demonstrated to be a sign of tumour aggravation (see p. 60). Nevertheless, recorded progressive improvement in the physical signs of brain, cranial nerve, or spinal nerve involvement during endocrine therapy is generally to be accepted as a manifestation of tumour growth remission.

Relief of pain is often quoted as an indicator of response to endocrine therapy in late breast cancer (Neal, 1966). While it undoubtedly represents desirable palliation, it cannot be regarded as a biological index of hormone response. It is well established that the pain of bone metastases can be relieved by placebos, by steroid therapy or by endocrine ablation, even when there is evidence of progressing bone destruction (see p. 79). An example is the case of hypophyseal ablation, where relief of pain within twenty-four or forty-eight hours is commonly noted, but its duration may be only a few days, weeks or months, without associated objective signs of healing in destroyed bone (see p. 93).

PROTOCOL OF LARGE SCALE TRIALS

In an attempt to overcome the lack of uniformity in criteria of hormonal response, an inter-hospital Co-operative Breast Cancer Group was set up under the National Institute of Health, Bethesda, USA. A uniform protocol for admission of breast cancer cases was insisted on, and the trials of steroids were randomised with control material (often placebos) in a double-blind fashion. As an example of this protocol, evidence of objective remission in breast cancer is defined by the Co-operative Breast Cancer Group (1961) as:

> 'All demonstrable tumour masses diminish measurably in size.
> or More than 50 per cent of non-osseous lesions decrease in size, although all bone lesions are static.
> or More than 50 per cent of all lesions improve while the remainder are static.'

THE AUTHOR'S PROTOCOL

The protocol used for many years by the author in the hormonal therapy of breast cancer is best summarised in the following extract from a published paper (Stoll, 1963b):

'Nathanson's classical specification of objective remission from hormone therapy is adopted—namely a measurable decrease in size of specified lesions, while at the very least, all other lesions are static and no new lesions appear.

The criteria for objective tumour growth remission in specific areas are:

1. *Osseous*. Recalcification in parts not previously treated by radiotherapy. Fall in serum calcium is *not* accepted as a criterion of response.

2. *Local*. Decrease in size of breast tumour or ulceration, nodules, or regional nodes, measurable by a ruler, and confirmed wherever demonstrable by photographs. 'Arrested' disease is *not* included.

3. *Intrathoracic*. Decrease in size of radiological opacities in the lungs or of mediastinal nodes, or decrease in the size of a pleural or peritoneal effusion without paracentesis. Gross decrease in the rate of reaccumulation of a serious effusion is recorded, but *not* counted as objective control of disease.

4. *Visceral*. Decrease in size of metastatic hepatic enlargement or decrease in physical signs arising from cerebral metastases.

In all cases, the histological diagnosis is established previously. In all cases given previous therapy, new treatment is instituted only if there are unequivocal objective signs of progressing lesions. Patients who have received irradiation to the part under observation within the previous two months are excluded from hormone trial. Blood transfusions, paracentesis, and symptomatic treatment are carried out as necessary, and in all cases of inadequate nutrition, attempts are made to correct this by suitable diet.

All objective criteria are assessed beforehand by diagrams, photographs, radiographs, and blood analysis. Subjective benefit is, however, also recorded, and improvement in appetite, gain in weight, and improvement in "performance status" recorded as subjective improvement. Decrease in dyspnoea or of pain are recorded only as subjective improvement.'

12

Biological Determinants of Hormonal Response

It has been suggested in the immediately preceding chapters that the selection of hormonal therapy for the individual with advanced breast cancer can be guided by laboratory indices of hormonal responsiveness, and the results assessed by significant clinical criteria of hormonal response. The third guiding factor to be considered, involves the 'biological determinants' of hormonal response. These are the factors in the natural history of the disease which determine hormonal response in the individual.

FACTORS GOVERNING INDIVIDUAL RESPONSE

Endocrine therapy in late breast cancer can achieve tumour control in only about one third of patients. It is essential to add a corollary that in the treatment of late cancer, the individual who fails to respond favourably to a particular endocrine therapy, has not only failed to benefit but has also lost valuable months of life, which might have been used for a more successful trial. It is, therefore, of the greatest importance that the form of therapy should be selected specifically for the patient, as not all methods of endocrine therapy are equally effective in a group of patients with what might appear to be similar disease manifestations. Although it has been pointed out that practically all methods of endocrine therapy yield a similar overall percentage response rate, *it does not of necessity imply that the same individual patients would respond favourably to all methods.*

For selection of individualised therapy, we can assess the individual's likelihood of a favourable response to a particular form of treatment by considering the known biological determinants of hormonal response. Such determinants include age group in relation to the menopause, free-interval between mastectomy and recurrence, site of metastasis, size of metastasis, pretreatment hormonal background of the patient, previous response to

endocrine manipulation, and possibly also the histological characteristics of the tumour (*see later*). Fairgrieve (1965) and Edelstyn *et al.* (1965) in an attempt at a rational approach to the selection of patients for bilateral adrenalectomy and hypophysectomy, took some of these factors into account.

Segaloff, having instigated, organised, and supervised numerous randomised trials in the endocrine therapy of breast cancer, now contemplates the future of hormonal agents in the treatment of the disease in the following words (Segaloff, 1966): 'This may require a series of agents, each most effective in a particular menopausal age group, a combination of hormones, or one particularly useful in a host with a certain type of hormonal excretion pattern.'

The recent trend to large randomised trials of endocrine therapy in breast cancer has resulted, finally, in only marginal differences in *overall* tumour remission rates between the major methods of endocrine therapy, but it has yielded valuable information on factors governing individual response to endocrine therapy. The inclusion of a patient in such randomised trials was ethically justified, only as long as we were ignorant of the biological factors favouring the choice of one method as against another in the individual patient.

UTILISATION OF BIOLOGICAL DETERMINANTS OF RESPONSE

A particular form of endocrine therapy in breast cancer should be selected for the individual, with the following biological determinants of hormonal response in mind.

AGE GROUP IN RELATION TO MENOPAUSE
Castration is probably less effective in premenopausal patients who are under the age of thirty-five, and it may therefore be useful to add androgen therapy to castration, in patients with disseminated

breast cancer who are in this age group (*see* p. 29). Hypophyseal ablation is probably more effective in premenopausal women and in women over sixty, than it is in other age groups (*see* p. 92). Bilateral adrenalectomy seems to be more effective in patients over fifty, than in those under fifty years of age (*see* p. 91).

Both androgen and oestrogen therapy are undoubtedly increasingly effective with increasing age past the menopause, although in the presence of bone metastases, benefit from androgen therapy appears less dependent on age group (*see* p. 38). Benefit from corticosteroid therapy in breast cancer seems to be relatively independent of age group (*see* p. 77), and the same probably applies to progestin therapy in the present state of our knowledge.

DURATION OF FREE INTERVAL BETWEEN
MASTECTOMY AND THE FIRST RECURRENCE
In the case of treatment by castration, bilateral adrenalectomy, or hypophyseal ablation, it seems probable that the longer the free interval between mastectomy and the first recurrence, the greater the likelihood of tumour growth remission (*see* pp. 25 and 89). If the free interval is short, surgical castration is to be preferred to radiation castration (*see* p. 24), because the rapid spread of the tumour does not permit of the delay necessary for radiation effects upon the ovary to manifest themselves.

In the case of oestrogen or androgen therapy also, the tumour remission rate is likely to be greater with a longer free interval between mastectomy and the first recurrence (*see* p. 55). A similar correlation has not been established for corticosteroid therapy in breast cancer. Tumours may alter their behaviour pattern in the body even when well established (Smithers, 1968) and a long free interval may signify temporary slowing of growth associated with sensitivity to intrinsic hormonal changes.

SITE SENSITIVITY
For treatment by castration, bilateral adrenalectomy, or hypophyseal ablation, the site sensitivity of breast cancer metastases to endocrine therapy appears to be, in descending order of sensitivity—bone, soft tissue, and viscera (*see* p. 27). For androgen therapy, the order appears to be the same (*see* p. 37). However, for oestrogen therapy, the order appears to be the soft tissue, viscera, and bone (*see* p. 55).

The controlling effect of oestrogen therapy in bone metastases is not as good as that of the other modalities mentioned. On the other hand, androgen therapy induces a favourable response in the case of widespread bone metastases, possibly because of a specific effect on calcium metabolism (*see* p. 17).

Hypophyseal ablation is the method of endocrine treatment which leads to the highest tumour remission rate—subjective and objective—in the case of bone metastases. Progestins and corticosteroids are both disappointing in their controlling effect upon such metastases (*see* p. 79).

Oestrogen therapy sometimes induces remarkable tumour growth remissions in the case of extensive soft tissue, lung, or pleural metastases (*see* p. 55). Progestin therapy although inferior in this respect to oestrogen therapy, also shows its best controlling effect in the case of soft tissue metastases (*see* p. 69). Corticosteroid therapy shows its most remarkable benefits in brain, lung, and liver metastases although such tumour growth remissions are very temporary. These are sites where bilateral adrenalectomy is least useful as a palliative treatment (*see* p. 91), and this observation is interesting because the use of corticosteroids in this disease has been termed a 'medical adrenalectomy' by some authors.

SIZE OF METASTASIS
It would seem that the size of breast cancer metastases may also influence the response to endocrine therapy. Smaller lesions respond better than larger lesions, probably because of defective vascularity in the latter lesions. This generalisation applies to all forms of endocrine therapy, but there are site variations. In the case of soft tissue lesions, corticosteroid or androgen therapy tends to cause regression only of smaller lesions (*see* pp. 40 and 74), while oestrogen therapy appears to control larger lesions equally as well (*see* p. 56).

It is generally agreed that major endocrine ablation therapy gives poor results in the case of large metastases in the liver or brain (*see* p. 91), although corticosteroid therapy may be useful in such cases. In the case of bone metastases, large lesions seem to heal as well as do smaller lesions with all forms of endocrine therapy, if sclerotic changes in the radiograph are accepted as an index of healing.

PRETREATMENT HORMONAL BACKGROUND
The sex hormone pattern of the patient with breast cancer may be reflected in the cytohormonal assay of the vaginal or urethral smear (*see* p. 107), the urinary oestrogen excretion (*see* p. 106), androgen metabolite excretion (*see* p. 109), gonadotropin excretion (*see* p. 108), and prolactin excretion (*see* p. 109). These patterns have been variously suggested as being possible indices for predicting response to castration, bilateral adrenalectomy, hypophyseal ablation, oestrogen, progestin, or androgen therapy. The response to corticosteroid therapy appears to be unrelated to such pretreatment assays.

TUMOUR HISTOLOGY

It was suggested by Haddow *et al.* (1944), that highly cellular breast cancer is more likely to respond to oestrogen therapy, whereas Wolff (1957) reports the opposite finding. Huggins and Dao (1953) and Galante *et al.* (1957) suggested that more differentiated tumours are the most likely to show a beneficial response to adrenalectomy, but other authors, including Smith and Emerson (1954), Peters (1956), Cade (1958), Pyrah (1958), and Swyer *et al.* (1961) were unable to confirm any correlation between histological grading and response to endocrine therapy.

Previous X-ray therapy to a part prejudices the likelihood of a favourable hormonal response because of the impaired vascular supply.

PREVIOUS RESPONSE TO ENDOCRINE MANIPULATION

It has been noted (*see* p. 27) that following tumour growth remission from castration in breast cancer, subsequent favourable response to androgen therapy may occur in 30 per cent of cases according to Escher (1958), or to oestrogen or androgen therapy in 23 per cent of cases according to Hall *et al.* (1963*b*). Again, following tumour growth remission from castration there is a 44·7 per cent likelihood of a subsequent favourable response from major endocrine ablation therapy according to McDonald (1962). Of castration non-responders, only 11 per cent will respond favourably to a major ablative procedure.

There is disagreement as to whether tumour growth remission from oestrogen or androgen therapy by breast cancer predicts a favourable response to major endocrine ablation. Douglas (1957), Jessiman *et al.* (1959), Pearson and Ray (1960), Byron *et al.* (1962), and Dao and Nemoto (1965) claim that it does, while Atkins *et al.* (1966), and Ahlquist *et al.* (1968) could find no correlation between response to previous steroid therapy, and subsequent benefit from major endocrine ablation (*see* p. 89). The issue is clouded because some authors (Kimel *et al.*, 1957; Edelstyn *et al.*, 1965) regard a failure of response to oestrogen therapy as being a sign of 'oestrogen dependence'. Furthermore, Cade (1958) suggests that previous tumour 'aggravation' by sex hormones or palliation by corticosteroids, is likely to predict a favourable response to bilateral adrenalectomy.

Tumour growth remission from secondary oestrogen therapy is seen in 20 per cent of breast cancer cases after previous remission from androgen therapy (*see* p. 59). Secondary androgen therapy yields a further tumour growth remission in 22 per cent of cases after previous remission from oestrogen therapy (*see* p. 39). The benefit from secondary progestin therapy or corticosteroid therapy seems to bear no relation to previous response to oestrogens or androgens (*see* pp. 69 and 77).

PHYSICAL APPEARANCE

There is no evidence to support the belief (Cornil, 1949; Green, 1966) that the choice of a steroid for therapy in late breast cancer can be based upon the physical appearance of the patient. It has been suggested on an empirical basis that patients with a female configuration are better treated by androgens, while patients with a moderate hirsutism should be treated by oestrogens. This observation has not been correlated with hormonal excretion studies.

Principles of Sequential Endocrine Therapy

TODAY, APPROXIMATELY twenty years after the introduction of oestrogens, androgens, corticosteroids, bilateral adrenalectomy, and hypophyseal ablation into the clinical management of advanced breast cancer, there are still large trials of endocrine therapy being reported, which attempt to demonstrate the *overall* superiority of one method over another.

In a balanced survey of the place of endocrine ablation therapy in the management of advanced breast cancer, Juret (1966) writes of such therapy:

'A demonstration of the efficacy of a procedure does not indeed fully justify its routine use, nor resolve all problems concerning its application. It is also imperative to be sure that similar results could not be obtained by less offensive means . . . These uncertainties result in different treatments for similar lesions according to the centre where the patient has decided to take advice.'

The following sections survey some examples of these 'uncertainties'.

ADRENALECTOMY VERSUS CASTRATION

The proportion of tumour growth remissions and the average duration of remission from combined adrenalectomy and ovariectomy in the premenopausal patient are not conclusively shown to be any greater than those from radiation or surgical castration alone (Tables 4.1 and 9.1). There is, therefore, no reason to advise the combined procedure as the initial form of therapy in premenopausal cases. Furthermore, following a favourable response to surgical or radiation castration, the likelihood of a similar response to bilateral adrenalectomy is about 40 per cent (*see* p. 88). The length of remission from the two procedures separately is at least as great as, and almost certainly greater than, that from the combined procedures. If, on the other

hand, there has been no response to castration, adrenalectomy is not advised. This major operation can thus be avoided in the majority of patients, although hypophyseal ablation may still yield benefit in some of these cases (*see* p. 89).

ADRENALECTOMY VERSUS STEROID THERAPY

In earlier years, it was considered that bilateral adrenalectomy was indicated in the management of advanced breast cancer, only after failure of less drastic hormonal methods. However, in a recent review by Cade (1966), he concludes that 'adrenalectomy should be undertaken as soon as metastases are diagnosed and not as a last resort'. Similar views have been expressed by Irvine *et al.* (1961), Nelson and Dragstedt (1961), and Dao and Nemoto (1965). The reasons given for this opinion are, first, that the frequency and duration of tumour growth remissions are higher after bilateral adrenalectomy than they are after oestrogen, androgen, or other steroid therapy, and, second, that late adrenalectomy is less effective than early adrenalectomy in the endocrine control of breast cancer. The latter proposition is probably well substantiated, but the former needs further discussion.

A randomised trial by Dao and Nemoto (1965) compared the results of bilateral adrenalectomy with those of androgen therapy in postmenopausal patients with breast cancer. They noted that the former method was followed by a 45 per cent tumour remission rate, the latter by only a 16 per cent remission rate. In this trial the choice of androgen as the hormone for comparison was an unfortunate one. In a randomised comparison of oestrogen therapy and androgen therapy in postmenopausal patients by Kennedy and Brown (1965), oestrogen therapy was followed by a 45·5 per cent tumour remission rate, compared to a 13·6 per cent remission rate for androgen therapy.

It appears, therefore, that the *overall* use of oestrogen therapy in postmenopausal patients would probably provide a similar tumour remission rate to that arising from the overall use of bilateral adrenalectomy, although such a randomised trial has not yet been reported. Moreover, if treatment is *individualised*, giving oestrogen therapy to those postmenopausal patients with soft tissue and intrathoracic metastases, androgen therapy to those with bone metastases, and corticosteroid therapy to those with brain or liver metastases, the overall tumour remission rate in the author's experience is even higher than that from the overall use of oestrogen therapy only (*see also* p. 39).

ENDOCRINE ABLATION VERSUS 'CONSERVATIVE' THERAPY

McCalister *et al.* (1961) have suggested that hypophysectomy should be carried out at the first sign of recurrence in patients with breast cancer, and similar views have been expressed by Jessiman *et al.* (1959). The former authors suggest that it is 'reasonable to suppose that the longer the disease is left untreated, the more likely it is to become independent of hormonal control'. There is no evidence to support this suggestion, and, in fact, hormonal control is more likely when clinical evidence of recurrence takes longer to appear (*see* p. 89). Furthermore, 'prophylactic' bilateral adrenalectomy at the time of mastectomy does not improve the prognosis (*see* p. 88).

A recent trial has been reported by Atkins *et al.* (1966) comparing, on a random selection basis, the effect of 'conservative' therapy with that of major endocrine ablation therapy in advanced breast cancer. The first group of patients was treated initially by localised radiotherapy and also by steroid hormones—androgen therapy for those patients premenopausal or up to five years postmenopausal, and oestrogen therapy for the older patients. Patients in this group were referred for major endocrine ablation only if, and when, conservative therapy failed.

The second group was referred directly for major endocrine ablation, without any attempt at prior hormone therapy. It will be noted in the results of therapy (Table 13.1) that the proportion of patients showing remission of tumour growth, and the mean survival times, are very similar for both groups. Atkins and his group conclude from the trial that there is no clinical advantage to be gained in advising bilateral adrenalectomy or hypophysectomy at the first sign of recurrence after mastectomy. Furthermore, as a result of conservative therapy, over half

of the successful cases could be spared a major operation, with no difference in palliative results.

It should further be noted, that in this reported trial, 'conservative' therapy did not include castration for the premenopausal, or early postmenopausal women. Castration undoubtedly yields a higher tumour remission rate than does androgen therapy in these groups (*see* p. 25) and patients responding favourably to castration have a high likelihood of achieving a second remission of tumour growth from bilateral adrenalectomy or hypophysectomy (*see* p. 88). A preliminary trial of castration in the younger patients, should, therefore, yield an even

TABLE 13.1

Tumour Remission from Primary Steroid Therapy Followed by Major Endocrine Ablation, Compared to that from Immediate Endocrine Ablation in Breast Cancer (after Atkins *et al.*, 1966)

	'Operation' group	'Conservative' group
Remission from hormones	—	16%
Remission from operation	30%	12% (together 28%)
Mean survival	14·94 months	15·46 months
Mean period of remission (successful cases)	25·5 ,,	21·0 ,,

longer duration of tumour growth remission in the 'conservative' therapy group.

Although hypophyseal ablation should, in theory, provide a remission of tumour growth summating in its duration those from all lesser procedures added together, there is no evidence that it does so. In fact, most cancer therapists prefer the sequential method of endocrine management in breast cancer and postpone hypophyseal ablation (Stoll, 1956*a*; Randall, 1960; Hortling *et al.*, 1961; Dobson, 1962; Juret, 1966; Donegan, 1967; Tagnon *et al.*, 1967 and Edelstyn *et al.*, 1968). The disadvantages of early hypophyseal ablation are the complications of diabetes insipidus, the danger of adrenocortical insufficiency under stress, and the problem that when the tumour reactivates, favourable response to further hormone therapy is rare (Escher and Kaufman, 1961).

SEQUENCE OF HORMONAL THERAPY IN BREAST CANCER

The following methods of hormonal control are practised in the management of advanced breast cancer. The methods are used in an ordered sequence (Table 13.2), according to whether the tumour is found to be hormone sensitive or not, according to whether there is evidence of oestrogen secretion or not, and according to the stage and rapidity of progression of the tumour. (The detailed management of the individual patient by sequential therapy is described in the next chapter.)

Each step is followed in the sequence shown. If the is not transected by the operation. A similar procedure is possible for the removal of a mobile mass of breast tumour, recurring after a previous local excision. Dissection of mobile axillary nodes which may appear after a simple mastectomy, has been shown to control the disease locally for a prolonged period (Ackland, 1968). Decompression laminectomy is indicated as an emergency operation on the appearance of symptoms suggesting pressure from metastases upon the spinal cord, radiation therapy being postponed until after the operation.

Radiotherapy should always be utilised for the control of localised, slowly growing manifestations

TABLE 13.2

Suggested Scheme of Sequential Management of Advanced Breast Cancer

Treatment stage	Hormone sensitive		Hormone insensitive	
	Oestrogen present	Oestrogen absent	Oestrogen present	Oestrogen absent
1 (Localised)	Radiotherapy			
2 (Disseminated)	Surgical castration	Oestrogen ℞	Ovarian irradiation inc. Corticosteroid ℞ and corticosteroid ℞	
3	Androgen or progestin ℞ or bilateral adrenalectomy			
4	Hypophyseal ablation (surgical)		Hypophyseal ablation (radiation)	
5	Progestin-oestrogen ℞		Cytotoxic agent ℞	

Note (*a*) Check hormone sensitivity after each stage of treatment
     (*b*) If hormone sensitivity changes after stages 2, 3 or 4, read the opposite side of table
     (*c*) In stage 3 choose treatment according to biological determinant
     (*d*) If disease is progressing rapidly after stage 2, omit stage 3

disease is obviously progressing, and if the indices of tumour activity show a rising level, the next method in sequence is proceeded to. It is useful to check the hormone sensitivity of the tumour before every change in treatment.

PRELIMINARY SURGERY OR RADIOTHERAPY

Both surgery and radiation therapy have a part to play in the management of recurrent and inoperable breast cancer, and such treatment may even be concomitant with endocrine therapy. Mention is made of the most common applications.

Palliative simple mastectomy is useful for the removal of a mobile ulcerated breast tumour in the presence of metastases, as long as malignant tissue of breast cancer particularly if they are causing symptoms (Taylor and Morris, 1951; Segaloff, 1960; Dobson, 1962). Practically all types of soft tissue deposits, such as the primary tumour, skin nodules, parasternal recurrence, axillary and supraclavicular nodes, can be controlled for periods usually ranging from six to twenty-four months. Bone metastases liable to pathological fracture should be irradiated urgently. The pain of bone metastases is almost invariably relieved within two or three weeks of radiation, and subsequent recalcification of bone metastases is not uncommon. Pressure symptoms, due to cerebral or mediastinal metastases, can be controlled for a period of six months or longer.

Endocrine therapy is reserved until the disease becomes disseminated.

1. CASTRATION

This is carried out surgically in urgent or hormone sensitive cases, but by irradiation of the ovaries combined with corticosteroid administration, in hormone insensitive cases. Castration is advised in all cases if the patient is premenopausal, and also after the menopause if persistent oestrogen secretion of ovarian origin is shown to be likely (*see* p. 25).

2. OESTROGEN THERAPY

This is advised in hormone sensitive cases if the patient is more than five years postmenopausal, or earlier than that, if cessation of oestrogen secretion is demonstrated (*see* p. 55).

3. ANDROGEN THERAPY: 4. PROGESTIN THERAPY: 5. BILATERAL ADRENALECTOMY

These methods of treatment are advised in hormone sensitive cases when methods (1) or (2) have failed or lost their effect, as long as the patients' symptoms are not urgent. Selection of one of these methods, is based upon the individual's biological determinants of response (*see* p. 115).

6. CORTICOSTEROID THERAPY

This is advised in primarily hormone insensitive cases, or after the development of autonomy in the tumour. Favourable response to such treatment is usually limited in time, and a small proportion of these patients may still respond to hypophyseal ablation later.

7. PROGESTIN/OESTROGEN THERAPY

Recent reports by Landau *et al.* (1963) and Kennedy (1965*b*) suggest that a combination therapy of high doses of progestin with low doses of oestrogen, may lead to tumour control even after hypophyseal ablation. Reports by the author (Stoll, 1967*a*) suggest that the addition of a progestin may sensitise breast cancer to the effect of oestrogen, after previous failure of control to this hormone. Trial of such a combination is thus indicated in an apparently hormone insensitive case of breast cancer, either before or after hypophyseal ablation.

8. HYPOPHYSEAL ABLATION

Whether carried out by surgery or by irradiation, hypophyseal ablation has a place in the treatment of apparently hormone insensitive as well as in hormone sensitive tumours. If symptoms are urgent, it is indicated after methods (1) or (2) have failed, but if symptoms are not urgent, it is postponed until after a trial of methods (3) to (7). Ablation of hypophyseal function by irradiation is preferred for apparently hormone insensitive tumours, because of its relatively minor morbidity.

9. CYTOTOXIC THERAPY

This is reserved for patients showing reactivation of the disease after hypophyseal ablation. Favourable response to such treatment is usually very limited in time, and therefore a preliminary trial of a combination of progestin and oestrogen therapy is usually indicated, if the patient's symptoms are not urgent.

14

Scheme of Individualised Hormonal Management

THE AUTHOR has emphasised for many years (Stoll, 1958*b*), that future developments in the endocrine therapy of breast cancer must include steps to individualise treatment in a rational manner. In our present state of knowledge, this can be achieved in many cases with the aid of biochemical indices to measure both the activity of the tumour, and the hormonal sensitivity of the tumour. Such criteria need to be established repeatedly, in relation to measurements of the shifting hormonal environment of the tumour.

Possible indices of this kind have been discussed in Chapter Eleven, and a selected group of the more simple procedures can be used in clinical practice to indicate the three major guiding factors which relate the tumour to its hormonal environment during endocrine therapy. The tests selected are all within the scope of the average hospital laboratory. (When the results are found to be equivocal, selection of treatment can be based only upon the biological determinants of response, and therefore, reference to these also is made in the following sections.)

1. *Tumour activity* as reflected by the levels of phosphohexose isomerase and lactic dehydrogenase in the serum (*see* p. 104); also by the serum alkaline phosphatase and calcium levels, if bone metastases are present (*see* p. 101).

2. *Tumour sensitivity to hormones* as reflected by the response of the serum phosphohexose isomerase level to steroid provocation or inhibition (*see* p. 103).

3. *The hormonal environment* of the tumour as reflected by serial estimations of the oestrogen excretion level in the urine (*see* p. 106), and by cyto-hormonal assessment of serial vaginal smears (*see* p. 107).

The result of the urinary 'discriminant function' (*see* p. 109) is claimed in some retrospective series to be correlated with the likelihood of favourable response to major endocrine ablation therapy. Although under trial, results have not yet been significant in a prospective series. As the result is not significant if the patient has recently been castrated or has received steroid therapy, the estimation of the 'discriminant function' must be carried out at the patient's *first* attendance, if it is to be used in a prospective fashion to select patients for major endocrine ablation.

PROPHYLACTIC CASTRATION

The value of prophylactic castration has been discussed earlier (*see* p. 29). In the author's opinion, it is indicated at the time of mastectomy only in Stage 2 cases (i.e. in the presence of axillary node metastases). Whether at this stage, castration is surgical or radio-therapeutic, is a matter of convenience, as either is effective (*see* p. 24).

1. INITIAL THERAPY IN ADVANCED CASES

The initial form of endocrine therapy in advanced breast cancer is decided by the presence or absence of measurable oestrogen secretion in the body. It is assumed present in premenopausal women, but, if menses have ceased, weekly assays of the urinary oestrogen excretion, or of the vaginal smear, are carried out for a month. Cyclical fluctuation in oestrogen excretion, or persistent oestrogen secretion after dexamethasone suppression, are suggestive of persistent ovarian secretion (*see* p. 107).

The tumour activity is assessed by serial estimations of the phosphohexose isomerase and the lactic dehydrogenase levels in the serum. If bone metastases are present, serial serum calcium and serum alkaline phosphatase estimations are carried out in addition. The tumour sensitivity to hormones is assessed by the effect of steroid provocation or inhibition upon the isomerase level. Management of the patient is then as follows:

(a) PREMENOPAUSAL OR WITH PERSISTENT OVARIAN SECRETION

Therapeutic castration is indicated as the initial method of endocrine treatment for all premenopausal patients with advanced breast cancer or with recurrence after mastectomy. It is indicated as the initial method of treatment also for postmenopausal patients with persistent ovarian secretion, and for all patients within two years of the menopause, if the results of the vaginal smear examination, or oestrogen excretion assessment are equivocal.

If *sensitivity to hormones* is shown by the enzyme assay method, castration by surgery is advised, and further management is as described later in Section 2(a). If the result of the test is equivocal, surgical castration is advised in the case of clinical urgency, including the presence of hypercalcaemia, painful bone metastases, or of lung, pleural, brain or liver metastases. Castration by surgery is indicated also in other types of metastasis, if tumour growth is rapid. Radiation castration is equally as effective in ablating oestrogen secretion, but slower in its action (*see* p. 24).

A short course of corticosteroid therapy before surgical castration may be usefully associated in the patient with hypercalcaemia (*see* p. 77), or in the very ill patient (*see* p. 29). Added androgen therapy, started immediately after castration, is advised in the presence of bone metastases, or in the case of patients under thirty-five years of age (*see* p. 29).

If *insensitivity to hormones* is shown by the enzyme assay method, or suggested by a short recurrence-free period, treatment is by a combination of ovarian irradiation and corticosteroid therapy. Apart from clinical observations on the progress of the tumour, serial monthly indices of tumour activity, and serial monthly oestrogen excretion levels are then estimated. The vaginal smear will yield no useful information at this stage, as its pattern will be influenced by the costicosteroid therapy.

In the absence of urgent symptoms, four to six months should be allowed for evidence of tumour remission to manifest after the combined therapy. If after that time, there is no objective evidence of tumour regression, and the indices of tumour activity continue to rise, the enzyme tests of hormone sensitivity are repeated. If they now show sensitivity to be present, a course of progestin or androgen therapy is advised, selecting the steroid by consideration of the biological determinants of response as in Section 3(a) later. Otherwise, an attempt is made at hypophyseal ablation by radiation, especially if the original urinary 'discriminant function' was positive.

(b) POSTMENOPAUSAL WITH CESSATION OF OESTROGEN SECRETION

If *sensitivity to hormones* is shown by the enzyme assay method in the absence of demonstrable oestrogen secretion by the ovaries, oestrogen therapy is advised and its management is as described in Section 2(b). It is also advised in patients more than five years postmenopausal, if the results of oestrogen excretion are equivocal. Oestrogen therapy causes a higher proportion of tumour remissions in older postmenopausal women, than any other method of endocrine therapy.

In patients between two and five years following the menopause, if the results of the vaginal smear examination and oestrogen excretion assessment are equivocal, androgen therapy is indicated as the initial method of treatment. Oestrogen therapy in this group may cause tumour growth stimulation. Favourable response to androgens is common in the presence of bone metastases (*see* p. 38) but rare for other sites. In the presence of hypercalcaemia, liver or brain metastases, corticosteroid therapy is preferred to androgen therapy.

In the presence of bone metastases, the addition of an alkylating agent (*see* p. 45) or of radioactive phosphorus (*see* p. 45) to androgen therapy is said to increase the likelihood of a favourable response. The author prefers to withhold the additional therapy until response from androgen therapy alone is lost.

If *insensitivity to hormones* is shown by the enzyme assay method, or suggested by a short recurrence-free period, treatment is by corticosteroid therapy. This is continued for at least three months, with serial monthly examinations of the indices of tumour activity (*see* Section 3(a) later). If these continue to rise and there is no objective evidence of tumour regression, enzyme assays of hormone sensitivity are repeated. If hormone sensitivity is now shown a course of oestrogen therapy is administered as in Section 2(b) later. Otherwise an attempt at tumour control is made by hypophyseal ablation especially if the original urinary 'discriminant function' was positive. A radiation ablation method is preferred to surgical ablation in hormone insensitive cases because of its relatively minor morbidity.

(2) CASTRATION OR OESTROGEN THERAPY

(a) SURGICAL CASTRATION

If hormonal sensitivity is shown by enzyme assays in the patient with persistent oestrogen secretion, surgical castration is advised. Following castration, serial estimations of urinary oestrogen secretion are carried out. In addition to clinical observations on the progress of the disease, serial monthly indices of tumour activity are measured in order to assess the duration of tumour control. It should be taken into account that in the presence of bone metastases, the serum alkaline phosphatase level may show an initial 'flare' before demonstrating a slow fall towards normal. Further treatment is as described in section 3(*a*).

(*b*) OESTROGEN THERAPY

If hormonal sensitivity is shown, in the absence of oestrogen secretion, oestrogen therapy is advised. The likelihood of response to oestrogen therapy increases with advancing postmenopausal age (*see* p. 55). The best results of oestrogen therapy are in the presence of metastases in soft tissue, bone, lung or pleura (*see* p. 55). Oestrogen therapy is also indicated following loss of response or absence of response to androgen therapy (*see* section 4 later). In the presence of hypercalcaemia, liver or brain metastases, corticosteroid therapy is preferred to oestrogen therapy.

In the patient receiving oestrogen therapy, serial monthly examination of vaginal smears is carried out. By this means is determined the lowest possible dose of oestrogen for the patient, compatible with achieving a Karyo-pyknotic (cornification) index in the vaginal smear of 50 per cent or more (*see* p. 107). It is usually found that the KPI level of the smear tends to fall progressively in the monthly assay, even if the same level of oestrogen dosage is maintained. This is due to the progressive decrease in sensitivity of the vaginal mucosa, which is commonly associated with long-term oestrogen administration.

In such cases there is no need to increase the dose of oestrogen, as long as the disease appears clinically to be under control and indices of tumour activity remain low. If however, serial observations show a rising trend in the level of these indices, and the KPI level of the smear falls below 50 per cent, then the dose of oestrogen should be increased (taking into account the patient's cardiovascular condition). A rise in the KPI level to 50 per cent or more is aimed at, and if this cannot be achieved by repeated increments in the dose of oral oestrogen, then parenteral forms of oestrogen therapy, such as oestradiol monobenzoate, Honvan or Estradurin may be tried.

Indices of tumour activity are measured monthly during oestrogen therapy in conjunction with observations on clinical progress, in order to assess the duration of tumour control. Further treatment is as described in section 3(*b*).

3. RELAPSE AFTER CASTRATION OR OESTROGEN THERAPY

(*a*) AFTER CASTRATION

The following management applies whether or not there has been a favourable response to castration. The mechanism of relapse after a previous favourable response to castration has been discussed previously (*see* p. 3). In the majority of patients, clinical evidence of relapse occurs within twelve to eighteen months of castration. If, when it occurs, not only are the indices of tumour activity rising, but also at the same time the oestrogen excretion level is rising, then tumour autonomy need not necessarily be the cause of the relapse. It is advisable in such cases to assess the hormonal sensitivity of the tumour by the steroid provocation or inhibition test.

If *insensitivity to hormones* is shown by enzyme assays, or suggested by a short recurrence-free period after mastectomy or by failure of response to castration, treatment is generally by corticosteroids. This treatment is almost always beneficial in the presence of hypercalcaemia or of lung, pleural, peritoneal, liver or brain metastases, whether or not there has been a response to previous castration (*see* p. 77). In the presence of hypercalcaemia, subsequent major endocrine ablation therapy (usually by hypophyseal ablation), is indicated after control of the serum calcium level is achieved. The addition of alkylating agent therapy to corticosteroids may be useful in the presence of brain, lung, pleural, or peritoneal metastases (*see* p. 79). Corticosteroid therapy is indicated also as an alternative to major endocrine ablation therapy in patients who are very ill. This would apply especially if the original 'discriminant function' was negative.

A good response to corticosteroid therapy is often followed by an attempt at hypophyseal ablation by radiation. This applies especially if the original 'discriminant function' was positive, even if there has been no response to castration. According to McDonald (1962), 11 per cent of castration non-responders will still show favourable response to major endocrine ablation therapy.

If, however, *sensitivity to hormones* is still present, management depends on the urgency of symptoms. If the patient's symptoms are urgent, and especially if the original 'discriminant function' was positive, a trial of bilateral adrenalectomy or of hypophyseal ablation is advised. These are indicated whether or not there was a response to previous castration, although remission is more likely in those patients previously responding favourably to castration. An exception is made for patients with hypercalcaemia, brain or liver metastases who are selected for corticosteroid therapy as noted above.

Hypophyseal ablation is preferred to bilateral adrenalectomy in younger women (under fifty years of age) and those with painful bone metastases (*see* p. 92). Neither method gives good results in the presence of large metastases or a short recurrence-free period (*see* p. 89). Hypophyseal ablation by irradiation is preferred in cases who have not previously responded to castration or those in poor condition.

If the patient's symptoms are not urgent, a trial of androgen or progestin therapy is indicated, selecting the steroid after consideration of the biological determinants of response. Androgen therapy is preferred after loss of response to therapeutic castration, especially in the presence of a long free interval between mastectomy and recurrence (*see* p. 38). Androgen therapy is especially useful in the presence of painful bone metastases except in the presence of hypercalcaemia when corticosteroid therapy is indicated (*see* p. 77). In the presence of bone metastases, the addition of alkylating agent therapy (*see* p. 45) or of radioactive phosphorus (*see* p. 45) is said to increase the likelihood of a favourable response. The author prefers to withhold the additional therapy unless response from androgen therapy alone is lost.

In patients having responded favourably to castration, a further tumour growth remission for androgen therapy is achieved in about 30 per cent of cases, according to Escher (1958). However, patients not having responded favourably to castration very rarely respond to subsequent androgen therapy, and progestin therapy is preferred in such cases. Progestin response is not related to previous sex hormone response, in the author's experience (Stoll, 1966), and progestin therapy is especially useful in the presence of soft tissue metastases (*see* p. 69).

(*b*) AFTER OESTROGEN THERAPY

The following management applies whether or not there has been a favourable response to oestrogens. Clinical evidence of relapse usually occurs within two years of a response to oestrogen therapy. When reactivation of tumour occurs, merely stopping the oestrogen administration will yield a withdrawal response in approximately 30 per cent of cases (*see* p. 59). Advantage should be taken of such a possibility, watching the objective and biochemical criteria of tumour activity. Except in cases of emergency, therefore, at least two months should be allowed after temporary tumour control from oestrogen therapy, before proceeding to another form of endocrine therapy. Endocrine management after oestrogen therapy is otherwise similar to that described in section 3(*a*) above.

If *insensitivity to hormones* is shown by enzyme assays, or suggested by a short recurrence-free period following mastectomy or failure of response to oestrogen therapy, treatment is generally by corticosteroids. This treatment is especially indicated in the presence of hypercalcaemia or of lung, pleural, peritoneal, liver, or brain metastases. In the case of hypercalcaemia, subsequent major endocrine ablation therapy (usually by hypophyseal ablation), is indicated after control of the serum calcium level is achieved. Corticosteroid therapy is indicated also as an alternative to major endocrine ablation therapy in patients who are very ill, especially if the original 'discriminant function' was negative. The addition to corticosteroid therapy of alkylating agents may be useful in the case of brain, lung, pleural or peritoneal metastases.

A good response to corticosteroid therapy is often followed by an attempt at hypophyseal ablation by irradiation. This would apply especially if the original 'discriminant function' was positive, and tumour remission is possible even if there was no tumour remission from oestrogen therapy.

If however, *sensitivity to hormones* is still present as shown in the enzyme assay test, management depends on the urgency of the symptoms. If the patient's symptoms are urgent, and especially if the original 'discriminant function' was positive, bilateral adrenalectomy or ablation of the hypophysis is advised. The latter is preferred for patients with painful bone metastases, or those previously not showing response to oestrogens. Generally, corticosteroid therapy is preferred in patients with hypercalcaemia, brain or liver metastases.

If the patient's symptoms are not urgent, a trial of androgen or progestin therapy is suggested, selecting the steroid as described in section 3(*a*) above. In patients who have responded favourably to oestrogen therapy, a similar response to androgen therapy is achieved in about 30 per cent of cases according to Escher and Kaufman (1961) and Witt *et al.* (1963). The likelihood of response to androgen therapy increases with advancing postmenopausal age. In patients not responding previously to oestrogen therapy, favourable response to androgen therapy is seen in about 5 per cent of cases according to Escher and Kaufman (1961), and such a response is seen mainly in patients with bone metastases.

Progestin therapy is indicated especially in the presence of soft tissue metastases, before proceeding to major endocrine ablation therapy. This applies whether or not there was a previous response to oestrogen or androgen therapy. A combination of progestin and oestrogen may achieve a remission in patients previously not responding to oestrogen therapy (*see* p. 69).

4. RELAPSE AFTER ANDROGEN OR PROGESTIN THERAPY

If the indices of tumour activity begin to rise and clinical evidence of relapse occurs, a further estimation of hormonal sensitivity by enzyme assay is necessary to decide if autonomy has occurred in the tumour.

If *sensitivity to hormones* is still present, bilateral adrenalectomy can be considered before hypophyseal ablation, if the general condition of the patient warrants it, and after consideration of the biological determinants of response. Prolonged tumour growth remission from bilateral adrenalectomy is particularly common in patients who have previously responded favourably to castration.

However, in those cases treated primarily by androgens (*see* section 1(*b*) above) a trial of oestrogen therapy is indicated before major endocrine ablation is considered. Secondary oestrogen therapy will lead to tumour remission in 20 per cent of cases following previous favourable response to androgen therapy, the likelihood of response being greater with advancing postmenopausal age (*see* p. 59).

If *insensitivity to hormones* is shown by enzyme assays or suggested by a short recurrence-free period following mastectomy, or failure of response to sex steroid therapy, a course of corticosteroid therapy is advised. Finally, hypophyseal ablation is indicated after consideration of the original urinary 'discriminant function'. Hypophyseal ablation by surgery is undertaken if the latter was positive and the patient's general condition permits it. Radiation ablation is preferred if there was no previous response to sex hormone therapy, or the urinary 'discriminant function' was negative or the patient is in poor general condition.

5. RELAPSE AFTER HYPOPHYSEAL ABLATION

Failure to show favourable response to hypophyseal ablation does not preclude the possibility of hormonal sensitivity, if evidence of pituitary secretion persists after the operation. When tumour reactivation occurs after hypophyseal ablation, there is often functional evidence of residual pituitary gland secretion, such as, for example, persistent urinary gonadotropin excretion (*see* p. 92). A course of progestin and oestrogen in combination may yield a favourable response in some cases (particularly those with soft tissue metastases) or a course of fluoxymesterone in others (particularly those with bone metastases). In the absence of hormonal sensitivity, localised radio-therapy or the use of cytotoxic agents, are the only forms of therapy likely to control tumour growth.

Comparison with other schemes of Endocrine Therapy

It will be noted that the scheme of endocrine control presented in this chapter differs in several major respects from others exemplified by those of Pearson and Lipsett (1956), Kennedy (1965*a*), Juret (1966), and Donegan (1967).

1. Selection of treatment method is based upon preliminary determination of tumour sensitivity to hormones, *and* the determination of the presence of measurable oestrogen secretion in the body. Both these determinations are repeated before every change in treatment. In the postmenopausal female, surgical castration should be advised in the presence of persistent ovarian secretion, or oestrogen therapy in the presence of an atrophic smear but in either case, *only if hormonal sensitivity is shown.*

2. Selection of androgen or progestin therapy is based upon biological determinants of response in the individual. As a result, in non-urgent cases, hypophyseal ablation can be postponed until the benefit of administering these steroids is observed.

3. A decision to change treatment is based upon rising biochemical indices of tumour activity, in addition to objective evidence of advancing disease. Rise in the level of these indices may considerably antedate evidence of clinical relapse, and, thus, permits change in treatment to occur more promptly.

4. Corticosteroid therapy is preferred to adrenalectomy in the presence of hypercalcaemia or of metastases in the lungs, pleura, peritoneum, brain, or liver. Such treatment may render the patient suitable for later hypophyseal ablation.

5. Progestin therapy can be used in an attempt to sensitise breast cancer to the effect of oestrogen therapy, either before or after hypophyseal ablation.

6. If hormonal sensitivity is demonstrated in a relapse after hypophyseal ablation, treatment is by a combination of progestin and oestrogen, or else by fluoxymesterone.

15

Breast Cancer in the Male

THE INCIDENCE of breast cancer in the male is only about 1 per cent of that in the female. In most reported series the commonest age group for its appearance is the decade between fifty and sixty, somewhat older than the commonest presenting age group in the female.

The prognosis, even in Stage 1 cases, is relatively worse in the male than in the female, and blood borne metastases are common. It is likely that the disease is already disseminated in the vast majority of patients before curative therapy is attempted, although the metastases may not manifest clinically for many years. Hormonal therapy is, therefore, of considerable importance in the management of male breast cancer.

HORMONAL INFLUENCES IN THE DEVELOPMENT OF MALE BREAST CANCER

The presence of long continued, high oestrogen levels in the blood has been suggested as a cause of breast cancer developing in the male. The clinical manifestation of the disease after oestrogen therapy for prostatic cancer, was reported by Abramson and Warshawski (1948) and by Howard and Grosjean (1949). More recently, it has been suggested that the majority of such cases are instances of prostatic cancer metastasis in breast tissue, hyperplastic as a result of oestrogen therapy. Campbell et al. (1962) confirmed the metastatic nature of such tumours, by demonstrating the high acid phosphatase content in a biopsy of the breast tumour.

It must be emphasised that the development of breast cancer may well reflect a hormonal imbalance existing ten to fifteen years before the clinical onset of the disease (Bulbrook, 1966). If due to an excess of oestrogen, such an abnormality could arise either from changes in anterior pituitary or adrenocortical secretion, or from abnormal metabolism of the sex steroids or decrease in their breakdown by the liver.

A shift in the oestrogen-androgen ratio would result from such changes. Alternatively, breast cancer could arise from an abnormal susceptibility of breast tissue to normal concentration of oestrogens.

It has been suggested by Davies (1949) that the high incidence both of gynaecomastia and of breast cancer in Bantu males is due to the failure of oestrogen inactivation by a damaged liver associated with vitamin B deficiency in these races. The peak incidence of male breast cancer is about ten years later than that of gynaecomastia, according to Bonser et al. (1961) and this time period would be compatible with a causal relationship.

The coexistence of gynaecomastia has been reported in an unusually high proportion of some male breast cancer series—19 per cent of that of Gilbert (1933) and 12·5 per cent of that of Liechty et al. (1967). Such gynaecomastia is usually unilateral and characterised microscopically by proliferation of both acinar and stromal elements, associated with the presence of epithelial hyperplasia. On the other hand, some reported series of male breast cancer, such as that of Treves (1959), find associated gynaecomastia to be a rare occurrence.

THEORETICAL BASIS OF HORMONAL THERAPY IN MALE BREAST CANCER

The Sertoli cells of the testis are thought to secrete oestrogens, and the Leydig cells, androgens. Hyperplasia of either group of cells can be associated with the development of gynaecomastia (Collins and Cameron, 1964; Collins and Symington, 1964). According to Teilum (1950) there is a relative predominance of lipochrome pigments in the Sertoli cells after the age of sixty years and this may explain why oestrogen secretion persists longer.

According to Burrows and Horning (1952), excessive oestrogenic stimulation is responsible for the development of breast cancer in the male. Once established, however, the continued growth of the tumour may depend more upon androgen secretion (Fig. 15.1).

On the basis of this hypothesis, it is suggested that hormone sensitive breast cancer in males retains androgen dependence, and the beneficial results of orchidectomy follow from withdrawal of testicular androgens. Even in the minority of patients who do not show a clinical response to orchidectomy, it is possible that there is a phase when the tumour is hormone dependent, although this phase may be so

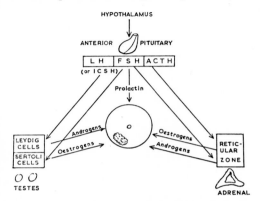

FIGURE 15.1 Diagrammatic representation of the hormonal factors which influence the growth of breast cancer in the male

→ denotes a controlling effect
(Figure modified from Valk and Owen, 1954)

short lived that it is not clinically discernible. After a shorter or longer period, all male breast cancers finally become autonomous and independent of hormonal control.

The exacerbating influence of androgens on the tumour (*see* p. 129) can be explained on the basis of the foregoing hypothesis. The palliative effect of oestrogen therapy in occasional cases, has been variously explained on the basis either of pituitary inhibition, or of direct antagonism to androgens at the target organ, or of a direct effect upon the metabolism of the tumour cells (*see* p. 15). However, there is no doubt that oestrogen therapy is a relatively less successful form of contrasexual hormone therapy in the male, than is androgen therapy in the female. In both cases, it is possible that such therapy acts by upsetting the normal androgen-oestrogen balance existing in the body, the environment of which the tumour finds favourable for growth.

CASTRATION IN MALE BREAST CANCER

As in the female, radiation therapy is the first step in the treatment of localised metastases in the skin,

nodes, or skeleton which are causing symptoms. The beneficial results of castration in advanced cancer of the breast in males, were early reported by Farrow and Adair (1942). The clinical palliation from such treatment is usually more striking than that resulting in the female from similar therapy. This may be because of the lesser complexity of sex hormone control in the male (Fig. 15.1).

According to Treves (1959), objective evidence of breast cancer regression is seen in 68 per cent of male patients who are castrated—approximately twice the proportion seen in the female. Regression in the size of skin or node metastases is the most common, but recalcification of bone metastases is not unusual. The average duration of such tumour growth remission is 29·6 months, and prolongation of life in such patients, compared to untreated patients, is undoubted.

To counteract the emotional resistance of patients to castration, subcapsular orchidectomy is widely practised—the operation cavity eventually filling with fibrosed blood clot. It is important, however, that subcapsular orchidectomy should ensure removal of *all* testicular tissue. Persistent androgen secretion in response to gonadotropin stimulation has been reported by O'Conor *et al.* (1963), in the majority of a group of patients treated by subcapsular orchidectomy. In these cases, the androgen secretion was later abolished by total orchidectomy.

X-ray irradiation of the testes of patients with male breast cancer leads to atrophy of the seminiferous tubules. The interstitial Leydig cells of the testicular tissue, and even more, the Sertoli cells are more resistant to irradiation (Collins and Pugh, 1964). Irradiation is followed by decrease in the urinary androgen excretion level, but very rarely by complete suppression of the hormone secretion. The latter requires very high dosage which would not be practicable, because the skin of the scrotal wall does not tolerate irradiation well.

Bone is the most frequent site of metastasis from breast cancer in the male, as it is in the female, and castration results in almost complete relief of pain in the vast majority of patients so treated. Pain relief is not uncommonly maintained in the male for four to five years after castration, although tumour regression in soft tissue and visceral metastases is rarely maintained for over two years. According to Treves (1959), the longer the interval between mastectomy and recurrence, the longer the period of tumour growth remission following castration. As in the female, there is no correlation between the histological grading of the breast cancer, and the likelihood of tumour growth remission from castration.

PROPHYLACTIC CASTRATION

By analogy with female breast cancer, the use of prophylactic castration at the time of mastectomy has been suggested also for the male. The indication for such treatment is even greater than in the female, because of the higher likelihood of tumour recurrence in the male. Subcapsular orchidectomy as a prophylactic measure, is therefore advised especially in Stage 2 cases (those with invaded axillary nodes) aged over sixty-five. Even if it does not actually prolong life, it should provide a high likelihood of delaying the onset of recurrence, thus giving the patient a longer period of physical and psychological well-being.

MAJOR ENDOCRINE ABLATION THERAPY

The practice of bilateral adrenalectomy or hypophyseal ablation has been suggested after castration has lost its control of tumour activity. On the other hand, Treves (1959) as a result of wide experience in the management of male breast cancer, considers corticosteroid therapy to be more efficacious than major endocrine ablation in such cases.

Because of the rarity of breast cancer in males, the reports of major endocrine ablation therapy are on very small groups of patients, and its place in management is, therefore, difficult to evaluate. Dao and Huggins (1957) and Cade (1958) were among the first to report tumour growth remission following bilateral adrenalectomy in occasional cases. McLaughlin *et al.* (1965) reviewed the literature, and reported objective evidence of tumour regression following bilateral adrenalectomy in eight out of twelve cases. According to Ray and Pearson (1956) and to Luft *et al.* (1958), favourable response may be seen also following hypophysectomy in occasional cases.

CORTICOSTEROID THERAPY

This is the form of endocrine treatment advised by Treves (1959) in all male patients with breast cancer reactivating after castration, but other authors prefer to reserve corticosteroid therapy only for such patients as are unfit for major endocrine ablation therapy. The palliative results of corticosteroid therapy in male breast cancer are similar to those seen in the female (*see* p. 74). Objective evidence of tumour regression, such as healing of ulcerated tumour or of lytic bone metastases, is rarely seen, but subjective benefit and relief of pain are seen in the majority of patients. Like the benefit from castra-tion, corticosteroid-induced palliation seems to be more prolonged in the male, than in the female with similar disease. Control of metastatic bone pain for two years or more in the male, is not uncommon in the author's experience.

The recommended dosage of prednisolone or prednisone is 30 mg daily, increased to 100 mg daily in the presence of urgent symptoms (*see* p. 77). Reduction of the dosage to 20 mg daily may be attempted once control is established, but more often it is found necessary to increase the dose in order to maintain control over a long period. The risk of increase in side-effects must be accepted if no alternative method of treatment is likely to help.

OESTROGEN THERAPY

Oestrogen therapy is rarely effective in the management of advanced male breast cancer, and castration is preferred as the primary method of endocrine treatment. Nevertheless, Huggins and Taylor (1955) reported occasional cases of clinical benefit from oestrogen treatment. Treves (1959) reported favourable response to oestrogen therapy in only two out of fourteen patients treated by 15 mg stilboestrol or 1·5 mg ethinyl oestradiol daily. He considers that, as the results of oestrogen therapy are poor and unpredictable, corticosteroid therapy is the preferred form of treatment after clinical control of tumour activity has been lost from castration. He has noted no benefit from the addition of oestrogen therapy to castration, in the primary treatment of disseminated cancer of the breast in the male.

ANDROGEN THERAPY

Farrow and Adair (1942) early reported that androgen administration is likely to cause exacerbation of pain in the presence of bone metastases from male breast cancer and Huggins (1954) confirmed this observation. Androgen-induced exacerbation of objective manifestations of the disease has not been reported clinically, but exacerbation has been demonstrated biochemically in the following manner.

A series of testosterone propionate injections 100 mg daily for three days can establish the existence of hormone sensitivity in male breast cancer, after control of the tumour growth has been lost from castration. If the injections of androgen lead to an increase in the serum level of phosphohexose isomerase (*see* p. 103) it will suggest sex hormone sensitivity, and, therefore, the choice of either oestrogen therapy, bilateral adrenalectomy, or hypophyseal ablation, in preference to corticosteroid therapy.

TO SUMMARISE

Castration as the primary method of treatment in advanced male breast cancer yields striking palliative benefit, both objective and subjective, which may be prolonged for years. When clinical control of tumour activity is lost, the choice is between major endocrine ablation therapy and corticosteroid therapy. Oestrogen therapy is of minor benefit in this disease, either by itself or in association with castration, as primary treatment.

16

The Place of Cytotoxic Chemotherapy

AT FIRST sight, the relevance of this chapter to a book on hormonal therapy may not be obvious. However, there are several stages in the evolution of breast cancer, when cytotoxic therapy presents itself either as an alternative, or as a concomitant method, to hormonal control. Examples of the latter application which have been mentioned previously are the combination of an alkylating agent with corticosteroid therapy or with androgen therapy (*see* pp. 45 and 79). Such a combination of a steroid and a cytotoxic agent may block several pathways of tumour metabolism at the same time, and provides a possibility of synergic action.

As an alternative to hormones, it is claimed that in patients who are less than one year postmenopausal, the administration of 5 fluoro-uracil is more likely to lead to a remission of tumour growth than is the use of hormonal agents (Segaloff, 1967*b*). The selection of the most suitable stage of the disease for cytotoxic therapy, alone or in combination, and a knowledge of the benefit and toxicity liable to result from the administration of different agents, becomes essential for the clinician controlling the hormonal palliation of late breast cancer.

PROPHYLAXIS BY CYTOTOXIC AGENTS

Malignant cells have been demonstrated in the blood of patients with apparently localised breast cancer. A sharp rise in their number in the venous system during radical surgery for cancer, led to the suggestion of prophylactic systemic chemotherapy at the time of, and just after, surgery. Various agents have been tried, and from a nation-wide controlled trial in the USA, Noer *et al.* (1964) concluded that thioTEPA administration led to a decrease in the tumour recurrence rate following mastectomy for breast cancer (Table 16.1).

Such an effect has been assumed to result from a cytotoxic effect upon malignant cells liberated at

operation, but in the case of breast cancer it could also be due to an indirect endocrine effect. The report showed that the major improvement occurred in *premenopausal* Stage 2 cases, and it has been shown by Sears *et al.* (1960) that thioTEPA administration will cause amenorrhoea even before it causes systemic toxicity. Therefore, an effect on ovarian secretion has been suggested as the possible mechanism of breast cancer control in these cases (Stoll, 1964*a*).

TABLE 16.1

Percentage Recurrence Rate at Eighteen Months Following Mastectomy. Effect of ThioTEPA at Low Dosage Given Prophylactically at Mastectomy (Noer *et al.*, 1964)

	Total cases	% recurrence at 18 months	Significance
Treated group	49	18%	Difference
Control group	102	21%	sig.
			$p = 0.10$

The ovaries, adrenals and pituitary glands show a higher concentration of radioactively labelled thioTEPA than does the tumour itself after thioTEPA administration to breast cancer bearing patients (Fletcher *et al.*, 1965). Bateman and Carlton (1960) have shown ovarian atrophy to follow thioTEPA therapy in premenopausal women, and a clinical trial is at present comparing the relative clinical benefit from prophylactic oophorectomy with that from prophylactic thioTEPA, in premenopausal patients with breast cancer. It has previously been pointed out that incomplete or temporary castration can cause a remission of tumour growth in breast cancer (*see* p. 24).

PALLIATION BY CYTOTOXIC AGENTS

Currently available cytotoxic agents are capable of inducing objective evidence of tumour growth regression in between 20–30 per cent of patients with advanced breast cancer (Table 16.2). Lesions involving soft tissue show a favourable response more often than do lesions of bone, or viscera such as the brain, lung, or liver. It is interesting to note that all known cytotoxic agents effective in palliating breast cancer growth, achieve objective regression of tumour in practically the same percentage of patients, when the

agents. In their effect on soft tissue metastases, regression of tumour masses is rarely complete, and the periods of tumour growth remission achieved are very brief. Again, unlike steroidal agents, their use is rarely associated with a subjective feeling of well-being. Although it is stated by Bateman and Carlton (1960) that no form of endocrine therapy is as useful for cerebral metastases as intravenous thioTEPA, the author has found corticosteroid therapy to be more consistently beneficial.

Toxicity is much more easily induced by cytotoxic agents than by hormonal methods, and is of more serious danger to life. Bone marrow depression, alopecia, ulceration of the mouth, nausea, vomiting, and diarrhoea (with consequent electrolyte changes)

TABLE 16.2

Major Reports of Favourable Clinical Response to Cytotoxic Agent Therapy in Patients with Breast Cancer

Author		Cases with regressing tumour	Percentage with regressing tumour	Average duration of tumour regression
Conference, 1958	Alkylating agents	724	26%	4 months
Ansfield and Curreri, 1963	5 Fluorouracil	158	29%	6 months
Dao and Grinberg, 1963	5 Fluorodeoxyuridine	101	34%	
Nevinny, 1964				
Wright *et al.*, 1959	Methotrexate	53	28%	5 months
Greening, 1961				
Goldenberg, 1963	Vinblastine	79	17%	3 to 4 months
Frei, 1963	Vincristine	135	29%	

agent is given at a dose compatible with systemic tolerance, i.e. moderate haemopoietic or gastro-intestinal toxicity.

Although it has been reported that a patient resistant to the effect of one cytotoxic agent may occasionally respond favourably to another of the same group, the author has not seen a convincing example of this if both agents are given at *optimal* dosage. Nor is it his experience that increasing the dose to a level that induces extreme toxicity is more likely to secure a remission of tumour growth in breast cancer than a more moderate dose (Stoll, 1962a). It seems likely that a proportion of about one quarter of all breast cancers may have a clinical sensitivity to known cytotoxic agents.

A 20–30 per cent tumour remission rate from cytotoxic agents should make them potential rivals of hormone therapy in the management of breast cancer. However, although cytotoxic agents carry no danger of exacerbating the growth of breast cancer, they are less effective *qualitatively* than hormonal

are not uncommon signs of toxicity. In the author's opinion, it is important to avoid overburdening an already sick patient with added side effects of this nature.

SELECTION OF PATIENTS FOR CHEMOTHERAPY

The same problems must be faced in selecting cytotoxic chemotherapy for the individual with breast cancer as have been stressed for hormonal therapy. Suitable criteria must be decided for the following factors.

1. *Evidence of tumour activity.* Advancing disease must be selected for treatment, and time must be allowed for the effects of previous therapy to have passed off. Biochemical indices of tumour activity should be taken into account (*see* p. 101).

2. *Recognition of clinical response.* Objective evidence of tumour regression must be differentiated from subjective benefit, and a significant decrease in

measurable size of all lesions for a reasonable time period should be established (*see* p. 112).

3. *Biological characteristics of the individual tumour.* There is a wide range of histology, vascularity, and metabolic activity in the same type of tumour occurring in different patients. As a result, the response of breast cancer to cytotoxic chemotherapy is different from patient to patient, and no satisfactory method is available for predicting the response of a tumour before clinical trial. Nevertheless, as in the hormonal therapy of breast cancer, there are certain 'biological determinants of response'.

It has been suggested that beneficial response to cytotoxic agents is more likely, if previous attempts at endocrine therapy have been successful. According to Hurley *et al.* (1961), of seventy breast cancer patients responding favourably to stilboestrol therapy, 83 per cent subsequently responded in a similar fashion to cytotoxic agents. Previous favourable response to hypophysectomy or to androgen therapy predicts a similar response to thioTEPA therapy (Edelstyn *et al.*, 1968). On the other hand, Ravdin and Eisman (1967) could establish no correlation between response to endocrine therapy, and subsequent response to cyclophosphamide or 5 fluorouracil therapy.

According to Hurley *et al.* (1961), cytotoxic therapy, like endocrine therapy, yields better results, the longer the free-interval before recurrence. Again, Ravdin and Eisman (1967) claim that this does not apply to 5 fluorouracil therapy. It is generally agreed that previous X-ray irradiation of the part decreases the likelihood of a favourable response, presumably because of interference with the tumour vascularity. Recent previous chemotherapy of any type will reduce the tolerance of the bone marrow to further cytotoxic therapy.

It is agreed that cytotoxic therapy used late in breast cancer is less likely to be effective than if used earlier in the disease. This probably reflects the greater likelihood of tumour control in the presence of a smaller number of malignant cells. The histological grading of breast cancer cannot be correlated with the likelihood of favourable response. According to Hurley *et al.* (1961), patients over fifty years of age have twice the likelihood of responding favourably to cytotoxic therapy as would younger patients. Metastases in liver, lung, or brain show remission of tumour growth much less frequently than do soft tissue and bone metastases (Hurley *et al.*, 1961).

The clinical benefit from cytotoxic agents in the treatment of breast cancer is temporary, and tumour resistance soon develops to the agent used. This may result from proliferation of surviving resistant cells in the tumour, or it is possible that blocked enzymatic pathways in metabolism tend to be circumvented by alternative pathways of nucleoprotein synthesis. It is said that clinical sensitivity to the action of a different cytotoxic agent may manifest at this stage, but this is rare in the author's experience.

SELECTION OF METHOD OF CHEMOTHERAPY

Cytotoxic therapy is used in the treatment of advanced breast cancer by two major methods; intracavitary and systemic therapy.

INTRACAVITARY THERAPY

Cytotoxic agents are particularly useful when instilled into a serous cavity, in the control of recurrent accumulation of fluid due to tumour deposits on a serous surface. Decrease in the rate of reaccumulation of fluid follows in about 70 per cent of treated cases. In combination with corticosteroids, treatment is especially useful (*see* p. 79). Failure to respond favourably in such a case suggests that the fluid results from transudation, liver cirrhosis, hypoalbuminaemia, or other cause.

According to Bonte *et al.* (1952) and Weisberger (1959), intracavitary nitrogen mustard therapy is as effective as colloidal radioactive gold instillation in controlling metastatic pleural effusions, and involves a much less complicated procedure. Nitrogen mustard is not, however, recommended for intraperitoneal instillation, as its local irritant effect, useful in causing plastic adhesions in the pleural cavity, might cause complications in the peritoneal cavity. Intrapleural therapy by these agents may lead to survival of patients for two years or longer. Pleurodesis by talc insufflation has been suggested in such cases, but in the author's experience, is likely to lead to the appearance of malignant infiltration at the site of intercostal catheterisation.

ThioTEPA can be used either in the pleural or peritoneal cavities and can be given in repeated doses with only slight toxicity and no local discomfort, whereas nitrogen mustard almost invariably causes severe nausea, and can cause severe local irritation unless well diluted. The place of these two alkylating agents has hardly been challenged in this field for many years, although intracavitary quinacrine may be useful in the presence of a damaged bone marrow. Used intracavitarily the local concentration of an agent is high, and because of the slower absorption from the serous cavities, approximately twice the dose can be given as by the parenteral route, for the same degree of systemic toxicity.

SYSTEMIC THERAPY

Systemic administration of cytotoxic agents is used in the presence of extensive local recurrence or of distant metastases not amenable to radiation therapy, or to hormonal therapy. Cytotoxic agents exert an antimitotic effect on the normal dividing cells of the body as well as on the tumour cells, and the intention is to achieve preferential concentration in the more rapidly dividing tumour cells.

The only way to increase the differential effect on the tumour in practice, is to increase both the concentration of the agent in the tumour bed, and the time for which the tumour cells are exposed to it. Continuous therapy for a period of days is theoretically preferable, because it is believed that those nuclei which are in a resting phase are less sensitive to chemotherapeutic agents. However continuous perfusion with a cytotoxic agent can be applied only to an isolated part, and in the case of systemic therapy, either a single dose or fractionated dosage are generally used. Cyclophosphamide and phenylalanine mustard are often given orally for long periods of time.

AGENTS USED IN SYSTEMIC CHEMOTHERAPY

The non-steroidal cytotoxic agents that are effective in the treatment of breast cancer fall into three main categories; alkylating agents, antimetabolites and antibiotics.

ALKYLATING AGENTS

Nitrogen mustard was the first of the cytotoxic agents to be introduced into clinical practice in 1946, and still maintains an important place in cancer chemotherapy. In the treatment of breast cancer, useful related agents are *thioTEPA, Triethylene melamine* (TEM), *Cyclophosphamide* (Endoxan, Cytoxan), *Phenylalanine mustard* (Melphalan), *Chlorambucil* (Leukeran), *Mannomustine* (Degranol) and *Nitrogen mustard oxide* (Nitromin). Alkylating agents are both cytotoxic and nucleotoxic, interfering with nucleoprotein synthesis and the duplication of chromosomes. Signs of toxicity affect mainly the bone marrow, causing leucopenia, thrombocytopenia, and a tendency to haemorrhages, but in addition, nausea, vomiting, or alopecia result from some of the agents.

The benefit from therapy by alkylating agents in the palliation of advanced breast cancer is well documented, and a review of 724 collected cases reported at a Conference (1958) noted objective evidence of tumour regression in 26 per cent of the total number. It was suggested that thioTEPA might be a more effective agent clinically than nitrogen mustard in breast cancer therapy, but Gold *et al.* (1962),

following a random controlled trial, reported that it induced no higher a proportion of tumour regression. In spite of widely differing tumour remission rates in numerous reports, it is likely that using uniform criteria of response, and dosage taken to optimal levels, the choice between the various members of the group noted above is merely one of convenience and side effects.

ThioTEPA has the advantage that it does not cause nausea or vomiting to any extent, but occasionally manifests a sudden and unpredictable depressing effect on the marrow, in the author's experience. Cyclophosphamide can be given orally and demonstrates a thrombocyte sparing effect, but unfortunately it tends to cause alopecia, most marked when high dosage is given parenterally (Stoll and Matar, 1961).

Phenylalamine mustard can be given orally and induced tumour growth regression in 11 per cent of a small group of patients reported by Silva *et al.* (1959), with severe marrow depression as the major sign of toxicity. Nitrogen mustard oxide can also be given orally with almost no side effects apart from moderate marrow depression as noted in the author's series (Stoll 1956c, 1960d). Therapy by a combination of alkylating agents and corticosteroids in the presence of thoracic metastases or serous effusions has been referred to elsewhere (*see* p. 79). The use of androgens to counteract bone marrow depression by thioTEPA or cyclophosphamide has also been mentioned (*see* p. 45).

Tumour regression from the use of alkylating agents in advanced breast cancer usually takes six to eight weeks to manifest. Tumour shrinkage is often incomplete, and has an average duration of about four months (Plates 7 and 8).

ANTIMETABOLITES

Vitamins, co-enzymes, and intermediary products of nucleoprotein synthesis such as purines and pyrimidines, may be chemically altered, so that they act as competitive inhibitors of essential metabolic processes in the rapidly dividing malignant cell.

5 Fluorouracil and 5 Fluorodeoxyuridine. Ansfield and Curreri (1963) reported that 5 fluorouracil induced tumour growth remission in breast cancer in 29 per cent of 158 patients, and Hurley *et al.* (1961) reported a remission in 51 per cent of 82 patients. 5 fluorodeoxyuridine was reported by Ansfield and Curreri (1963) to induce remission of tumour growth in 48 per cent of 46 patients, and by Dao and Grinbery (1963), and Nevinny (1964) in 12 per cent and 29 per cent of patients respectively. The two agents appear overall to induce an equivalent proportion of tumour growth remission in breast cancer, when allowance is made for different criteria of response.

In this respect Ansfield and Curreri (1962) accept a 25 per cent reduction in size of a lesion for two months as evidence of favourable response.

The average duration of tumour growth remission is somewhat longer from these agents than from the alkylating agents, being over six months in half the patients. The toxicity from these agents is also greater than from the alkylating agents, the treatment mortality rate being about 5 per cent. Signs of toxicity include marrow depression, diarrhoea, stomatitis, nausea, and vomiting. According to Silva *et al.* (1965), response to 5 fluorouracil is possible, even after failure of other cytotoxic agents.

Amethopterin (Methotrexate). This antimetabolic agent inhibits the conversion of folic acid into citrovorum factor. Introduced into clinical cancer therapy by Farber (1949), it is used most successfully in the treatment of chorioncarcinoma. In the treatment of breast cancer, early reports were those of Wright *et al.* (1959) and Greening (1961) who reported regression in 28 per cent of fifty-three patients with advanced breast cancer. Using less strict criteria, Vogler *et al.* (1968) reported tumour growth remission in 41 per cent of thirty-seven patients but in a randomised comparison of methotrexate with the pyrimidine analogues, Nevinny (1964) reported objective evidence of tumour regression in only 17 per cent of breast cancer patients from methotrexate therapy.

The use of a combination of chemotherapeutic agents has been advised by Goldin and Mantel (1957) from the results of their experimental work. Its importance was stressed by the author (Stoll, 1955, 1959b) as a means of blocking more than one pathway of tumour metabolism, and thus delaying the onset of drug resistance. Recent reports by Greenspan (1964, 1965) note a favourable response in 60 per cent of brain, lung, or soft tissue metastases, in a series of 106 patients treated by a combination of methotrexate and thioTEPA. An average remission period of over five months is claimed, but it should be noted that androgen therapy was added in all patients, and corticosteroid therapy, also in a large proportion. The high tumour remission rate can hardly be credited to the cytotoxic agents alone.

Vinblastine. Vinblastine is a plant alkaloid, which is included among the anti-metabolites, because experimentally, its cytotoxic effects can be reversed by administration of co-enzyme A and various amino acids. Goldenberg (1963) reported not a single response from its administration in twenty-three women with advanced breast cancer, but according to Frei (1965), vinblastine therapy induced objective evidence of tumour regression in 23 per cent of fifty-six patients with breast cancer for an average period of three to four months. Toxicity is mainly directed against the bone marrow but is sometimes gastro-intestinal. Fortunately, recovery of the marrow occurs fairly rapidly.

Vincristine. Vincristine is an alkaloid related to vinblastine. It is claimed that favourable response to this agent occurs within three to four weeks of starting treatment, and may occur in the absence of favourable response to previous cytotoxic therapy (Goldenberg, 1964). It has been reported by Gailani (1963) Mittelman *et al.* (1963) and Frei (1965) to yield remission of tumour growth in 29 per cent of 135 patients. Toxicity from this agent is severe, and includes alopecia, leucopenia, gastro-intestinal symptoms, and neurological symptoms which include paraesthesiae and motor weakness.

ANTIBIOTICS

A number of antibiotics have demonstrated mild oncolytic activity and in most cases, the effect upon breast cancer has been to cause partial regression in the size of tumour and then only for short periods.

Mitomycin 'C'. The use of this antibiotic in a series of breast cancer patients was reported by Colsky *et al.* (1960) and by the author (Stoll, 1960b). Remission of tumour growth in 45 per cent of twenty patients was noted. A review of collected reports by Frank and Osterburg (1960) reported remission of tumour growth in 42 per cent of twenty-six breast cancer cases. The severe toxic effect of the agent upon the marrow has tended to limit the clinical use of Mitomycin outside Japan, where it originated. Other toxic effects are alopecia and gastrointestinal upset.

Carzinophilin. This antibiotic, like the previous one, is derived from soil fungi. It was reported by Kurokawa and Saito (1959) to have a palliative effect upon advanced cancer, but the author (Stoll, 1960a) reported no benefit from its administration in breast cancer. Its toxic side effects upon the bone marrow were found to be low, and its use in the treatment of breast cancer is still being reported from Japan.

Actinomycin 'F'. Actinomycin 'D'. This agent was introduced into the therapy of cancer by Farber and his group (1956), and has been used most successfully in the treatment of Wilm's tumour in children. While reporting poor response to Actinomycin D, Tan *et al.* (1957) reported that 30 per cent of thirty patients with breast cancer showed favourable response to Actinomycin F, a newer derivative. Toxic effects from the latter include gastro-intestinal symptoms, oral ulceration, but only rarely marrow depression.

TO SUMMARISE

Systemic chemotherapy by cytotoxic agents yields objective evidence of tumour regression in 20–30 per cent of patients with advanced breast cancer. The use of thioTEPA or 5 fluorouracil is generally advised, their results being fairly similar. The palliation from cytotoxic agents is generally incomplete and transient. Such a response must be weighed against the toxic side effects common to these agents, in order to avoid further burdening of an already sick patient. Nevertheless, there are accepted indications for cytotoxic chemotherapy including the palliation of malignant serous effusions by intracavitary instillation of the agent.

Cytotoxic Therapy

ILLUSTRATIVE CASE HISTORIES

Patient T.B.E. Short-term Regression of Soft Tissue Tumour from Cyclophosphamide and from a Combination of Prednisolone and Nitrogen Mustard Oxide. No Control from Androgen, Oestrogen, Corticosteroid or Progestin Therapy

A premenopausal woman aged thirty-nine, presented in October 1953 with a carcinoma of the right breast. Primary treatment was by radical mastectomy, but thirty-nine months later, metastatic tumour appeared in the left parasternal area. This was associated with the appearance of recurrent skin nodules in the region of the mastectomy scar.

X-ray therapy was given to the soft tissue tumours, and endocrine therapy was begun by carrying out surgical castration. Within eight months, new skin nodules had appeared in the region of the mastectomy scar. A trial of Sublings testosterone 10 mg qid was prescribed for two months, but the skin nodules continued to grow, and a malignant left pleural effusion appeared. After an interval, a course of prednisolone 10 mg tds was prescribed for three months and with it was associated a course of nitrogen mustard oxide 750 mg orally. This combined treatment resulted in regression of the skin nodules for a period of eight months.

When recurrence of activity appeared, successive trials of medroxyprogesterone 100 mg qid, dexamethasone 1·6 mg qid, and stilboestrol 5 mg tds were prescribed, each for a period of two months. Each was tried in succession with an interval between, but without clinical evidence of benefit. Finally, a single intravenous dose of cyclophosphamide 50 mg/kilo was given and was followed by remarkable regression in the widespread area of skin nodulation. It lasted only for six months, and the patient finally died three and a half years after her first recurrence.

Patient C.N.E. Short-term Regression of Soft Tissue Tumour and Pleural Effusion from a Combination of Androgen and ThioTEPA. No Control from Oestrogen Therapy Previously

A woman aged fifty with a history of a hysterectomy eleven years previously, presented in July 1957 with a carcinoma of the right breast. Primary treatment was by radical mastectomy. Within seven months of the operation, recurrent cutaneous nodules appeared in the vicinity of the mastectomy scar, and were treated by a palliative course of X-ray therapy. When the nodules reactivated nine months later, hormonal therapy was begun with a course of stilboestrol 5 mg tds. It was prescribed for four months without clinical evidence of response, and after this time a malignant right pleural effusion appeared.

A course of testosterone propionate 100 mg intramuscularly three times a week was prescribed for three months, and with this was associated an intramuscular course of thioTEPA to haemopoietic tolerance levels. This resulted in regression of the soft tissue tumour, and control of the pleural effusion for a period of six months. The tumour then reactivated, with evidence of spread to the opposite breast and metastatic enlargement of the liver, and the patient died two months later.

Patient D.A.L. Short-term Regression of Soft Tissue Tumour from Mitomycin and from Androgen Therapy

A premenopausal patient aged thirty-seven, presented in September 1956 with a Stage 1 carcinoma of the right breast. Primary treatment was by radical mastectomy, followed by a prophylactic course of X-ray therapy to the axillary, supraclavicular, and internal mammary draining node areas. Within twelve months of the operation, recurrent skin nodules appeared in the region of the mastectomy scar.

Endocrine therapy was begun by carrying out X-ray castration, delivering 1,000 roentgens in four days to the region of the ovaries. At the end of ten months, new evidence of tumour spread was found in the opposite breast and axillary nodes. This was soon followed by the appearance of bone pains found to be associated with multiple lytic areas of metastasis in bone, and also of multiple nodular opacities suggestive of metastasis, in the lung fields.

A course of testosterone propionate 100 mg intramuscularly three times a week was prescribed and continued for six months, during which time the skin and lung nodules regressed in size. At the end of six months, reactivation of the nodules occurred and a course of Mitomycin was given—60 mg intravenously in two months. Again regression of skin nodules resulted for five months, although bone and lung metastases showed no control. The patient died one month later.

Patient E.C.O.W. Short-term Regression of Soft Tissue Tumour and Pleural Effusion from ThioTEPA and from Oestrogen Therapy. No Control from Androgen Therapy, or from a Combination of Prednisolone and Nitrogen Mustard Oxide
A woman aged fifty-six and eight years postmenopausal, gave a history of radical mastectomy ten years previously for carcinoma of the left breast. She then presented in January 1958 with recurrent skin nodules near the mastectomy scar, complaining also of dyspnoea associated with the presence of a malignant pleural effusion.

Hormonal treatment was initiated with a course of prednisolone 10 mg tds for three months and with this was associated a course of 750 mg nitrogen mustard oxide orally. Clinical benefit was not achieved. After an interval a course of ethinyl oestradiol 0·5 mg tds was prescribed for five months, and this led to regression in the size of the nodules and of the pleural effusion. When control was lost after five months, an intramuscular course of thioTEPA was given to haemopoietic tolerance levels. Again regression resulted, this time for a period of seven months. A final attempt at steroid therapy, with fluoxymesterone 10 mg tds for four months, was not followed by clinical benefit, and the patient died one month later.

Patient B.S.I. Short-term Regression of Soft Tissue Tumour from Cyclophosphamide. No Control from either Oestrogen or Androgen Therapy Previously
A woman aged sixty-three, and fourteen years postmenopausal, presented in February 1958 with an advanced carcinoma of the right breast associated with enlarged metastatic supraclavicular nodes. A 'toilet' mastectomy was carried out, and followed by a postoperative course of X-ray therapy to the mastectomy scar, axillary and supraclavicular areas. Within seventeen months of the operation, tumours were palpable in the opposite breast, axilla, and supraclavicular area, and recurrent skin nodules appeared in the vicinity of the mastectomy scar.

Hormonal therapy was initiated with a course of stilboestrol 5 mg tds for three months, but without clinical signs of response. This was followed by a trial of testosterone propionate 100 mg intramuscularly three times a week for two months, again

without benefit. At this stage, a single dose of cyclophosphamide 50 mg/kilo was given intravenously, and resulted in regression of the soft tissue tumour for a period of three months. Nevertheless, the patient developed bilateral malignant pleural effusions one month later and died.

Patient E.C.O.S. Short-term Regression of Soft Tissue Tumour from a Combination of Androgen and ThioTEPA. No Control from either Cyclophosphamide Alone or from Androgen Therapy Alone Subsequently
A woman aged sixty-eight, and eighteen years postmenopausal, presented in October 1952 with a Stage 1 cancer of the breast. Because of her poor cardiac condition, it was decided to treat the tumour primarily by X-ray therapy, and a tumour dose of 4,000 roentgens in twenty-seven days was given to the breast, axillary, and supraclavicular node areas. Regression of the tumour followed the X-ray therapy and was maintained for thirty-four months, after which the tumour slowly reactivated.

Trials of oestrogen therapy, both with stilboestrol and with ethinyl oestradiol were attempted, but were not tolerated because of nausea and vomiting. A course of testosterone propionate 100 mg intramuscularly three times a week was then prescribed for three months, and with it was associated an intramuscular course of thioTEPA to haemopoietic tolerance levels. Regression of the soft tissue tumour resulted for four months. When reactivation occurred a single intravenous dose of Cyclophosphamide 50 mg/kilo was given but without clinical evidence of response. This was followed by a course of fluoxymesterone 10 mg tds for three months, again without clinical benefit. The patient died of cardiac failure six months later.

Patient I.B.R. Short-term Regression of Soft Tissue Tumour from Mannomustine. No Control from Oestrogen or Androgen Therapy Previously
A woman aged fifty-four and eight years postmenopausal, presented in July 1956 with carcinoma of the right breast invading the pectoralis muscles. Primary treatment was by radical mastectomy followed by a prophylactic course of X-ray therapy to the axillary, supraclavicular, and internal mammary draining node areas. Within twelve months of mastectomy, recurrent skin nodules appeared in the region of the mastectomy scar and were treated by a palliative course of X-ray therapy.

When reactivation occurred seven months later, a course of ethinyl oestradiol 0·5 mg tds was prescribed for five months but without clinical evidence of response. When enlarged metastatic nodes appeared in the opposite axilla, a three months course of fluoxymesterone 10 mg tds was prescribed, but again without clinical benefit. At this stage, an intravenous course of mannomustine was prescribed to haematological tolerance levels. Regression of soft tissue tumour occurred within two months, but five months later, while mannomustine therapy was being maintained, a sudden unexpected fall in the platelet level occurred, and the patient died following massive haemorrhages.

Patient T.S.T. Short-term Regression of Soft Tissue Tumour from a Combination of Androgen and ThioTEPA. Response to Castration Previously

A premenopausal patient aged thirty-eight, presented in January 1956 with a Stage 2 carcinoma of the right breast. Primary treatment was by radical mastectomy, but seventeen months after operation, she developed recurrent skin nodules near the mastectomy scar. Endocrine therapy was initiated by carrying out X-ray castration, and regression of nodules was apparent within two months of castration.

At the end of twenty-one months, bone pain appeared and multiple bone metastases of a mixed lytic-sclerotic type were visible in the radiographs. Shortly afterwards, the patient developed enlarged metastatic nodes in both inguinal regions. A course of testosterone propionate 100 mg intramuscularly three times a week was given, and with this was associated an intramuscular course of thioTEPA to haemopoietic tolerance levels. Regression of soft tissue tumour resulted, and bone pains were relieved for a total period of eleven months. At this stage, clinical examination showed irregular and gross enlargement of the liver due to metastases, and the patient died one month later.

Patient M.T.O. Short-term Regression of Soft Tissue Tumour from Cyclophosphamide after Failure of Control from Castration or from Androgen Therapy. Subsequent Oestrogen Therapy Induced Hypercalcaemia

A premenopausal woman aged thirty-eight, presented in May 1958 with a Stage 2 carcinoma of the left breast. Primary treatment was by radical mastectomy, but seven months after the operation she developed recurrent skin nodules near the mastectomy scar. With this, was associated metastatic enlargement of the left supraclavicular nodes, and a left parasternal tumour presumed to be arising in the internal mammary chain. A malignant left pleural effusion was also present.

Endocrine therapy was initiated by carrying out X-ray castration, delivering a dose of 1,500 roentgens in seven days to the region of the ovaries. Regression of the soft tissue tumour did not occur, and at the end of ten months the radiographs showed multiple

sclerotic areas of metastasis in bone. At this stage a course of fluoxymesterone 10 mg tds was instituted for three months, but again without clinical evidence of response.

A single intravenous dose of cyclophosphamide 50 mg/kilo was then given, and this led to relief of pain for five months, and recalcification of the bone metastases. When reactivation of pain occurred, a trial of stilboestrol 5 mg tds was attempted, but hypercalcaemia developed within two weeks of administration. The hypercalcaemia persisted in spite of intensive prednisolone therapy, and the patient died within two weeks.

Patient E.C.U. Short-term Regression of Soft Tissue Tumour and Malignant Ascites from a Combination of Androgen and ThioTEPA

A woman aged seventy-one presented in December 1957 with a carcinoma of the left breast. Primary treatment was by radical mastectomy, followed by a prophylactic course of X-ray therapy to the axillary, supraclavicular, and internal mammary draining node areas. Within sixteen months of the operation, metastatic enlargement of the left supraclavicular and infraclavicular nodes was palpable, and this was soon followed by the appearance of malignant ascites.

Hormonal therapy was initiated with a course of testosterone propionate 100 mg intramuscularly three times a week. It was continued for three months, and with it was associated an intramuscular course of thioTEPA to haemopoietic tolerance levels. This combination treatment resulted in regression of the metastatic nodes, and control of ascites for a period of four months. The tumour then showed signs of reactivation, and the patient died four months later.

Patient A.M.A. Short-term Regression of Soft Tissue Metastases from Cyclophosphamide. No Control from either Progestin, Androgen, or Oestrogen Therapy

A premenopausal patient aged thirty-nine, presented in May 1958 with a Stage 2 carcinoma of the right breast. Primary treatment was by radical mastectomy, and, at the same time, prophylactic castration was carried out by surgery. In addition, the mastectomy was followed by a prophylactic course of X-ray therapy to the axillary, supraclavicular, and internal mammary draining node areas. Nevertheless, within only five months of the operation, recurrent skin nodules appeared near the mastectomy scar, and nine months later, enlarged metastatic nodes were palpable in the left axilla and above the right clavicle.

Hormonal therapy was begun with a course of medroxyprogesterone 100 mg qid given for three months, but without any clinical signs of benefit. A single intravenous dose of cyclophosphamide 50 mg/kilo was then given, and this caused regression of soft tissue tumour for a period of four months. When control was lost, a course of fluoxymesterone 10 mg tds for four months and one of stilboestrol 5 mg tds for two months were tried, but both without evidence of clinical benefit.

Patient C.W.I. Short-term Regression of Soft Tissue Tumour from Androgen Therapy Alone and from its Combination with ThioTEPA. No Control from Corticosteroid Therapy or from Bilateral Adrenalectomy Subsequently

A premenopausal patient aged thirty-six, presented in July 1958 with a carcinoma of the left breast. Primary treatment was by radical mastectomy, followed by a prophylactic course of X-ray therapy to the mastectomy scar, axillary, and supraclavicular draining node areas. Within only four months of the operation, recurrent skin nodules appeared in the vicinity of the mastectomy scar.

Endocrine therapy was initiated by carrying out X-ray castration, delivering 1,200 roentgens to the region of the ovaries in twelve days. Clinical benefit did not result, and six months later a course of fluoxymesterone 10 mg tds was prescribed for five months. As a result, the metastatic nodules disappeared rapidly, but after five months new enlarged nodes were palpable in the left supraclavicular region. With this, was associated the development of a malignant pleural effusion on the same side. Fluoxymesterone was continued for a further six months, and concurrently an intramuscular course of thioTEPA was added to haemopoietic tolerance levels. The enlarged nodes and the pleural effusion both regressed in size as a result of the combined treatment.

At the end of eleven months androgen therapy, the soft tissue tumour again reactivated. It responded neither to a two months trial of prednisolone 10 mg tds, nor to the operation of bilateral adrenalectomy and oophorectomy. The patient died four months after stopping therapy.

Patient N.J.A. Short-term Regression of Soft Tissue and Bone Metastases from Cyclophosphamide and from Androgen Therapy, but No Control from Corticosteroid Therapy

A postmenopausal woman aged sixty, and twelve years postmenopausal, presented in January 1957 with a Stage 2 carcinoma of the right breast. Primary treatment was by radical mastectomy, but twenty-one months after the operation she developed recurrent skin nodules in the region of the mastectomy scar. She also complained of bone pain, and this was found to be associated with multiple lytic areas of metastases in bone. Soon after, she developed evidence of new tumour in the left breast, axillary, and supraclavicular nodes.

Hormonal treatment was begun with a course of dexamethasone 1·6 qid given for four months, but without any clinical signs of benefit from the corticosteroid therapy. After an interval, a course of fluoxymesterone 10 mg tds was prescribed for four months. This led to regression of the soft tissue metastases and relief of pain, and recalcification was visible in radiographs of the bone metastases. When the soft tissue tumour reactivated three months later, a single intravenous dose of cyclophosphamide 50 mg/kilo was given, and this again led to a short period of tumour regression. Nevertheless, the patient's condition deteriorated and she died three months later.

Bibliography

Abrams, H. L., Spiro, R. and Goldstein, N. (1950) 'Metastases in carcinoma: analysis of 1000 autopsied cases'. *Cancer (Phil.)*, **3**, 74.

Abramson, W. and Warshawsky, H. (1948) 'Cancer of the breast in the male, secondary to estrogenic administration; report of a case'. *J. Urol.*, **59**, 76.

Ackland, T. H. (1968) Personal communication.

Adair, F. E. (1947) 'The use of the male sex hormone in women with breast cancer'. *Surg. Gynec. Obstet.*, **84**, 719.

Adair, F. E., Treves, N., Farrow, J. H. and Scharnagel, I. M. (1945) 'Clinical effects of surgical and X-ray castration in mammary cancer'. *J. Amer. Med. Assoc.*, **128**, 161.

Adams, J. B. and Wong, M. S. F. (1968) 'Para-endocrine behaviour of human breast carcinoma. *In vitro* transformation of steroids to physiologically active hormones'. *J. Endoc.*, **41**, 41.

Ahlbom, H. (1930) 'Castration by roentgen rays as an auxiliary treatment in the radiotherapy of cancer mammae at Radiumhemmet, Stockholm'. *Acta Radiol.*, **11**, 614.

Ahlquist, K. A., Jackson, A. W. and Stewart, J. C. (1968) 'Urinary steroid values as a guide to prognosis in breast cancer'. *Brit. Med. J.*, **i**, 217.

Ahren, K. and Hamberger, L. (1962) 'Direct action of testosterone propionate on the rat mammary gland'. *Acta Endoc. (Kobn.)*, **40**, 265.

Albert, A. (1956) 'Human urinary gonadotropin'. *Recent Progress in Hormone Research*, **12**, 227.

Allaben, G. R. and Owen, S. E. (1939) 'Adenocarcinoma of the breast coincidental with strenuous endocrine therapy'. *J. Amer. Med. Assoc.*, **112**, 1933.

Altmann, F. P. and Chayen, J. (1967) 'A study of breast cancer by techniques of cellular biology and multiphase biochemistry', in *Cambridge Symposium on the Treatment of Carcinoma of the Breast*, p. 56, Ed. A. S. Jarrett. Excerpta Medica Foundation.

AMA Committee on Research (1960) 'Androgens and estrogens in the treatment of disseminated mammary carcinoma'. *J. Amer. Med. Assoc.*, **172**, 1271.

Anderson, E., Reed, S. C., Huseby, R. A. and Oliver, C. P. (1950) 'Possible relationship between menopause and age at onset of breast cancer'. *Cancer (Phil.)*, **3**, 410.

Anstield, D. (1967) In 'Symposium on cancer of the breast'. *Cancer (Phil.)*, **20**, 1065.

Ansfield, F. J. and Curreri, A. R. (1963) 'Further clinical comparison between 5 fluorouracil and 5 fluorodeoxyuridine'. *Cancer Chemother. Rep.*, **32**, 101.

Arslan, M. (1966) 'Ultrasonic hypophysectomy'. *J. Laryng*, **80**, 73.

Atkin, N. B. (1967) 'Sex chromatin in female breast cancer'. *Lancet*, **ii**, 1145.

Atkins, H. J. B., Falconer, M. A., Hayward, J. L., Maclean, K. S., Schurr, P. H. and Armitage, P. (1960) 'Adrenalectomy and hypophysectomy for advanced cancer of the breast'. *Lancet*, **i**, 1148.

Atkins, H., Falconer, M. A., Hayward, J. L., Maclean, K. S. and Schurr, P. H. (1966) 'The timing of adrenalectomy and of hypophysectomy in the treatment of advanced breast cancer'. *Lancet*, **i**, 827.

Auchinloss, H. and Haagensen, C. D. (1940) 'Cancer of the breast possibly induced by estrogenic substances'. *J. Amer. Med. Assoc.*, **114**, 1517.

Bacigalupo, C. (1959) 'Certain aspects and results of hormone therapy in oncology'. *Prob. Oncol. (N.Y.)*, **5**, No. 8, 51.

Backwinkel, K. and Jackson, A. S. (1964) 'Some features of breast cancer and thyroid deficiency'. *Cancer (Phil.)*, **17**, 1174.

Baggett, B., Engel, L. L., Savard, K. and Dorfman, R. I. (1956) 'The conversion of testosterone-3-C14 to C14-Estradiol-17β by human ovarian tissue'. *J. Biol. Chem.*, **221**, 931.

Barrett, R. J., Friesen, H. and Astwood, E. B. (1961) 'Electrophoresis of pituitary hormones in starch gel'. *Fed. Proc.*, **20**, 183.

Bateman, G. H. (1962) 'Transsphenoidal hypophysectomy'. *J. Laryng.*, **76**, 442.

Bateman, J. C. and Carlton, H. (1960) 'The role of chemotherapy in the treatment of breast cancer'. *Surgery*, **47**, 895.

Bauld, W. S. (1956) 'A method for the determination of estriol, estrone, and estradiol-17β in human urine by partition chromatography and colorimetric estimation'. *Biochem. J.*, **63**, 488.

Beatson, G. T. (1896) 'On the treatment of inoperable cases of carcinoma of the mamma. Suggestion for a new method of treatment with illustrative cases'. *Lancet*, **ii**, 104, 162.

Beck, J. C., Blair, A. J., Griffiths, M. M., Rosenfeld, M. W. and McGarry, E. E. (1966) 'In search of hormonal factors as an aid in predicting the outcome of breast carcinoma'. *Canad. Cancer Conf.*, **6**, 3.

Beckett, V. L. and Brennan, M. J. (1959) 'Treatment of advanced breast cancer with fluoxymesterone (Halotestin)'. *Surg. Gynec. Obstet.*, **109**, 235.

Biden, W. M. (1943) 'Stilboestrol for breast cancer'. *Brit. Med. J.*, **ii**, 57.

Birke, G., Diczfalusy, E., Franksson, C., Hellstrom, J., Hultberg, S., Plantin, L. and Westman, A. (1958) 'On the correlation between steroid excretion and clinical response to oophorectomy plus adrenalectomy in breast cancer', in *Endocrine Aspects of Breast Cancer*, p. 213, Eds A. R. Currie and C. F. W. Illingsworth, Edinburgh; E. & S. Livingstone.

Bisel, H. F. (1964) 'Treatment of advanced breast cancer with delta-testololactone'. *Acta Un. Int. Contra Canc.*, **20**, 429.

Bishop, P. M. F. (1960) 'Hormones and cancer'. *Clin. Obst. Gynec.*, **31**, 1109.

Blackburn, C. M. and Childs, D. S. (1959) 'Use of 2α methyl dihydrotestosterone in the treatment of advanced cancer of the breast'. *Proc. Mayo Clin.*, **34**, 113.

Bleasel, K. and Lazarus, L. (1965) 'Cryogenic hypophysectomy'. *Med. J. Aust.*, **2**, 148.

Bleehen, N. M. and Bryant, T. H. E. (1967) '*In vivo* studies of radioactive phosphorus in malignant tumours'. *Clin. Radiol.*, **18**, 237.

Block, G. E., Lampe, I., Vial, A. B. and Coller, F. A. (1960) 'Therapeutic castration for advanced mammary cancer'. *Surgery*, **47**, 877.

Block, G. E., Vial, A. B., McCarthy, J. D., Porter, C. W. and Coller, F. A. (1959) 'Adrenalectomy in advanced mammary cancer'. *Surg. Gynec. Obstet.*, **108**, 651.

Block, G. E., Vial, A. B. and Pullen, F. W. (1958) 'Estrogen excretion following operative and irradiation castration in cases of mammary cancer'. *Surgery*, **43**, 415.

Bloom, H. J. G. (1950) 'Further studies on prognosis of breast cancer'. *Brit. J. Cancer*, **4**, 347.

Bloom, H. J. G. (1955) 'Clinicopathological investigations; (a) Carcinoma of the breast'. *Brit. Emp. Cancer Camp. Ann. Rep.*, **33**, 30.

Bodansky, O. (1954) 'Serum phosphohexose isomerase in cancer: II. As an index of tumour growth in metastatic carcinoma of the breast'. *Cancer (Phil.)*, **7**, 1200.

Boesen, E., Radley-Smith, E. J. and Baron, D. N. (1961) 'Further experience with hypophysectomy in advanced breast cancer'. *Brit. Med. J.*, **ii**, 790.

Bohle, A. (1965) 'Significance of Barr bodies in mammary carcinoma'. *Med. Welt.*, **23**, 1266. English abstract in *Cancer Chemother. Rep.*, **6**, 1345.

Bond, W. H. and Arthur, K. (1966) 'Some observations on the use of cytotoxic drugs and anabolic steroids in the treatment of breast carcinomatosis', in *The Value of Cytotoxic Agents and Anabolic Steroids in the Treatment of Advanced Malignant Disease*, p. 57, Ed M. Abrahamson, London; Parcener Press.

Bonser, G. M., Dossett, J. A. and Jull, J. W. (1961) 'Selection of patients for hypophysectomy or adrenalectomy', in *Human and Experimental Breast Cancer*, p. 450, Springfield; Charles C. Thomas.

Bonte, F. J., Storaasli, J. P. and Weisberger, A. S. (1956) 'Comparative evaluation of radioactive colloidal gold and nitrogen mustard in the treatment of serous effusions of neoplastic origin'. *Radiology*, **67**, 63.

Bosboom, B. J. M., Meischke-De Jongh, M. L. and Gerbrandy, J. (1960) quoted by R. Nissen-Meyer (1964).

Boyd, S. (1900) 'On oophorectomy in cancer of the breast'. *Brit. Med. J.*, **ii**, 1161.

Boyland, E., Godsmark, B., Greening, W. P., Rigby-Jones, P., Stevenson, J. J. and Abul Fadl, M. A. M. (1958) 'The effect of irradiation of the pituitary on gonadotrophin excretion in women with advanced mammary cancer', in *Endocrine Aspects of Breast Cancer*, p. 170, Eds A. R. Currie and C. F. W. Illingsworth, Edinburgh; E. & S. Livingstone.

Brennan, M. J. (1966) 'Indices of response to breast cancer therapy', in *Clinical Evaluation in Breast Cancer*, p. 141, Eds J. L. Hayward and R. D. Bulbrook, London; Academic Press.

Briggs, M. H., Caldwell, A. D. S. and Pitchford, A. G. (1967) 'The treatment of cancer by progestogens'. *Hosp. Med.*, **1**, 63.

Brindley, C. O. and Francis, F. L. (1963) 'Serum lactic dehydrogenase and glutamic-oxalacetic transaminase correlations with measurements of tumour masses during therapy'. *Cancer Res.*, **23**, 112.

Brinkley, D. M. and Kingsley-Pillers, E. (1960) 'Treatment of advanced carcinoma of the breast by bilateral oophorectomy and prednisone'. *Lancet*, **i**, 123.

Brown, J. B. (1955) 'A chemical method for the determination of oestriol, oestrone and oestradiol in human urine'. *Biochem. J.*, **60**, 185.

Brown, J. B. (1967) Personal communication.

Brown, J. B. and Strong, J. A. (1962) 'The metabolism of oestrogens in relation to thyroid function'. *Acta Endoc. (Kobn.) Suppl.*, **67**, 90.

Brown, P. S., Wells, M. and Cunningham, F. J. (1964) 'A method for studying the mode of action of oral contraceptives'. *Lancet*, **ii**, 446.

Browne, P. A. (1966) 'The treatment of secondary deposits in bone from carcinoma of the breast with P32 and Durabolin', in *The Value of Cytotoxic Agents and Anabolic Steroids in the Treatment of Advanced Malignant Disease*, Ed M. Abrahamson, London; Parcener Press.

Bucalossi, P., Dipietro, S. and Gennari, L. (1963) 'Hormonal treatment of metastatic breast carcinoma with a synthetic progestin—methyl acetoxy progesterone'. English abstract in *Practitioner*, **191**, 702.

Bulbrook, R. D. (1966) 'Hormonal factors in the etiology and treatment of breast cancer'. *Canad. Cancer Conf.*, **6**, 36.

Bulbrook, R. D. (1967) 'Studies on the endocrinology of breast cancer', in *Cambridge Symposium on the Treatment of Carcinoma of the Breast*, p. 40, Ed A. S. Jarrett: Excerpta Medica Foundation.

Bulbrook, R. D. and Greenwood, F. C. (1957) 'Persistence of urinary oestrogen excretion after oophorectomy and adrenalectomy'. *Brit. Med. J.*, **i**, 662.

Bulbrook, R. D., Greenwood, F. C., Hadfield, G. J. and Scowen, E. F. (1958) 'Oophorectomy in breast cancer. An attempt to correlate clinical results with oestrogen production'. *Brit. Med. J.*, **ii**, 7.

Bulbrook, R. D., Greenwood, F. C. and Hayward, J. L. (1960a) 'Selection of breast cancer patients for adrenalectomy or hypophysectomy by determination of urinary 17 hydroxycorticosteroids and aetiocholanolone'. *Lancet*, **i**, 1154.

Bulbrook, R. D., Hayward, J. L. and Thomas, B. S. (1964a) 'The relation between the urinary 17 hydroxy corticosteroids and 11 deoxy 17 oxosteroids and the fate of patients after mastectomy'. *Lancet*, **i**, 945.

Bulbrook, R. D., Greenwood, F. C. and Williams, P. C. (1960b) 'Comparison of biological and chemical estimations of urinary oestrogens: II Urine from patients with breast cancer maintained on cortisone after oophorectomy, adrenalectomy, or hypophysectomy'. *J. Endoc.*, **20**, 220.

Bulbrook, R. D. and Hayward, J. L. (1962) 'Steroid hormones and prognosis in human breast cancer'. *Acta Unio Int. Contra Canc.*, **18**, 893.

Bulbrook, R. D., Thomas, B. S. and Utsunomiya, J. (1964b) 'Urinary 11-deoxy-17 oxosteroids in British and Japanese women with reference to the incidence of breast cancer'. *Nature*, **201**, 4915.

Burnett, W., McAllister, R. A. and Shields, R. (1963) 'The use of serum glycoprotein levels in the selection of patients with advanced breast cancer for endocrine surgery'. *Scot. Med. J.*, **8**, 197.

Burrows, H. and Horning, E. S. (1952) *Oestrogens and Neoplasia*, Oxford; Blackwell Scientific Publications.

Byron, R., Yonemoto, R. H., Bashore, R., Bierman, H. R., Cronemiller, P. and Masters, H. (1962) 'Bilateral adrenalectomy in advanced breast cancer'. *Surgery*, **52**, 725.

Cade, S. (1950) *Malignant Disease and its Treatment by Radium*, Vol. 3, p. 74, Bristol; John Wright.

Cade, S. (1958) 'Adrenalectomy in cancer of the breast', in *Endocrine Aspects of Breast Cancer*, p. 2, Eds A. R. Currie and C. F. W. Illingsworth, Edinburgh; E. & S. Livingstone.

Cade, S. (1966) 'Adrenalectomy for disseminated breast cancer', *Brit. Med. J.*, **ii**, 613.

Campbell, J. H., Cummins, S. D., Kirk, D. L. and Mathews, W. R. (1962) 'Secondary breast cancer of prostatic origin'. *J. Amer. Med. Assoc.*, **179**, 458.

Cantino, T. J. and Gordan, G. S. (1967) 'High dosage delta-testololactone therapy of disseminated carcinoma of the breast'. *Cancer (Phil.)*, **20**, 458.

Carter, A. C., Feldman, E. B., and Schwartz, H. L. (1960) 'Levels of serum PBI in patients with metastatic carcinoma of the breast'. *J. Clin. Endoc.*, **20**, 477.

Castellanos, H., Fairgrieve, J., O'Morchoe, P. J. and Moore, F. D. (1963) 'Corticotropin stimulation of urethral cornification'. *J. Amer. Med. Assoc.*, **184**, 295.

Castellanos, H. and Sturgis, S. H. (1958) 'Cytology of human urinary sediment. Diagnostic value of the non nucleated cell'. *J. Clin. Endoc.*, **18**, 1369.

Clemmesen, J. (1948) 'Carcinoma of breast. Results from statistical research'. *Brit. J. Radiol.*, **21**, 583.

Clemmesen, J. (1951) 'On the etiology of some human cancers'. *J. Nat. Cancer Inst.*, **12**, 1.

Clemmesen, J. (1965) 'Statistical studies in the aetiology of malignant neoplasms: I Review and results'. *Acta Path. Microbiol. Scand. Suppl.* 174, **1**, 254.

Cole, M. P. (1964) 'The place of radiotherapy in the management of early breast cancer. A report of two clinical trials'. *Brit. J. Surg.*, **51**, 216.

Collins, D. H. and Cameron, K. M. (1964) 'Interstitial cell tumours', *Brit. J. Urol. Suppl.* (The pathology of testicular tumours), 36, 2, p. 62.

Collins, D. H. and Pugh, R. C. B. (1964) 'Classification and frequency of testicular tumours', *Brit. J. Urol. Suppl.* (The pathology of testicular tumours), **36**, 2, p. 1.

Collins, D. H. and Symington, T. (1964) 'Sertoli cell tumours', *Brit. J. Urol. Suppl.* (The pathology of testicular tumours), **36**, 2, p. 52.

Colsky, J., Escher, G. C., Evans, A., Mitus, A., Li, M. C., Roath, S., Sullivan, R. D., Sykes, M. P. and Tan, C. T. C. (1960) 'Preliminary clinical pharmacology of Mitomycin C'. Personal communication.

Conference (1958) 'Comparative clinical and biological effects of alkylating agents'. *Ann. N.Y. Acad. Sci.*, **68**, 657.

Connor, T. B., Hopkins, T. R., Thomas, W. C. Jr., Carey, R. H. and Howard, J. E. (1956) 'The use of cortisone and ACTH in hypercalcemic states'. *J. Clin. Endoc.*, **16**, 945.

Cook, H. H., Gamble, C. J. and Satterthwaite, A. P. (1961) 'Oral contraception by norethynodrel'. *Amer. J. Obstet. Gynec.*, **82**, 437.

Co-operative Breast Cancer Group (1961) 'Progress report—results of studies by the Co-operative Breast Cancer group'. *Cancer Chemother. Rep.*, **11**, 109.

Co-operative Breast Cancer Group (1962) 'Testosterone propionate therapy of breast cancer. A progress report'. *Cancer Chemother. Rep.*, **16**, 273.

Co-operative Breast Cancer Group (1964) 'Testosterone propionate therapy in breast cancer'. *J. Amer. Med. Assoc.*, **188**, 106.

Cornil, L. (1949) 'The value of oestrogen treatment in postmenopausal epithelioma of the breast with late virilism,' English abstract in *Excerpta Medica Sect.* 3 (1950), **4**, 389.

Cree, I. C. (1960) 'Toxic marrow failure after treatment of carcinoma with cytotoxic drugs'. *Brit. Med. J.*, **ii**, 1499.

Crowley, L. G., Demetriou, J. A., McDonald, I., Kotin, P., Kushinsky, S. and Donovan, A. J. (1962) 'Levels of exogenous estrogens in tissues in human mammary carcinoma'. *Surg. Forum*, **13**, 103.

Crowley, L. G. and McDonald, I. (1965) 'Delalutin and estrogens for the treatment of advanced mammary carcinoma in the postmenopausal women'. *Cancer (Phil)*, **18**, 346.

Curreri, A. R. and McIver, F. A. (1956) 'OPSPA with and without corticosteroids in the treatment of human cancer'. *Proc. Amer. Assoc. Cancer Res.*, **2**, 101.

Curwen, S. (1963) 'The value of norethisterone acetate in the treatment of advanced carcinoma of the breast'. *Clin. Radiol.*, **14**, 445.

Daicoff, G. R., Harmon, R. and Van Prohaska, J. (1962) 'Effect of adrenalectomy on mammary carcinoma.' *Arch. Surg.*, **85**, 800.

Dao, T. L. Y. (1953) 'Estrogen excretion in women with mammary cancer before and after adrenalectomy'. *Science*, **118**, 21.

Dao, T. L. Y. (1962) 'Site of metastases and response to therapy in women with cancer of the breast'. *Acta Unio Int. Contra Canc.*, **18**, 928.

Dao, T. L. Y. and Grinberg, R. (1963) 'Fluorinated pyrimidines in the treatment of breast cancer patients with liver metastases'. *Cancer Chemother. Rep*, **27**, 71.

Dao, T. L. Y. and Huggins, C. (1955) 'Bilateral adrenalectomy in the treatment of cancer of the breast'. *Arch. Surg.*, **71**, 645.

Dao, T. L. Y. and Nemoto, T. (1965) 'An evaluation of adrenalectomy and androgen in disseminated mammary carcinoma'. *Surg. Gynec. Obstet.*, **121**, 1257.

Dao, T. L. Y., Tan, E. and Brooks, V. (1961) 'A comparative evaluation of adrenalectomy and cortisone in the treatment of advanced mammary carcinoma'. *Cancer (Phil.)*, **14**, 1259.

Dargent, M., Berger, M. and Lahneche, B. (1962) 'Thyroid function in breast cancer patients'. *Acta Unio Int. Contra Canc.*, **18**, 915.

Davies, J. N. P. (1949) 'Sex hormone upset in Africans'. *Brit. Med. J.*, **ii**, 676.

De Carvalho, S. (1963) 'Preliminary experimentation with specific immuno-therapy of neoplastic disease in man'. *Cancer (Phil.)*, **16**, 306.

Dekker, A. and Russfield, A. B. (1963) 'Pituitary tropic hormone studies and morphological observations in carcinoma of the prostate'. *Cancer (Phil.)*, **16**, 743.

Delarue, N. C. (1955) 'Fundamental concepts determining a philosophy of treatment in mammary carcinoma'. *Canad. Med. Assoc. J.*, **73**, 597.

Deshpande, N., Bulbrook, R. D. and Ellis, F. G. (1963) 'An apparent selective accumulation of testosterone by human breast tissue'. *J. Endoc.*, **25**, 555.

Deshpande, N., Jensen, V., Bulbrook, R. D. and Doouss, T. W. (1967) '*In vivo* steroidogenesis by the human adrenal gland'. *Steroids*, **9**, 393.

Diczfalusy, E. (1965) 'Probable mode of action of oral contraceptives'. *Brit. Med. J.*, **ii**, 1394.

Diczfalusy, E., Notter, G., Edsmyr, F. and Westman, A. (1959) 'Estrogen excretion in breast cancer patients before and after ovarian irradiation and oophorectomy'. *J. Clin. Endoc.*, **19**, 1230.

Dobriner, K., Lieberman, S., Hariton, L., Sarett, L. H. and Rhoads, C. P. (1947) 'The isolation of delta-9-etiocholenolone from human urine'. *J. Biol. Chem.*, **169**, 221.

Dobson, L. (1962) 'The management of metastatic breast cancer'. *Surg. Clin. N. America*, **42**, 861.

Donegan, W. L. (1967) 'Endocrine ablation, hormone therapy, and chemo-therapy', in *Cancer of the Breast*, Eds J. S. Spratt and W. L. Donegan, Philadelphia; W. B. Saunders.

Dorfman, R. I., Baba, S., Abe, O., Harada, T. and Rooks, W. H. (1967) 'The influence of drostalone on a transplantable rat mammary fibroadenoma and carcinogen induced adenocarcinoma', in *Cambridge Symposium on the Treatment of Carcinoma of the Breast*, p. 15, Ed A. S. Jarrett: Excerpta Medica Foundation.

Douglas, M. (1952) 'The treatment of advanced breast cancer by hormone therapy'. *Brit. J. Cancer*, **6**, 32.

Douglas, M. (1957) 'Indications for adrenalectomy and hypophysectomy in advanced breast cancer'. *Acta Endoc. (Kobn.) Suppl.*, **31**, 307.

Douglas, M., Falconer, C. W. A., Strong, J. A. and Loraine, J. A. (1961) 'Urinary excretion of gonadotropins in relation to treatment of mammary carcinoma by bilateral adrenalectomy and oophorectomy', in *Human Pituitary Gonadotropins*, p. 249, Ed A. Albert, Springfield; Charles C. Thomas.

Edelstyn, G., Gleadhill, C. and Lyons, A. (1965) 'A rational approach to hypophysectomy'. *Brit. J. Surg.*, **52**, 953.

Edelstyn, G., Gleadhill, C. and Lyons, A. (1968) 'Total hypophysectomy for advanced breast cancer'. *Clin. Radiol.*, **19**, 426.

Edelstyn, G. A., Lyons, A. R. and Welbourn, R. B. (1958) 'Thyroid function in patients with mammary cancer'. *Lancet*, **i**, 670.

Eisalo, A., Jarvinen, P. A. and Luukkainen, T. (1964) 'Hepatic impairment during the intake of contraceptive pills: clinical trial with postmenopausal women'. *Brit. Med. J.*, **ii**, 426.

Eley, A. and Riddell, V. (1960), 'Treatment of advanced carcinoma of the breast by oophorectomy and prednisone'. *Lancet*, **i**, 278.

Ellerker, A. G. (1956) 'Thyroid disorders and breast cancer—a causal connection'? *Med. Press*, **235**, 280.

Ellis, F. and others (1944) 'Discussion on advanced cases of carcinoma of breast treated by stilboestrol'. *Proc. Roy. Soc. Med.*, **37**, 731.

Ellis, F., Hoch Ligeti, C. and Oliver, R. (1961) 'Investigation of the effect of X-radiation on the localisation of radioactive phosphorus in breast tumours'. *Brit. J. Cancer*, **5**, 45.

Emerson, K. and Jessiman, A. G. (1956) 'Hormonal influences on the growth and progression of cancer: Tests for hormone dependency in mammary and prostate cancer'. *New Engl. J. Med.*, **254**, 252.

Emerson, W. J., Kennedy, B. J., Graham, J. N. and Nathanson, I. T. (1953) 'Pathology of primary and recurrent carcinoma of the human breast after administration of steroid hormones'. *Cancer (Phil.)*, **6**, 641.

Emerson, W. J., Kennedy, B. J. and Taft, E. B. (1960) 'Correlation of histological alterations in breast cancer with response to hormone therapy'. *Cancer (Phil.)*, **13**, 1047.

Emery, E. S. and Trotter, W. R. (1963) 'Tri-iodothyronine in advanced breast cancer'. *Lancet*, **i**, 358.

Escher, G. (1958) 'Panel discussion', in *Breast Cancer*, p. 225, Ed A. Segaloff, St. Louis; C. V. Mosby.

Escher, G. (1967) 'Early versus late castration', in *Current Concepts in Breast Cancer*, p. 316, Eds A. Segaloff, K. K. Meyer and S. Debakey, Baltimore; Williams and Wilkins.

Escher, G. C. and Kaufman, R. J. (1961) 'Current views on the management of metastatic mammary carcinoma'. *Med. Clin. N. Amer.*, **45**, 613.

Escher, G. C. and Kaufman, R. J. (1963) 'Advanced breast carcinoma—factors influencing survival'. *Acta Unio Int. Contra Canc.*, **19**, 1039.

Fairgrieve, J. (1965) 'Selective criteria for surgical removal of the endocrine glands in advanced breast cancer'. *Surg. Gynec. Obstet.*, **120**, 371.

Falls, J. L. (1955) 'Accessory adrenal cortex in the broad ligament: Incidence and functional significance'. *Cancer (Phil)*, **8**, 143.

Farber, S. (1949) 'Some observations on the effect of folic acid antagonists in acute leukaemia and other forms of incurable cancer'. *Blood*, **4**, 160.

Farber, S., Maddock, C. and Swaffield, M. (1956) 'Studies of the carcinolytic and other biological activity of Actinomycin D'. *Proc. Amer. Assoc. Cancer Res.*, **2**, 104.

Farrow, J. H. and Adair, F. E. (1942) 'Effect of orchidectomy on skeletal metastases from cancer of male breast'. *Science*, **95**, 654.

Ferguson, K. A. and Wallace, A. L. C. (1961) 'Starch gel electrophoresis of anterior pituitary hormones'. *Nature*, **190**, 629.

Fifth International Congress on Geographical Pathology (1954). Reported in *Brit. Med. J.*, **ii**, 981.

Finley, J. W. and Bogardus, G. M. (1960) 'Breast cancer and thyroid disease'. *Quart. Rev. Surg. Obstet. Gynec.*, **17**, 139.

Fishman, J., Hellman, L., Zumoff, B. and Gallagher, T. F. (1962) 'Influence of thyroid hormone on estrogen metabolism in man'. *J. Clin. Endoc.*, **22**, 389.

Flaxel, J. and Wellings, S. R. (1963) 'Toxic effects of testosterone on organ cultures of mammary carcinoma cells of C3H/CRGL mice'. *Fed. Proc.*, **22**, 331.

Fletcher, W. S., Dennis, D. L. and Ross, H. B. (1965) 'Distribution and possible mechanism of action of thioTEPA in experimental breast cancer'. *Cancer (Phil.)*, **18**, 1437.

Fluhmann, C. F. and Murphy, K. M. (1939) 'Estrogenic and gonadotropic hormones in the blood of climacteric women and csatrates'. *Amer. J. Obstet. Gynec.*, **38**, 778.

Folca, P. J., Glascock, R. F. and Irvine, W. T. (1961) 'Studies with tritium labelled hexoestrol in advanced breast cancer'. *Lancet*, **ii**, 796.

Foley, J. F. and Aftonomos, B. T. (1965) 'Growth of human breast neoplasms in cell culture'. *J. Nat. Cancer Inst.*, **34**, 217.

Ford, H. T. (1959) 'Durabolin and Deca-Durabolin in the treatment of advanced mammary cancer'. *Brit. Emp. Cancer Camp. Ann. Rep.*, **37**, 267.

Forrest, A. P. M. (1965) 'Endocrine treatment of breast cancer'. *Israel J. Med. Sci.*, **1**, 259.

Foss, G. L. and Simpson, S. L. (1959) 'Oral methyltestosterone and jaundice', *Brit. Med. J.*, **i**, 259.

Foss, G. L. and Simpson, S. L. (1959) 'Oral methyltestosterone and jaundice'. *Brit. Med. J.*, **i**, 259.

Fracchia, A. A., Holleb, A. I., Farrow, J. H., Treves, N. E., Randall, H. T., Finkbeiner, J. A. and Whitmore, Jr., W. F. (1959) 'Results of bilateral adrenalectomy in the management of incurable breast cancer'. *Cancer (Phil.)*, **12**, 58.

Frank, W. and Osterberg, A. E. (1960) 'Mitomycin C—an evaluation of the Japanese reports'. *Cancer Chemother. Rep.*, **9**, 114.

Freckman, H. A., Fry, H. L., Mendez, F. L. and Maurer, E. R. (1964) 'Chlorambucil, Prednisolone therapy for disseminated breast cancer'. *J. Amer. Med. Assoc.*, **189**, 23.

Frei, E. (1965) 'Chemotherapy of breast cancer'. *Ann. Int. Med.*, **63**, 334.

Furth, J. and Clifton, K. H. (1958) 'Experimental observations on mammotropes and the mammary gland', in *Endocrine Aspects of Breast Cancer*, p. 276, Eds A. R. Currie and C. F. W. Illingsworth, Edinburgh; E. & S. Livingstone.

Gailani, S. (1963) 'Phase II studies on Vincristine in human cancer'. *Proc. Amer. Assoc. Cancer Res.*, **4**, 21.

Galante, M., Fournier, D. J. and Wood, D. A. (1957) 'Adrenalectomy for metastatic breast carcinoma'. *J. Amer. Med. Assoc.*, **163**, 1011.

Galicich, J. H., French, L. A. and Melby, J. C. (1961) 'Use of dexamethasone in the treatment of cerebral oedema resulting from brain tumours and brain surgery'. *J. Lancet*, **81**, 46.

Gardner, F. H. and Pringle, J. C., Jr. (1961) 'Androgens and erythropoiesis: I Preliminary clinical observations'. *Arch. Int. Med.*, **107**, 846.

Gardner, B., Thomas, A. N. and Gordan, G. S. (1962) 'Anti-tumor efficacy of prednisone and sodium liothyronine in advanced breast cancer'. *Cancer (Phil.)*, **15**, 334.

Gennes, L. De (1966) Quoted in *Endocrine Surgery in Human Cancers*, p. 163, Ed P. Juret, Springfield; Charles C. Thomas.

Gerbrandy, J. and Hellendorn, H. B. A. (1957) 'The diagnostic value of calciuria during hormonal treatment of metastasised mammary carcinoma'. *Acta Endoc. (Kobn.) Suppl.*, **31**, 275.

Gilbert, J. (1933) 'Carcinoma of the male breast'. *Surg. Gynec. Obstet.*, **57**, 451.

Gilse, H. A. Van (1962) 'Long-term treatment with corticosteroids of patients with metastatic breast cancer'. *Cancer Chemother. Rep.*, **16**, 293.

Gold, G. L., Salvin, L. G. and Shnider, B. I. (1962) 'A comparative study with 3 alkylating agents: Mechlorcthamine, cyclophosphamide, and Uracil Mustard'. *Cancer Chemother. Rep.*, **16**, 417.

Goldenberg, I. S. (1963) 'Vinblastine sulphate therapy of women with advanced breast cancer'. *Cancer Chemother. Rep.*, **29**, 111.

Goldenberg, I. S. (1964) 'Vincristine therapy of women with advanced breast cancer'. *Cancer Chemother. Rep.*, **41**, 7.

Goldenberg, I. S. and Hayes, M. A. (1959) 'Hormonal therapy of metastatic female breast carcinoma: I 9α-bromo-11-ketoprogesterone'. *Cancer (Phil.)*, **12**, 738.

Goldenberg, I. S. and Hayes, M. A. (1961) 'Hormonal therapy of metastatic female breast carcinoma: II 2α methyl dihydrotestosterone propionate'. *Cancer (Phil.)*, **14**, 705.

Goldin, A. and Mantel, N. (1957) 'The employment of combinations of drugs in the chemotherapy of neoplasia—a review'. *Cancer Res.*, **17**, 635.

Goldsmith, R. S. and Ingbar, S. H. (1966) 'Inorganic phosphate treatment of hypercalcemia of diverse etiologies'. *New Engl. J. Med.*, **274**, 1.

Goldzieher, J. W. (1964) 'Newer drugs in oral contraception'. *Med. Clin. N. Amer.*, **48**, 529.

Gomez, E. T. and Turner, C. W. (1938) 'Further evidence for a mammogenic hormone in the anterior pituitary'. *Exper. Biol. and Med.*, **37**, 607.

Gordon, D., Horwitt, B. N., Segaloff, A., Murison, P. J. and Schlosser, J. V. (1952) 'Hormonal therapy in cancer of the breast: III Effect of progesterone on clinical course and hormonal excretion'. *Cancer (Phil.)*, **5**, 275.

Gordon, D. L. and Segaloff, A. (1958) 'Castration as a palliative therapy for advanced breast cancer', in *Breast Cancer*, p. 187, Ed A. Segaloff, St. Louis; C. V. Mosby.

Graham, L. S. (1953) 'Celiac accessory adrenal glands'. *Cancer (Phil.)*, **6**, 149.

Green, A. (1961) 'Hormone control of breast cancer'. *Lancet*, **ii**, 828.

Green, A. (1966) 'General discussion', in *The Value of Cytotoxic Agents and Anabolic Steroids in the Treatment of Advanced Malignant Disease*, p. 93, Ed M. Abrahamson, London; Parcener Press.

Greenberg, E. (1962) 'Prognosis of patients with liver metastasis from breast cancer undergoing hypophysectomy'. *Acta Unio Int. Contra Canc.*, **18**, 949.

Greening, W. P. (1961) 'Symposium on Methotrexate in the treatment of cancer'. *Brit. Med. J.*, **ii**, 954.

Greening, W. P., Ramsay, G. S., Stevenson, J. J., Boyland, E., Rigby-Jones, P. C., and Godsmark, B. (1960) 'Results in the treatment of cancer of the breast by interstitial irradiation of the pituitary'. *Brit. J. Cancer*, **14**, 627.

Greenspan, E. M. (1964) 'Combinations of methotrexate, thioTEPA and 5-fluorouracil in advanced breast carcinoma'. *Proc. Amer. Assoc. Cancer Res.*, **5**, 23.

Greenspan, E. M. (1965) 'Results of four drug sequential combination chemotherapy of breast carcinoma in relation to predominant organ metastases'. *Proc. Amer. Assoc. Cancer Res.*, **6**, 24.

Greenwood, F. C. and Bulbrook, R. D. (1957) 'Effect of hypophysectomy on urinary oestrogen in breast cancer.' *Brit. Med. J.*, **i**, 666.

Grice, O. D., Faircloth, S. and Thomas, C. G. (1966) 'The effect of hypopthyroidism on induced cancer of the breast'. *Proc. Amer. Assoc. Cancer Res.*, **7**, 26.

Griffith, M. M. and Beck, J. C. (1963) 'The value of serum phosphohexose isomerase as an index of metastatic breast carcinoma activity'. *Cancer (Phil.)*, **16**, 1032.

Gurling, K. J., Scott, G. B. D. and Baron, D. N. (1957) 'Metastases in pituitary tissue removed at hypophysectomy in women with mammary carcinoma'. *Brit. J. Cancer*, **11**, 519.

Haddow, A., Watkinson, J. M., Paterson, E. and Koller, P. (1944) 'Influence of synthetic oestrogens upon advanced malignant disease'. *Brit. Med. J.*, **ii**, 393.

Hadfield, G. (1957) 'The nature and origin of the mammotropic agent present in human female urine'. *Lancet*, **i**, 1058.

Hadfield, G. J. and Holt, J. A. G. (1956) 'The physiological castration syndrome in breast cancer'. *Brit. Med. J.*, **ii**, 972.

Halberstadter, L. (1905) 'Die einwirkung der Rontgenstrahlen auf Ovarien'. *Berl. Klin. Wochenschr.*, **42**, 64.

Hale, B. T. (1961) 'A technique for studying human tumour growth *in vivo*'. *Lancet*, **ii**, 345.

Hall, T. C., Dederick, M. M. and Nevinny, H. B. (1963a) 'Prognostic value of hormonally induced hypercalcemia in breast cancer'. *Cancer Chemother. Rep.*, **30**, 21.

Hall, T. C., Dederick, M. M., Nevinny, H. B. and Muench, H. (1963b) 'Prognostic value of response of patients with breast cancer to therapeutic castration.' *Cancer Chemother. Rep.*, **31**, 47.

Hayward, J. L. and Bulbrook, R. D. (1966) *Clinical Evaluation in Breast Cancer*. London; Academic Press.

Heller, C. G., Farney, J. P. and Myers, G. B. (1944) 'Development and correlation of menopausal symptoms, vaginal smear and urinary gonadotropin changes following castration in 27 women'. *J. Clin. Endoc.*, **4**, 101.

Hellman, L., Bradlow, H. L., Zumoff, B. and Gallagher, T. F. (1961) 'The influence of thyroid hormone on hydrocortisone production and metabolism'. *J. Clin. Endoc.*, **21**, 1231.

Hellstrom, J. and Franksson, C. (1958) 'Adrenalectomy in cancer of the breast', in *Endocrine Aspects of Breast Cancer*, p. 5, Eds A. R. Currie and C. F. W. Illingsworth, Edinburgh; E. & S. Livingstone.

Hems, G. (1967) 'Two types of breast cancer?' *Brit. Med. J.*, **iii**, 496.

Henderson, W. R. and Rowlands, I. W. (1938) 'The gonadotropic activity of the anterior pituitary gland in relation to increased intracranial pressure'. *Brit. Med. J.*, **i**, 1094.

Herman, G. E. (1900) 'Four cases of recurrent mammary carcinoma treated by oophorectomy and thyroid extract'. *Brit. Med. J.*, **ii**, 1167.

Herrell, W. E. (1937) 'The relative incidence of oophorectomy in women with and without carcinoma of the breast'. *Amer. J. Cancer*, **29**, 659.

Herrmann, J. B., Adair, F. E. and Woodard, H. Q. (1947) 'Use of testosterone propionate in the treatment of advanced carcinoma of the breast; treatment of osseous metastases'. *Surgery*, **22**, 101.

Hertz, S. (1950) 'The modifying effect of steroid therapy on human neoplastic tissue as judged by ^{32}P studies'. *J. Clin. Invest.*, **29**, 821.

Heuson, J. C. and Legros, N. (1963) '*In vitro* effect of testosterone and 17β-Estradiol on L-leucine ^{14}C incorporation into human breast cancer'. *Cancer (Phil.)*, **16**, 404.

Hiisi-Brummer, L., Hortling, H., Malmio, K. and Af Bjorkesten, G. (1960) 'The effect of hypophysectomy on the oestrogen effect in the body as measured by the vaginal smear technique in metastasising mammary cancer'. *Acta Endoc. (Kobn.)*, **33**, 81.

Hill, B. R. and Levi, C. (1954) 'Elevation of a serum component in neoplastic disease'. *Cancer Res.*, **14**, 513.

Hollander, V. P., Jonas, H. and Smith, D. E. (1958) 'Estradiol-sensitive isocitric dehydrogenase in non-cancerous and cancerous human breast tissue'. *Cancer (Phil.)*, **11**, 803.

Hollander, V. P., Smith, D. E. and Adamson, T. E. (1959) 'Studies on estrogen-sensitive transhydrogenase: the effect of estradiol 17β on α ketoglutarate production in non-cancerous and cancerous human breast tissue'. *Cancer (Phil.)*, **12**, 135.

Holleb, A. I. and Farrow, J. H. (1962) 'The relation of carcinoma of the breast and pregnancy in 283 cases'. *Surg. Gynec. Obstet.*, **115**, 65.

Horsley, J. S. (1944) 'Bilateral oophorectomy with radical operation for breast cancer'. *Surgery*, **15**, 590.

Horsley, G. W. (1957) 'Prophylactic oophorectomy in treatment of cancer of the breast'. *Amer. Surg.*, **23**, 396.

Hortling, H., Hiisi-Brummer, L. and Af Bjorkesten, G. A. (1959) 'Thyroid function in cases of mammary cancer'. *Ann. Med. Intern. Fenn.*, **48**, Suppl. 28, 50.

Hortling, H., Hiisi-Brummer, L., and Af Bjorkesten G. A. (1962) 'Endocrine therapy of metastasising breast cancer'. *Acta Med. Scand.*, **172**, Suppl. 385.

Hortling, H., Malmio, K. and Hiisi-Brummer, L. (1961) 'Norandrostenolone in the treatment of metastasising mammary cancer'. *Acta Endoc. (Kobn.) Suppl.*, **63**, 132.

Howard, R. R. and Grosjean, W. A. (1949) 'Bilateral mammary carcinoma in the male coincident with prolonged stilboestrol therapy'. *Surgery*, **25**, 300.

Huggins, C. (1952) 'Endocrine factors in cancer'. *J. Urol.*, **68**, 875.

Huggins, C. (1954) 'Endocrine methods of treatment of cancer of the breast'. *J. Nat. Cancer Inst.*, **15**, 1.

Huggins, C. and Bergenstal, D. M. (1952) 'Inhibition of human mammary and prostatic cancers by adrenalectomy'. *Cancer Res.*, **12**, 134.

Huggins, C. and Dao, T. L. Y. (1953) 'Adrenalectomy and oophorectomy in treatment of advanced carcinoma of the breast'. *J. Amer. Med. Assoc.*, **151**, 1388.

Huggins, C., Moon, R. C. and Morii, S. (1962) 'Extinction of experimental mammary cancer. 1. Estradiol 17β and progesterone'. *Proc. Nat. Acad. Sci.*, **48**, 379.

Huggins, C. and Taylor, G. W. (1955) 'Carcinoma of the male breast'. *Arch. Surg.*, **70**, 303.

Humphrey, L. J. and Swerdlow, M. (1964) 'The relationship of breast disease to thyroid disease'. *Cancer (Phil.)*, **17**, 1170.

Hurley, J. D., Trump, D. S., Flatley, T. J. and Riesch, J. D. (1961) 'A method of selecting patients for cancer chemotherapy'. *Arch. Surg.*, **83**, 611.

Huseby, R. A. (1958) 'The use of estrogen in the treatment of advanced human breast cancer', in *Breast Cancer*, p. 206, Ed A. Segaloff, St. Louis; C. V. Mosby.

Huseby, R. A. and Thomas, L. B. (1954) 'Histological and histochemical alterations in the normal breast tissues of patients with advanced breast cancer being treated with estrogenic hormones'. *Cancer (Phil.)*, **7**, 54.

Irvine, W. T., Aitken, E. H., Rendleman, D. L. and Folca, P. J. (1961) 'Urinary oestrogen measurements after oophorectomy and adrenalectomy for advanced breast cancer'. *Lancet*, **ii**, 791.

Jensen, E. V., Desombre, E. R. and Jungblut, P. W. (1967) 'Estrogen receptors in hormone responsive tissues and tumour', in *Endogenous Factors Influencing Host-tumor Balance*, Eds Wissler, Dao and Wood, Illinois; University of Chicago Press.

Jessiman, A. G. (1958) in *Endocrine Aspects of Breast Cancer*, p. 26, Eds A. P. Currie and C. F. W. Illingsworth, Edinburgh; E. & S. Livingstone.

Jessiman, A. G., Emerson, K., Shah, R. C. and Moore, F. D. (1963) 'Hypercalcemia in carcinoma of the breast'. *Ann. Surg.*, **157**, 377.

Jessiman, A. G., Matson, D. D. and Moore, F. D. (1959) 'Hypophysectomy in the treatment of breast cancer'. *New Engl. J. Med.*, **261**, 1199.

Joint Committee on Endocrine Ablative Procedures in Disseminated Mammary Carcinoma (1961). *J. Amer. Med. Assoc.*, **175**, 137, 787.

Jolles, B. (1962) 'Progesterone in the treatment of advanced malignant tumours of breast, ovary and uterus'. *Brit. J. Cancer*, **16**, 209.

Jonsson, U., Colsky, J., Lessner, H. E., Roath, O. S., Alper, R. G. and Jones, R. Jr., (1959) 'Clinical and pharmacological observations of the effects of 9α bromo-11β ketoprogesterone on patients with carcinoma of the breast'. *Cancer* (*Phil.*), **12**, 509.

Joplin, G. F. and Jegatheesan, K. A. (1962) 'Serum glycolytic enzymes and acid phosphatases in mammary carcinomatosis'. *Brit. Med. J.*, **i**, 827.

Jull, J. W. (1958) 'Hormonal mechanisms in mammary carcinogenesis', in *Endocrine Aspects of Breast Cancer*, p. 305, Eds A. R. Currie and C. F. W. Illingsworth, Edinburgh; E. & S. Livingstone.

Jull, J. W., Shucksmith, H. S. and Bonser, G. M. (1963) 'A study of urinary estrogen excretion in relation to breast cancer'. *J. Clin. Endoc.*, **23**, 433.

Juret, P. (1966) *Endocrine Surgery in Human Cancers*. Springfield; Charles C. Thomas.

Juret, P., Hayem, M. and Flaisler, A. (1964) quoted in *Endocrine Surgery in Human Cancers*, p. 215, Ed P. Juret, Springfield; Charles C. Thomas, 1966.

Juret, P., Hayem, M. and Thomas, M. (1962) quoted in *Endocrine Surgery in Human Cancers*, p. 237, Ed P. Juret, Springfield; Charles C. Thomas, 1966.

Karnofsky, D. A. and Burchenal, J. H. (1949) 'Clinical evaluation of chemotherapeutic agents in cancer', in *Evaluation of Chemotherapeutic Agents*, p. 101, Ed C. M. McLeod, New York; Columbia University Press.

Kaufman, R. J. and Escher, G. C. (1961) 'Rebound regression in advanced mammary carcinoma'. *Surg. Gynec. Obstet.*, **113**, 635.

Kaufman, R. J., Rothschild, E. O., Escher, G. C. and Myers, W. P. L. (1964) 'Hypercalcemia in mammary carcinoma following the administration of a progestational agent'. *J. Clin. Endoc.*, **24**, 1235.

Kellner, G. and Turcic, G. (1962) 'The importance of tissue culture for hormonal therapy of mammary carcinoma'. *Klin. Med.* (*Wien*), **17**, 83.

Kennedy, B. J. (1957) 'Present status of hormone therapy in advanced breast cancer'. *Radiology*, **69**, 330.

Kennedy, B. J. (1958) 'Fluoxymesterone therapy in advanced breast cancer'. *New Engl. J. Med.*, **259**, 673.

Kennedy, B. J. (1962a) 'Massive estrogen administration in premenopausal women with metastatic breast cancer'. *Cancer* (*Phil.*), **15**, 641.

Kennedy, B. J. (1962b) 'Stimulation of erythropoiesis by androgenic hormones'. *Ann. Int. Med.*, **57**, 917.

Kennedy, B. J. (1965a) 'Hormonal control of breast cancer'. *Ann. Int. Med.*, **63**, 329.

Kennedy, B. J. (1965b) 'Hormone therapy for advanced breast cancer'. *Cancer* (*Phil.*), **18**, 1551.

Kennedy, B. J. and Brown, J. H. (1965) 'Combined estrogenic and androgenic hormone therapy in advanced breast cancer'. *Cancer* (*Phil.*), **18**, 431.

Kennedy, B. J. and French, L. (1965) 'Hypophysectomy in advanced breast cancer'. *Amer. J. Surg.*, **110**, 411.

Kennedy, B. J., Mielke, P. W. and Fortuny, I. E. (1964) 'Therapeutic castration versus prophylactic castration in breast cancer.' *Surg. Gynec. Obstet.*, **118**, 524.

Kennedy, B. J., Nathanson, I. T., Tibbetts, D. M. and Aub, J. C. (1955) 'Biochemical alterations during steroid hormone therapy of advanced breast cancer'. *Amer. J. Med.*, **19**, 337.

Kennedy, B. J., Tibbetts, D. M., Nathanson, I. T. and Aub, J. C. (1953) 'Hypercalcemic complications of hormone therapy of advanced breast cancer'. *Cancer Res.*, **13**, 445.

Khazan, N., Primo, C. H., Danon, A., Assael, M., Sulman, F. G. and Winnik, H. Z. (1962) 'The mammotropic effect of tranquillising drugs'. *Arch. Int. Pharmacodyn.*, **141**, 29.

Kim, U. (1965) 'Pituitary function and hormonal therapy of experimental breast cancer'. *Cancer Res.*, **25**, 1146.

Kim, U., Furth, J. and Yannopoulos, K. (1963) 'Observations on hormonal control of mammary cancer: I Estrogen and mammotropes'. *J. Nat. Cancer Inst.*, **31**, 233.

Kimel, V. M. (1957) 'Clinical cytological correlations of mammary carcinoma based upon sex chromatin counts'. *Cancer* (*Phil.*), **10**, 922.

Kleinfeld, G., Haagensen, C. D. and Cooley, E. (1963) 'Age and menstrual status as prognostic factors in carcinoma of the breast'. *Ann. surg.*, **156**, 600.

Kofman, S., Garvin, J. S., Nagamani, D. and Taylor, S. G. III (1957) 'Treatment of cerebral metastases from breast carcinoma with prednisolone'. *J. Amer. Med. Assoc.*, **163**, 1473.

Koller, P. C. (1944) 'Addendum—cytology of serial biopsies from a case of carcinoma of the breast treated with stilboestrol'. *Brit. Med. J.*, **2**, 398.

Kolodziejska, H. (1959) 'Hormone treatment of patients with well advanced forms of cancer of the breast'. *Prob. Oncol. (N.Y.)*, **5**, No. 11, 45.

Kurokawa, T. and Saito, T. (1959) 'Chemotherapy of malignant tumours'. *Acta Unio Int. Contra Canc.*, **15**, (suppl.), 159.

Lacassagne, A. (1936a) 'Hormonal pathogenesis of adenocarcinoma of the breast'. *Amer. J. Cancer*, **27**, 217.

Lacassagne, A. (1936b) 'Attempts to modify by progesterone or testosterone the development in mice of mammary adenocarcinoma induced by oestrone'. *C.R. Soc. de Biol.*, **126**, 385.

Landau, R. L., Ehrlich, E. N. and Huggins, C. (1962) 'Estradiol benzoate and progesterone in advanced human breast cancer'. *J. Amer. Med. Assoc.*, **182**, 632.

Lane-Claypon, J. E. (1926) 'A further report on cancer of the breast with special reference to its associated antecedent conditions', in *Ministry of Health Report on Public Health and Medical Subjects*, No. 32, London; H.M.S.O.

Larionov, L. F. (1965) *Cancer Chemotherapy*, p. 459, Oxford; Pergamon Press.

Lazarev, N. J. (1960) 'New developments in the hormone therapy of malignant tumours', in *Cancer Progress* 1960, p. 204, Ed R. W. Raven, London; Butterworths.

Lees, J. C. and Park, W. W. (1949) 'The malignancy of cancer at different ages: a histological study'. *Brit. J. Cancer*, **3**, 186.

Lemon, H. M. (1957) 'Cortisone-thyroid therapy of metastatic mammary cancer'. *Ann. Int. Med.*, **46**, 457.

Lemon, H. M. (1959) 'Prednisone therapy of advanced mammary cancer'. *Cancer (Phil.)*, **12**, 93.

Lemon, H. M. (1961) Discussion of 'Hormonal therapy of breast cancer', in *Biological Activities of Steroids in Relation to Cancer*, p. 375, Eds G. Pincus and E. P. Vollmer, New York; Academic Press.

Lemon, H. M., Reynolds, M. D. and Wotiz, H. H. (1958) 'Anti-oestrogenic therapy of advanced mammary carcinoma with prednisone'. *Proc. Amer. Assoc. Cancer Res.*, **2**, 319.

Lerner, L. J. and Hilf, R. (1967) 'Biological activities of steroids and their relation to breast cancer therapy', in *Current Concepts in Breast Cancer*, p. 80, Eds A. Segaloff, K. K. Meyer and S. Debakey, Baltimore; Williams and Wilkins.

Lett, H. (1905) 'An analysis of 99 cases of inoperable carcinoma of the breast treated by oophorectomy'. *Lancet*, **i**, 227.

Lewin, I., Spencer, H. and Herrmann, J. (1959) 'Clinical and metabolic effects of 17α ethinyl–19 nortestosterone in mammary cancer'. *Proc. Amer. Assoc. Cancer Res.*, **3**, 37.

Lewison, E. F. (1965) 'Castration in the treatment of advanced breast cancer'. *Cancer (Phil.)*, **18**, 1558.

Lewison, E. F., Trimble, F. H. and Griffith, P. C. (1953) 'Result of surgical treatment of breast cancer at Johns Hopkins Hospital'. *J. Amer. Med. Assoc.*, **153**, 905.

Liechty, R. D., Davis, J. and Gleysteen, J. (1967) 'Cancer of the male breast'. *Cancer (Phil.)*, **20**, 1617.

Lilienfield, A. M. (1956) 'The relationship of cancer of the female breast to artificial menopause and marital status'. *Cancer (Phil.)*, **9**, 927.

Lipsett, M. B. and Bergenstal, D. M. (1960) 'Lack of effect of human growth hormone and ovine prolactin on cancer in man'. *Cancer Res.*, **20**, 1172.

Lipsett, M. B., Whitmore, W. F., Treves, N., West, C. D., Randall, H. T. and Pearson, O. H. (1957) 'Bilateral adrenalectomy in the palliation of metastatic breast cancer'. *Cancer (Phil.)*, **10**, 111.

Liu, W. (1957) 'Vaginal cytology in breast cancer patients'. *Surg. Gynec. Obstet.*, **105**, 421.

Loeser, A. (1939) 'Male hormone in the treatment of cancer of the breast'. *Acta Unio Int. Contra. Canc.*, **4**, 375.

Loeser, A. A. (1954) 'A new therapy for prevention of post-operative recurrences in genital and breast cancer'. *Brit. Med. J.*, **ii**, 1380.

Loraine, J. A., Strong, J. A. and Douglas, M. (1957) 'The value of pituitary gonadotrophin assays in patients with mammary carcinoma'. *Lancet*, **ii**, 575.

Low-Beer, B. V. A. and Green, R. B. (1952) 'Radio-phosphorus studies in breast tumours'. *Cardiologia*, **21**, 497.

Lucchini, A., Arraztoa, J. and Vargas, L. (1962) 'Metastalysis syndrome and effectiveness of subcutaneous implantation of hexestrol in the treatment of breast cancer metastases'. *Cancer (Phil.)*, **15**, 189.

Luehrs, W. (1961) Conference on 'Biochemistry of human cancer'. *Brit. Med. J.*, **i**, 1752.

Luft, R., Olivecrona, H., Ikkos, D., Nilsson, L. B. and Mossberg, H. (1958) 'Hypophysectomy in the management of metastatic carcinoma of the breast', in *Endocrine Aspects of Breast Cancer*, p. 27, Eds A. R. Currie and C. F. W. Illingsworth, Edinburgh; E. & S. Livingstone.

Lumb, G. and Mackenzie, D. H. (1959) 'The incidence of metastases in adrenal glands and ovaries removed for carcinoma of the breast.' *Cancer (Phil.)*, **12**, 521.

Lyons, A. and Edelstyn, G. (1962) 'ThioTEPA in treatment of advanced breast cancer'. *Brit. Med. J.*, **ii**, 1280.

McAllister, R. A., Sim, A. W., Hobkirk, R., Stewart, H., Blair, D. W. and Forrest, A. P. M. (1960) 'Urinary oestrogens after endocrine ablation'. *Lancet*, **i**, 1102.

McBride, J. M. (1957) 'Estrogen excretion levels in the normal postmenopausal woman'. *J. Clin. Endoc.*, **17**, 1440.

MacBryde, C. M. (1939) 'The production of breast growth in the human female'. *J. Amer. Med. Assoc.*, **112**, 1045.

McCalister, A. and Welbourn, R. B. (1962) 'Stimulation of mammary cancer by prolactin and the clinical response to hypophysectomy'. *Brit. med. J.*, **i**, 1669.

McCalister, A., Welbourn, R. B., Edelstyn, G. J. A., Lyons, A. R., Taylor, A. R., Gleadhill, C. A., Gordon, D. S. and Cole, J. O. Y. (1961) 'Factors influencing response to hypophysectomy for advanced cancer of the breast'. *Brit. Med. J.*, **i**, 613.

McCarthy, W. D. (1955) 'The palliation and remission of cancer with combined corticosteroid and nitrogen mustard therapy; report of 100 cases'. *New Engl. J. Med.*, **252**, 467.

McCullagh, E. P., Feldstein, M. A., Tweed, D. C. and Dohn, D. F. (1965) 'A study of pituitary function after intrasellar implantation of ^{90}Yt'. *J. Clin. Endoc.*, **25**, 832.

McDonald, I. (1962) 'Endocrine ablation in disseminated mammary carcinoma'. *Surg. Gynec. Obstet.*, **115**, 215.

McLaughlin, J. S., Hull, H. C., Oda, F. and Buxton, W. R. (1965) 'Metastatic carcinoma of the male breast: Remission by adrenalectomy'. *Ann. Surg.*, **162**, 9.

McMahon, B. and Feinleib, M. (1960) 'Breast cancer in relation to nursing and menopausal history'. *J. Nat. Cancer Inst.*, **24**, 733.

McWhirter, R. (1957) 'Some factors influencing prognosis in breast cancer'. *J. Fac. Radiol.*, **8**, 220.

Mandel, P. R. and Chiat, H. (1962) 'Radioactive phosphorus for carcinoma of the breast with diffuse metastatic bone disease'. *New York J. Med.*, **62**, 1970.

Marmorston, J. (1966) 'Urinary hormone metabolic levels in patients with cancer of the breast, prostate and lung'. *Ann. N.Y. Acad. Sci.*, **125**, 959.

Marques, P., Bru, A. and Espinasse, A. (1959) 'Role du fonctionement thyroidien dans le pronostic du cancer du sein'. *Bul. Assn. Franc. Cancer.*, **46**, 645.

Martin, F. I. R. (1964) 'Urinary gonadotropins in postmenopausal women with breast cancer.' *Brit. med. J.*, **ii**, 351.

Maximow, A. A. and Bloom, W. (1952) *A Text Book of Histology*, 6th ed., p. 114, Philadelphia; W. B. Saunders.

Meites, J. and Nicoll, C. S. (1966) 'Adenophyphysis, prolactin'. *Annual Rev. Physiol.*, **28**, 57.

Miller, H., Durant, J. A., Jacobs, A. G. and Allison, J. F. (1967) 'Alternative discriminating function for determining hormone dependency of breast cancer'. *Brit. med. J.*, **i**, 147.

Mioduszewska, O. (1968) In *Prognostic Factors in Breast Cancer*, Eds A. P. M. Forrest and P. B. Kunkler, p. 347, Edinburgh: E. & S. Livingstone.

Mittelman, A., Grinberg, R. and Dao, T. L. (1963) 'Clinical experiences with Vincristine in women with breast cancer'. *Proc. Amer. Assoc. Cancer Res.*, **4**, 44.

Mixner, J. P., Bergman, A. J. and Turner, C. W. (1942) 'Relation of mammogenic lobule-alveolar growth factor of the anterior pituitary to other anterior pituitary hormones'. *Endocrinology*, **31**, 461.

Montemurro, D. G. (1966) 'Neural relationships in pituitary function'. *Canad. Cancer Conf.*, **6**, 82.

Moon, W. J. (1968) Personal communication.

Moore, C. R. (1935) 'Hormones in relation to reproduction'. *Amer. J. Obstet. Gynec.*, **29**, 1.

Moore, K. and Barr, M. (1957) 'The sex chromatin in human malignant tissues'. *Brit. J. Cancer*, **11**, 384.

Muller, W. (1958) 'On the pharyngeal hypophysis', in *Endocrine Aspects of Breast Cancer*, p. 106, Eds A. R. Currie and C. F. W. Illingsworth, Edinburgh; E. & S. Livingstone.

Munguia, M. H., Pina, A., Franco, P. E., Rivadeneyra, G. J., Velasco Arce, H. J. M. and Montano, G. (1960) 'Vaginal cytology in advanced mammary cancer: I Selection of patients for oophorectomy'. English abstract in *Cancer Chemother. Abstracts*, 1961, 311.

Mustacchi, P. and Gordan, G. S. (1958) 'Frequency of cancer in estrogen treated osteoporotic women', in *Breast Cancer*, p. 163, Ed A. Segaloff, St. Louis; C. V. Mosby.

Myers, W. P. L. and Bodansky, O. (1957) 'Comparison of serum phosphohexose isomerase activity and urinary calcium excretion in patients with metatastatic mammary carcinoma'. *Amer. J. Med.*, **23**, 804.

Myers, W. P. L., West, C. D., Pearson, O. H. and Karnofsky, D. A. (1955) 'Androgen induced exacerbation of human breast cancer as measured by calcium excretion'. *Proc. Amer. Assoc. Cancer Res.*, **2**, 36.

Nabarro, J. D. N. (1960) 'Selection of breast cancer patients for adrenalectomy or hypophysectomy'. *Lancet*, **i**, 1293.

Nathanson, I. T. (1946) 'The effect of stilbestrol on advanced cancer of the breast'. *Cancer Res.*, **6**, 484.

Nathanson, I. T. (1947) 'Hormonal alteration of advanced cancer of the breast'. *Surg. Clin. N. Amer.*, **27**, 1144.

Nathanson, I. T. (1952) 'Clinical investigative experience with steroid hormones in breast cancer'. *Cancer (Phil.)*, **5**, 754.

Nathanson, I. T., Engel, L. L. and Kelley, R. M. (1951) 'The effect of ACTH on the urinary excretion of steroids in neoplastic disease'. In *Proceedings of the Second Clinical ACTH Conference*, p. 54, New York; Blakiston.

Nathanson, I. T., Engel, L. L., Kelley, R. M., Ekman, G., Spaulding, K. H. and Elliott, J. (1952) 'The effect of androgens on the urinary excretion of ketosteroids, non ketonic alcohols and estrogens'. *J. Clin. Endoc.*, **12**, 1172.

Nathanson, I. T. and Kelley, R. M. (1952) 'Hormonal treatment of cancer'. *New England J. Med.*, **246**, 135.

Nathanson, I. T., Rice, C. and Meigs, J. V. (1940) 'Hormonal studies in artificial menopause produced by roentgen rays'. *Amer. J. Obstet. Gynec.*, **40**, 936.

Neal, F. E. (1966) 'The choice of hormones in the treatment of advanced carcinoma of the breast', in *The Value of Cytotoxic Agents and Anabolic Steroids in the Treatment of Advanced Malignant Disease*, p. 38. Ed M. Abrahamson, London; Parcener Press.

Nelsen, T. S. and Dragstedt, L. R. (1961) 'Adrenalectomy and oophorectomy for breast cancer'. *J. Amer. Med. Assoc.*, **175**, 379.

Nevinny, H. B. (1964) 'Comparative study of 5 fluorouracil, 5 fluorodeoxyuridine and methotrexate in patients with advanced cancer'. *Proc. Amer. Assoc. Cancer Res.*, **5**, 47.

Nevinny, H. B., Dederick, M. M. and Hall, T. C. (1960) 'Effect of methotrexate on hormone induced hypercalcaemia'. *Clin. Res.*, **8**, 251.

Nevinny, H. B. and Hall, T. C. (1963) '*In situ* determination of the anti-tumour effect of chemotherapeutic compounds'. *2nd Int. Symp. Chemother. Naples*, **3**, 219.

Nicol, T. and Bilbey, D. L. J. (1957) 'Reversal by diethyl-stilboestrol of the depressant effect of cortisone on the phagocytic activity of the reticulo-endothelial system'. *Nature*, **179**, 1137.

Nicol, T., Bilbey, D. L. J., Charles, L. M., Cordingley, J. L. and Vernon Roberts, B. (1964) 'Oestrogen, the natural stimulant of body defence'. *J. Endoc.*, **30**, 277.

Nissen-Meyer, R. (1964) 'Prophylactic endocrine treatment in carcinoma of the breast'. *Clin. Radiol.*, **15**, 152.

Nissen-Meyer, R. and Sanner, T. (1963) 'The excretion of oestrone, pregnanediol, and pregnanetriol in breast cancer patients'. *Acta Endoc. (Kobn.)*, **44**, 334.

Nissen-Meyer, R. and Vogt, J. H. (1959) 'Cortisone treatment of metastatic breast cancer'. *Acta Unio Int. Contra Canc.*, **15**, 1140.

Noer, R. J., Moore, G. E. and others (1964) 'Chemotherapy as an adjuvant to radical mastectomy for mammary cancer'. *Bull. Soc. Int. de Chirurgie*, **22**, 36.

O'Conor, V. J., Chiang, S. P. and Grayhack, J. T. (1963) 'Is subcapsular orchidectomy a definitive procedure? Studies of hormone excretion before and after orchietomy'. *J. Urol.*, **89**, 236.

Olch, I. Y. (1937) 'The menopausal age in women with cancer of the breast'. *Amer. J. Cancer*, **30**, 563.

Palmer, J. D. and Hellstrom, J. (1962) 'The use of urinary estrogen estimations as a means of predicting response to oophorectomy and adrenalectomy in breast cancer'. *Canad. J. Surg.*, **5**, 180.

Parker, T. G. and Sommers, S. C. (1956) 'Adrenal cortical hyperplasia accompanying cancer'. *Arch. Surg.*, **72**, 495.

Paterson, R. and Russell, M. H. (1959) 'Breast cancer: value of irradiation of the ovaries'. *J. Fac. Radiol.*, **10**, 130.

Patey, D. H. (1960) 'Early (prophylactic) oophorectomy and adrenalectomy in carcinoma of the breast—an interim report'. *Brit. J. Cancer*, **14**, 457.

Pearson, O. H. (1957) 'Observations on the role of androgens and estrogens in body balance'. *Arch. Int. Med.*, **100**, 724.

Pearson, O. H. (1967) 'Hormone dependence of tumours in man', in *Modern Trends in Endocrinology*, Vol. 3, p. 242, Ed H. Gardiner Hill, London; Butterworth.

Pearson, O. H. and Lipsett, M. B. (1956) 'Endocrine management of metastatic breast cancer'. *Med. Clinics N. Amer.*, **40**, 761.

Pearson, O. H. and Ray, B. S. (1959) 'Results of hypophysectomy in the treatment of metastatic mammary carcinoma'. *Cancer (Phil.)*, **12**, 85.

Pearson, O. H. and Ray, B. S. (1960) 'Hypophysectomy in the treatment of metastatic mammary cancer'. *Amer. J. Surg.*, **99**, 544.

Pearson, O. H., West, C. D., Hollander, V. P. and Escher, G. C. (1952) 'Alterations in calcium metabolism in patients with osteolytic tumours'. *J. Clin. Edoc.*, **12**, 926.

Pearson, O. H., West, C. D., Hollander, V. P. and Treves, N. E. (1954) 'Evaluation of endocrine therapy of advanced breast cancer'. *J. Amer. Med. Assoc.*, **154**, 234.

Pearson, O. H., West, C. D., Li, M. C., McLean, J. P. and Treves, N. (1955) 'Endocrine therapy of metastatic breast cancer'. *Arch. Int. Med.*, **95**, 357.

Peck, F. C. and Olson, K. B. (1963) 'The treatment of advanced breast cancer by hypophysectomy'. *N.Y. State J. Med.*, **63**, 2191.

Perrault, M., Le Beau, J., Klotz, B., Sicard, J. and Clavel, B. (1952) 'Total hypophysectomy in the treatment of breast cancer: First French report and future of the technique'. Quoted in *Endocrine Surgery in Human Cancers*, p. 142, Ed P. Juret. Springfield; Charles C. Thomas, 1966.

Peters, M. V. (1956) 'The influence of hormone therapy on metastatic mammary carcinoma'. *Surg. Gynec. Obstet.*, **102**, 545.

Peters, M. V. (1963) 'Carcinoma of the breast associated with pregnancy and lactation'. *Proceedings of the Tenth Clinical Conference*, p. 161, Canada; Ontario Research Foundation.

Pincus, G., Garcia, C. R., Rock, J., Paniagua, M., Pendleton, A., Laraque, F., Nicolas, R., Borno, R. and Pean, V. (1959) 'Effectiveness of an oral contraceptive'. *Science*, **130**, 81.

Pincus, I. J., Rakoff, A. E., Cohn, E. M. and Tumen, H. J. (1951) 'Hormonal studies in patients with chronic liver disease'. *Gastroenterol*, **19**, 735.

Plimpton, C. H., and Gellhorn, A. (1956) 'Hypercalcemia in malignant disease without evidence of bone destruction'. *Amer. J. Med.*, **21**, 750.

Pommatau, E., Poulain, S., Dargent, M. and Mayer, M. (1963) 'FSH levels in the postmenopausal or castrated woman with advanced mammary cancer. Effect of adrenalectomy'. English abstract in *Cancer Chemother. Abstracts*, 1280.

Pommatau, E., Poulain, S., Maurel, C., Vauterin, C. and Olivier, L. (1961) 'Initial results of the treatment of advanced breast cancer with Nilevar (norethandrolone)'. English abstract in *Cancer Chemother. Abstracts*, 1961, 2664.

Poppe, H. and Gregl, A. (1961) Quoted by Hortling *et al.*, 1962.

Prudente, A. (1945) 'Postoperative prophylaxis of recurrent mammary cancer with testosterone propionate'. *Surg. Gynec. Obstet.*, **80**, 575.

Pundel, J. P. (1958) 'Does one need to gradually increase the dosage of administered estrogens in patients under long term estrogen therapy in order to maintain high proliferation?' *Acta Cytol.*, **2**, 377.

Pyrah, L. N. (1958) 'The results of adrenalectomy with gonadectomy in breast cancer', in *Endocrine Aspects of Breast Cancer*, p. 22, Eds A. R. Currie and C. F. W. Illingsworth, Edinburgh; E. & S. Livingstone.

Randall, H. T. (1960) 'Oophorectomy and adrenalectomy in patients with inoperable or recurrent carcinoma of the breast'. *Amer. J. Surg.*, **99**, 553.

Ratzkowski, E. and Hochman, A. (1961) 'Survival of patients with recurrent or inoperable carcinoma of the breast with special consideration of the effect of hormonal treatment'. *Cancer (Phil.)*, **14**, 300.

Ravdin, R. G. and Eixman, S. H. (1967) 'Disseminated breast cancer; relationship of response to endocrine manipulation, Cytoxan and Fluorouracil', in *Current Concepts in Breast Cancer*, p. 200, Eds A. Segaloff, K. K. Meyer and S. Debakey, Baltimore; Williams and Wilkins.

Raven, R. W. (1954) 'Hormone treatment of disseminated breast cancer'. *Brit. med. J.*, **i**, 1124.

Rawson, R. W. (1956) 'Today's thyroidologists and their beckoning frontiers—presidential address'. *J. Clin. Endoc.*, **16**, 1405.

Ray, B. S. and Pearson, O. H. (1956) 'Hypophysectomy in the treatment of advanced cancer of breast'. *Ann. Surg.*, **144**, 394.

Read, L. J. (1957) 'Metastatic breast cancer: hormonal manipulation in the palliative treatment'. *Virginia Med. Mth.*, **84**, 57.

Rees, E. D. and Huggins, C. (1960) 'Steroid influences on respiration, glycolysis, and levels of pyridine nucleotide-linked dehydrogenases of experimental mammary cancers'. *Cancer Res.*, **20**, 963.

Reeve, T. S., Rundle, F. F., Hales, I. B., Myhill, J. and Croydon, M. (1961) 'Thyroid function in the presence of breast cancer'. *Lancet*, **i**, 632.

Regele, H., Kaufmann, F. and Wasl, H. (1964) 'The problem of sex chromatin in tumors'. English abstract in *Cancer Chemother. Abstracts*, 1964, 2950.

Regele, H. and Vagacs, H. (1962) 'Hormone dependency in malignant tumours of the breast'. English abstract in *Cancer Chemother. Abstracts*, 1962, 4752.

Repert, R. W. (1952) 'Breast carcinoma study—relationship to thyroid disease and diabetes'. *J. Mich. Med. Soc.*, **51**, 1315.

Rice-Wray, E., Goldzieher, J. W. and Aranda-Rosell, A. (1963) 'Oral progestins in fertility control. A comparative study'. *Fertil. Steril.*, **14**, 402.

Richards, G. E. (1948) 'Mammary cancer, the place of surgery and of radiotherapy in its management'. *Brit. J. Radiol.*, **21**, 109.

Rider, W. D. (1960) 'Bradford approach to breast cancer'. *Brit. med. J.*, **i**, 1501.

Riddle, O. (1963) 'Prolactin in vertebrate function and organisation'. *J. Nat. Canc. Inst.*, **31**, 1039.

Rienits, K. G. (1959) 'The effects of estrone and testosterone on respiration of human mammary cancer *in vitro*'. *Cancer (Phil.)*, **21**, 958.

Rimm, A. A., Ahlstrom, J. K. and Bross, I. D. J. (1966) 'What is objective response?' *Proc. Amer. Assoc. Cancer Res.*, **7**, 59.

Riordan, D. J. and Browne, P. A. (1966) 'The treatment of secondary deposits in bone from carcinoma of the breast, with radiophosphorus and Durabolin'. *J. Irish Med. Assn.*, **49**, 40.

Rivera, E. M., Elias, J. J., Bern, H. A., Napalkov, N. P. and Pitelka, D. R. (1963) 'Toxic effects of steroid hormones on organ cultures of mouse mammary tumours'. *J. Nat. Canc. Inst.*, **31**, 671.

Rosemberg, E. and Engel, I. (1960) 'The influence of steroids on urinary gonadotropin excretion in a postmenopausal woman'. *J. Clin. Endoc.*, **20**, 1576.

Rowlands, I. W. and Sharpey-Schafer, E. P. (1940) 'Effect of oestradiol benzoate on the amount of gonadotrophin found in the pituitary gland and urine of postmenopausal women'. *Brit. med. J.*, **i**, 205.

Rubenstein, B. B. and Duncan, D. R. L. (1941) 'A technic for assay of estrogen by evaluation of human vaginal smears and comparison with urinary estrogen assay on the mouse uterus'. *Endocrinology*, **28**, 911.

Salmon, U. J. and Frank, R. T. (1956) 'Hormonal factors affecting vaginal smears in castrates and after the menopause'. *Proc. Soc. Exp. Biol. Med.*, **33**, 612.

Sandberg, H., Paulsen, C. A., Leach, R. B. and Maddock, W. O. (1958) 'Estrogen excretion in ovariectomised women receiving adrenocorticotropin'. *J. Clin. Endoc.*, **18**, 1268.

Scarff, R. W. (1948) 'Prognosis in carcinoma of the breast'. *Brit. J. Radiol.*, **21**, 594.

Schinzinger, A. (1889) 'Das karzinom der mamma'. *Munchen Med. Wchnschr.*, **52**, 1724.

Schweppe, J. S., Jungman, R. A. and Lewin, I. (1967) 'Urine steroid excretion in postmenopausal cancer of the breast'. *Cancer (Phil.)*, **20**, 155.

Scowen, E. F. (1955) 'Langdon Brown lecture' quoted by G. J. Hadfield and J. A. G. Holt, (1956) *Brit. med. J.*, **ii**, 972.

Scowen, E. F. (1958) 'Oestrogen excretion after hypophysectomy in breast cancer', in *Endocrine Aspects of Breast Cancer*, p. 208, Eds A. R. Currie and C. F. Illingsworth, Edinburgh; E. & S. Livingstone.

Sears, M. E., Eckles, N. and Kirschbaum, A. (1960) 'ThioTEPA induced amenorrhoea associated with prolonged regression of human breast cancer'. *Proc. Amer. Assoc. Cancer. Res.*, **3**, 150.

Segaloff, A. (1957) 'Testosterone and miscellaneous steroids in the treatment of advanced mammary cancer'. *Cancer (Phil.)*, **10**, 808.

Segaloff, A. (1958) 'The therapy of advanced breast cancer with androgens', in *Breast Cancer*, p. 203, Ed A. Segaloff, St. Louis; C. V. Mosby.

Segaloff, A. (1960) 'Testosterone propionate therapy of breast cancer—a report from the Co-operative breast cancer group', in *Biological Activities of Steroids in Relation to Cancer*, p. 355, Eds G. Pincus and E. P. Vollmer, New York; Academic Press.

Segaloff, A. (1966) 'Hormones and breast cancer'. *Recent Progress in Hormone Research*, **22**, 351.

Segaloff, A. (1967*a*) 'Pituitary hormones influencing breast cancer', in *Current Concepts in Breast Cancer*, p. 94, Eds A. Segaloff, K. K. Meyer and S. Debakey, Baltimore; Williams and Wilkins.

Segaloff, A. (1967*b*) 'Progress in the treatment of cancer', in *Cambridge Symposium on the Treatment of Carcinoma of the Breast*, p. 8, Ed A. S. Jarrett, Excerpta Medica Foundation.

Segaloff, A., Bowers, C. Y., Rongone, E. L., Murison, P. J. and Schlosser, J. (1958) 'Hormonal therapy in cancer of the breast: XIII The effect of fluoxymesterone therapy on clinical course and hormonal excretion'. *Cancer (Phil.)*, **11**, 1187.

Segaloff, A., Carabasi, R. A., Horwitt, B. N., Schlosser, J. V. and Murison, P. J. (1954*a*) 'Hormonal therapy in cancer of the breast: VI Effect of ACTH and cortisone on clinical course and hormonal excretion'. *Cancer (Phil.)*, **7**, 331.

Segaloff, A., Gordon, D., Carabasi, R. A., Horwitt, B. N., Schlosser, J. V. and Murison, P. J. (1954*b*) 'Hormonal therapy in cancer of the breast: VII Effect of conjugated estrogens (equine) on clinical course and hormonal excretion'. *Cancer (Phil.)*, **7**, 758.

Segaloff, A., Gordon, D., Horwitt, B. N., Schlosser, J. V. and Murison, P. J. (1951) 'Hormonal therapy in cancer of the breast: I The effect of testosterone propionate on clinical course and hormonal excretion'. *Cancer (Phil.)*, **4**, 319.

Segaloff, A., Weeth, J. B., Meyer, K. K., Rongone, E. L. and Cunningham, M. E. G. (1962) 'Hormonal therapy in cancer of the breast. Effect of oral administration of delta-testololactone on clinical course and hormonal excretion'. *Cancer (Phil.)*, **15**, 633.

Severinghaus, A. E. (1944) 'Cytology of anterior pituitary gland of postmenopausal women'. *J. Clin. Endoc.*, **4**, 583.

Sherlock, P. and Hartmann, W. H. (1962) 'Adrenal steroids and the pattern of metastases of breast cancer'. *J. Amer. Med. Assoc.*, **181**, 313.

Sherman, A. I. and Woolf, R. B. (1959) 'An endocrine basis for endometrial carcinoma'. *Amer. J. Obstet. Gynec.*, **77**, 233.

Shirley, R. L. (1967) 'The nuclear sex of breast cancer'. *Surg. Gynec. Obstet.*, **125**, 737.

Sicard, A. (1948) 'La frequence de metastases ovariennes des cancers du sein'. *Presse Med.*, **56**, 606.

Siegert, A. (1952) 'Castration and mammary carcinoma'. *Strahlentherapie*, **87**, 62.

Silva, A. R. M., Smart, C. R. and Rochlin, D. B. (1965) 'Chemotherapy of breast cancer'. *Surg. Gynec. Obstet.*, **121**, 494.

Sim, A. W., Hobkirk, R., Blair, D. W., Stewart, H. J. and Forrest, A. P. M. (1961) 'Accessory adreno-cortical function after adrenalectomy in patients with breast cancer'. *Lancet*, **ii**, 73.

Sinohara, H. and Sky-Peck, H. H. (1964) 'The effects of estradiol on acid mucopolysaccaride metabolism in oophorectomised rats'. *Arch. Biochem. Biophys.*, **106**, 138.

Smith, O. W. and Emerson, K. Jr. (1954) 'Urinary estrogens and related compounds in postmenopausal women with mammary cancer—effect of cortisone treatment'. *Proc. Soc. Exper. Biol. Med.*, **85**, 264.

Smith, G. V. and Smith, O. W. (1953) 'Carcinoma of the breast. Results and evaluation of X-radiation, and relation of age and surgical castration to length of survival'. *Surg. Gynec. Obstet.*, **97**, 508.

Smithers, D. W. (1968) 'Clinical assessment of growth rate in human tumours'. *Clin. Radiol.*, **19**, 113.

Smithers, D. W., Rigby-Jones, P., Galton, D. A. G. and Payne, P. N. (1952) 'Cancer of the breast—a review'. *Brit. J. Radiol. Suppl.*, **4**, 1.

Sommers, S. C. (1955) 'Endocrine abnormalities in women with breast cancer'. *Lab. Invest.*, **4**, 160.

Sommers, S. C. and Teloh, H. A. (1952) 'Ovarian stromal hyperplasia in breast cancer'. *Arch. Path.*, **53**, 160.

Sommers, S. C., Teloh, H. A. and Goldman, G. (1953) 'Ovarian influence upon survival in breast cancer'. *Arch. Surg.*, **67**, 916.

Southam, C. M. (1965) 'Evidence of immunological reactions to autochthonous cancer in man'. *Europ. J. Cancer*, **1**, 173.

Steinach, E. and Kun, H. (1937) 'Transformation of male sex hormones into a substance with the action of female hormone'. *Lancet*, **ii**, 845.

Stewart, J. G., Skinner, L. G. and O'Connor, P. J. (1965) 'Hormone therapy in metastatic breast cancer: clinical response and urinary gonadotropins'. *Acta Endoc. (Kobn.)*, **50**, 345.

Stocks, P. (1939) 'Distribution in England and Wales of cancer of various organs'. *Brit. Emp. Cancer Camp. Ann. Rep.*, 308.

Stoll, B. A. (1950) 'Hormone therapy in relation to radiotherapy in the treatment of advanced carcinoma of the breast'. *Proc. Roy. Soc. Med.*, **43**, 875.

Stoll, B. A. (1955) 'Chemotherapy in cancer'. *Med. J. Aust.*, **2**, 322.

Stoll, B. A. (1956a) 'Total adrenalectomy and oophorectomy for carcinoma of the breast'. *Med. J. Aust.*, **1**, 72.

Stoll, B. A. (1956b) 'p-Hydroxypropiophenone for advanced breast cancer'. *Med. J. Aust.*, **2**, 181.

Stoll, B. A. (1956c) 'Advanced cancer treated with Nitromin'. *Med. J. Aust.*, **2**, 882.

Stoll, B. A. (1958a) 'Fluoxymesterone in advanced breast cancer'. *Proc. 7th Internat. Cancer Cong.*, 382.

Stoll, B. A. (1958b) 'Endocrine factors in the aetiology and treatment of cancer of the breast and prostate', in *Modern Trends in Endocrinology*, p. 212, Vol. 1, Ed H. Gardiner Hill, London; Butterworth.

Stoll, B. A. (1959a) 'Fluoxymesterone (Halotestin) in advanced breast carcinoma'. *Med. J. Aust.*, **1**, 70.

Stoll, B. A. (1959b) 'Recent advances in the chemotherapy of cancer'. *Med. J. Aust.*, **2**, 240.

Stoll, B. A. (1960a) 'Carzinophilin in advanced breast cancer'. *Cancer (Phil.)*, **13**, 439.

Stoll, B. A. (1960b) 'Mitomycin C in advanced breast carcinoma—preliminary report'. *Asian Med. J.*, **3**, 1.

Stoll, B. A. (1960c) 'Dexamethasone in advanced breast cancer'. *Cancer (Phil.)*, **13**, 1074.

Stoll, B. A. (1960d) 'Nitromin and corticosteroids in the treatment of advanced cancer'. *Acta Un. Int. Contra Canc.*, **16**, 919.

Stoll, B. A. (1962a) 'Cyclophosphamide in disseminated malignant disease'. *Brit. Med. J.*, **i**, 475.

Stoll, B. A. (1962b) 'A clinical trial of tri-iodothyronine as a hormone potentiator in advanced breast cancer'. *Brit. J. Cancer*, **16**, 436.

Stoll, B. A. (1963a) 'ThioTEPA and breast cancer'. *Brit. med. J.*, **i**, 54.

Stoll, B. A. (1963*b*) 'Corticosteroids in the therapy of advanced mammary cancer'. *Brit. med. J.*, **ii,** 210.

Stoll, B. A. (1964*a*) 'Fact and fallacy in the hormonal control of breast cancer'. *Med. J. Aust.*, **1,** 980.

Stoll, B. A. (1964*b*) 'Hormones and breast cancer'. *Brit. med. J.*, **ii,** 755.

Stoll, B. A. (1964*c*) 'Oral contraceptives and breast cancer'. *Brit. med. J.*, **ii,** 875.

Stoll, B. A. (1965*a*) 'Progestogens and oestrogens in the treatment of breast cancer', in *Recent Advances in Ovarian and Synthetic Steroids,* Ed R. Shearman, Sydney; Globe.

Stoll, B. A. (1965*b*) 'Breast cancer and hypothyroidism'. *Cancer (Phil.)*, **18,** 1431.

Stoll, B. A. (1966) 'Therapy by progestational agents in advanced breast cancer'. *Med. J. Aust.*, **1,** 331.

Stoll, B. A. (1967*a*) 'Effect of Lyndiol, an oral contraceptive, on breast cancer'. *Brit. med. J.*, **i,** 150.

Stoll, B. A. (1967*b*) 'Vaginal cytology as an aid to hormone therapy in postmenopausal breast cancer'. *Cancer (Phil.)*, **20,** 1807.

Stoll, B. A. (1967*c*) 'Progestin therapy of breast cancer—comparison of agents'. *Brit. med. J.*, **ii,** 338.

Stoll, B. A. (1969) 'The sensitivity of breast cancer in organ culture to the effect of oestrogen and progestin'. Unpublished data.

Stoll, B. A., Andrews, J. T. and Motteram, R. (1966) 'Liver damage from oral contraceptives'. *Brit. med. J.*, **i,** 960.

Stoll, B. A., Andrews, J. T., Motteram, R. and Upfill, J. (1965) 'Oral contraceptives and liver damage'. *Brit. med. J.*, **i,** 723.

Stoll, B. A. and Burch, W. M. (1968) 'Surface detection of circadian rhythm in ^{32}P content of breast cancer'. *Cancer (Phil.)*, **21,** 193.

Stoll, B. A. and Ellis, F. (1953) 'Treatment by oestrogens of pulmonary metastases from breast cancer'. *Brit. med. J.*, **ii,** 796.

Stoll, B. A. and Matar, J. (1961) 'Cyclophosphamide in advanced breast cancer—a clinical and haematological appraisal'. *Brit. med. J.*, **ii,** 283.

Strong, J. A., Brown, J. B., Bruce, J., Douglas, M., Klopper, A. I. and Loraine, J. A. (1956) 'Sex hormone excretion after bilateral adrenalectomy and oophorectomy in patients with mammary carcinoma'. *Lancet*, **ii,** 955.

Struthers, R. A. (1956) 'Postmenopausal oestrogen production'. *Brit. med. J.*, **i,** 1331.

Swyer, G. I. M., Lee, A. E. and Masterton, J. P. (1961) 'Oestrogen excretion of patients with breast cancer'. *Brit. med. J.*, **1,** 617.

Tagnon, H. J., Coune, A., Heuson, J. C. and Van Rymenant, M. (1967) 'Problems in the treatment of disseminated cancer of the breast.

Selection of patients for hormone treatment', in *Recent Results in Cancer Research*, p. 126, Eds L. Manuila, S. Moles and P. Rentschnick, Berlin and New York; Springer.

Tan, C. T. C., Murphy, M. L., Dargeon, H. W. and Burchenal, J. H. (1957) 'Clinical effects of Actinomycin D'. *Proc. Amer. Assoc. Cancer Res.*, **2,** 254.

Taylor, D. M., Parker, R. P., Field, E. O. and Greatorex, C. A. (1968) 'An interpretation of the results of measurements of the uptake of ^{32}P in human tumours'. *Brit. J. Radiol.*, **41,** 432.

Taylor, G. W. (1939) 'Evaluation of ovarian sterilisation for breast cancer'. *Surg. Gynec. Obstet.*, **68,** 452.

Taylor, S. G. (1962) 'Endocrine ablation in disseminated mammary carcinoma'. *Surg. Gynec. Obstet.*, **115,** 443.

Taylor, S. G. and Morris, R. S. (1951) 'Hormones in breast metastasis therapy'. *Med. Clin. N. Amer.*, **35,** 51.

Taylor, S. G. and Perlia, C. P. (1960) 'Evaluation of endocrine ablative surgery in the treatment of mammary carcinoma: a preliminary study on survival', in *Biological Activities of Steroids in Relation to Cancer*, p. 343, Eds G. Pincus and E. P. Vollmer, New York; Academic Press.

Taylor, S. G., Perlia, C. P. and Kofman, S. (1958) 'Cortical steroids in the treatment of disseminated breast cancer', in *Breast Cancer*, p. 217, Ed A. Segaloff, St. Louis; C. V. Mosby.

Taylor, S. G., Slaughter, D. P., Smejkal, W., Fowler, E. F. and Preston, F. W. (1948) 'The effect of sex hormones on advanced carcinoma of the breast'. *Cancer (Phil.)*, **1,** 604.

Tchao, R., Easty, G. C., Ambrose, E. J., Raven, R. W. and Bloom, H. J. G. (1968) 'Effects of chemotherapeutic agents and hormones on organ cultures of human tumours'. *European J. Cancer*, **4,** 39.

Teilum, G. (1950) 'Oestrogen production by Sertoli cells in the etiology of benign senile hypertrophy of the human prostate'. *Acta Endoc.(Kobn.)*, **4,** 43.

Thalassinos, N. and Joplin, G. F. (1968) 'Phosphate treatment of hypercalcaemia due to carcinoma'. *Brit. med. J.*, **iv,** 14.

Thayssen, V. E. (1948) 'The influence of castration by roentgen on carcinoma of the breast'. *Acta Radiol.*, **29,** 189.

Thomas, A. N., Gordan, G. S., Goldman, L. and Lowe, R. (1962) 'Anti-tumor efficacy of 2α methyl dihydrotestosterone propionate in advanced breast cancer'. *Cancer (Phil.)*, **15,** 176.

Thomas, B. S., Bulbrook, R. D. and Hayward, J. L. (1967) 'Urinary steroid assays and response to endocrine ablation'. *Brit. med. J.*, **iii,** 523.

Thomson, A. (1902) 'Analysis of cases in which oophorectomy was performed for inoperable carcinoma of the breast'. *Brit. med. J.*, **ii**, 1538.

Treves, N. (1957) 'An evaluation of prophylactic castration in the treatment of mammary carcinoma'. *Cancer (Phil.)*, **10**, 393.

Treves, N. (1959) 'The treatment of cancer, especially inoperable cancer of the male breast, by ablative surgery (orchidectomy, adrenalectomy, and hypophysectomy) and hormone therapy (estrogens and corticosteroids)'. *Cancer (Phil.)*, **12**, 820.

Treves, N. and Finkbeiner, J. A. (1958) 'An evaluation of therapeutic surgical castration in the treatment of metastatic, recurrent and primary inoperable mammary carcinoma in women'. *Cancer (Phil.)*, **11**, 421.

Treves, N. and Holleb, A. I. (1958) 'A report of 549 cases of breast cancer in women 35 years of age or younger'. *Surg. Gynec. Obstet.*, **107**, 271.

Ulrich, P. (1939) 'Testosterone (hormone male) et son role possible dans le traitement de certains cancers du sein'. *Acta Unio Int. Contra Canc.*, **4**, 377.

Veterans Administration Co-operative Urological Research Group (1967) 'Treatment and survival of patients with cancer of the prostate'. *Surg. Gynec. Obstet.*, **124**, 1011.

Vogler, W. R., Furtado, V. P. and Huguley, C. M. (1968) 'Methotrexate for advanced cancer of the breast'. *Cancer (Phil.)*, **21**, 26.

Volk, H., Escher, G. C., Huseby, R. A., Tyler, F. H. and Cheda, J. (1960) 'Hormonal therapy in carcinoma of the breast: I Effect of oral progesterone on clinical course and metabolism of nitrogen and selected electrolytes and steroids'. *Cancer (Phil.)*, **13**, 757.

Wallach, S. and Henneman, P. H. (1959) 'Prolonged estrogen therapy in postmenopausal women'. *J. Amer. Med. Assoc.*, **171**, 1637.

Walpole, A. L. and Paterson, E. (1949) 'Synthetic oestrogens in mammary cancer'. *Lancet*, **ii**, 783.

Warren, S. and Witham, E. M. (1933) 'Studies on tumour metastasis: distribution of metastases in cancer of the breast'. *Surg. Gynec. Obstet.*, **57**, 81.

Watson, G. W. and Turner, R. L. (1959) 'Breast cancer. A new approach to therapy'. *Brit. med. J.*, **i**, 1315.

Weisberger, A. S. (1958) 'Direct instillation of nitrogen mustard in the management of malignant effusions'. *Ann. N.Y. Acad. Sci.*, **68**, 1091.

West, C. D., Damast, B. and Pearson, O. H. (1958) 'Adrenal estrogens in patients with metastatic breast cancer'. *J. Clin. Invest.*, **37**, 341.

West, C. D., Damast, B. L., Sarro, S. D. and Pearson, O. H. (1956) 'Conversion of testosterone to oestrogens in castrated adrenalectomised human females'. *J. Biol. Chem.*, **218**, 409.

West, C. D., Li, M. C., Maclean, J. P., Escher, G. C. and Pearson, O. H. (1954) 'Cortisone induced remissions in women with metastatic mammary cancer'. *Proc. Amer. Assoc. Cancer Res.*, **1**, No. 2, 51.

Westberg, S. V. (1946) 'Prognosis of breast cancer for pregnant and nursing women'. *Acta Obstet. Gyn. Scand.*, **25**, Suppl. No. 4, 239.

White, T. T. (1954) 'Carcinoma of the breast and pregnancy. Analysis of 920 cases collected from the literature and new cases'. *Ann. Surg.*, **139**, 9.

World Health Organisation Report (1966) *Clinical Aspects of Oral Gestagens.* (Technical Report, No. 326), p. 19, Geneva; W.H.O.

Wilkins, L., Gardner, L. I., Crigler, J. F., Silverman, S. H. and Migeon, C. J. (1952) 'Comparison of oral and intramuscular administration of cortisone with a note on the suppressive action of compounds F and B on the adrenal'. *J. Clin. Endoc.*, **12**, 257.

Wilson, C. B., Winternitz, W. W., Bertan, V. and Sizemore, G. (1966) 'Stereotaxic cryosurgery of the pituitary gland in carcinoma of the breast and other disorders'. *J. Amer. Med. Assoc.*, **198**, 587.

Wilson, H., Lipsett, M. B. and Butler, L. C. (1960) 'Steroid excretion in hypophysectomised women, and the initial effects of corticotropin. A study in urinary steroid patterns'. *J. Clin. Endoc.*, **20**, 534.

Wilson, R. A. (1962) 'The roles of estrogen and progesterone in breast and genital cancer'. *J. Amer. Med. Assoc.*, **182**, 327.

Wilson, R. E., Crocker, D. W., Fairgrieve, J., Bartholomay, A. F., Emerson, K. and Moore, F. D. (1967) 'Adrenal structure and function in advanced carcinoma of breast'. *J. Amer. Med. Assoc.*, **199**, 474.

Wilson, R. E., Jessiman, A. G. and Moore, F. D. (1958) 'Severe exacerbation of cancer of the breast after oophorectomy and adrenalectomy. Report of four cases'. *New Engl. J. Med.*, **258**, 312.

Wintz, H. (1926) 'Experiences in the irradiation of breast cancer'. *Brit. J. Radiol.*, **31**, 150.

Witt, J. A., Gardner, B., Gordan, G. S., Graham, W. P. and Thomas, A. N. (1963) 'Secondary hormonal therapy of disseminated breast cancer. Comparison of hypophysectomy, replacement therapy, estrogens, and androgens'. *Arch. Int. Med.*, **111**, 557.

Wolff, B. (1957) 'The differential cell count in cancer of the breast and response to hormone therapy'. *Guy's Hospital Rep.*, **106**, 53.

Woodard, H. Q., Escher, G. C. and Farrow, J. H. (1954) 'Changes in the blood chemistry of patients with disseminated carcinoma of the breast during endocrine therapy'. *Cancer (Phil.)*, **7**, 744.

Woolley-Hart, A., Twentyman, P., Corfield, J., Joslin, C., Morrison, R. and Fowler, J. F. (1968) 'Changes in ^{32}P counting rate in human and animal tumours'. *Brit. J. Radiol.*, **41**, 440.

Wright, J. C., Cobb, J. P., Golomb, F. M., Gumport, S. L., Lyall, D. and Safadi, D. (1959) 'Chemotherapy of disseminated carcinoma of the breast'. *Ann. Surg.*, **150**, 221.

Wroblewski, F. and Ladue, J. S. (1953) 'Lactic dehydrogenase activity in blood'. *Proc. Soc. Exp. Biol. Med.*, **90**, 210.

Wynder, E. L., Bross, I. J. and Hirayama, T. (1960) 'A study on the epidemiology of cancer of the breast.' *Cancer (Phil.)*, **13**, 559.

Young, S., Bulbrook, R. D. and Greenwood, F. C. (1957) 'The correlation between urinary estrogens and vaginal cytology'. *Lancet*, **i**, 350.

Index

THE LIBRARY
UNIVERSITY OF CALIFORNIA
San Francisco

THIS BOOK IS DUE ON THE LAST DATE STAMPED BELOW

Books not returned on time are subject to fines according to the Library Lending Code.

Books not in demand may be renewed if application is made before expiration of loan period.

15m-5,'70(N6489s4)4128—A33-9